D1622244

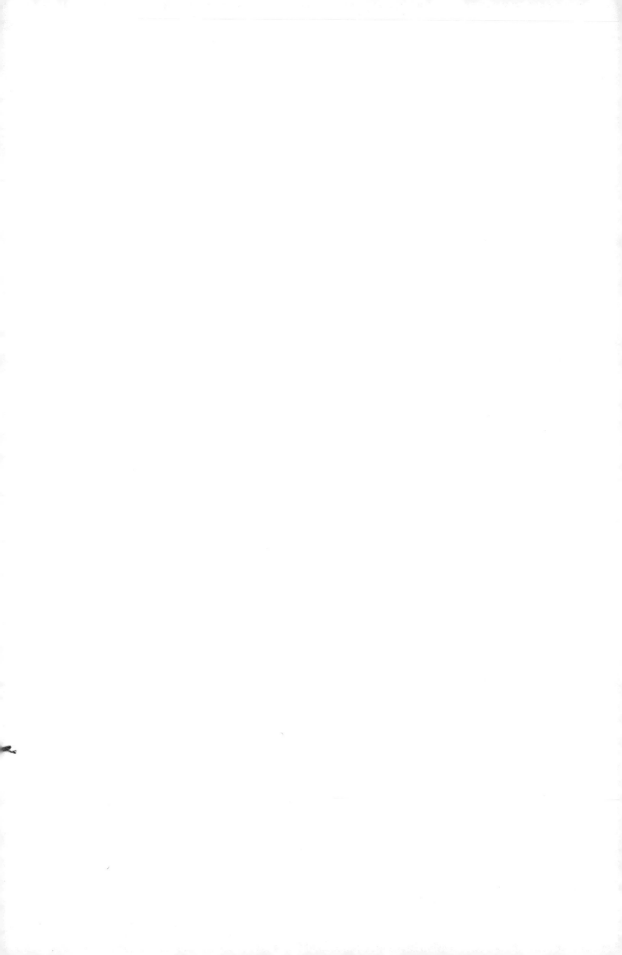

Nutrition Applied to Injury Rehabilitation and Sports Medicine

Luke R. Bucci

CRC Press
Boca Raton   Ann Arbor   London   Tokyo

Library of Congress Cataloging-in-Publication Data

Bucci, Luke.
    Nutrition applied to injury rehabilitation and sports medicine /
Luke R. Bucci.
      p.   cm. -- (Nutrition in exercise and sport)
    Includes bibliographical references and index.
    ISBN 0-8493-7913-X
    1. Sports injuries--Nutritional aspects. I. Title. II. Series.
RD97.B83   1994
615.8′54′088796--dc20

                                                                94-11109
                                                                  CIP

No claim to original U.S. Government works
International Standard Book Number 0-8493-7913-X
Library of Congress Card Number 94-11109
Printed in the United States of America   2 3 4 5 6 7 8 9 0
Printed on acid-free paper

SERIES PREFACE

The CRC series *Nutrition in Exercise and Sport* is designed to provide the setting for in-depth exploration of the many and varied aspects of nutrition and exercise, including sport. The topic of sports nutrition gained real interest among physiologists in the 1960s, and since then, numerous scientific studies have been performed, many of which have focused on the healthful benefits of good nutrition and exercise. As we move forward to the next century, scientists will search evermore for the elusive "optimum" nutritional preparation. As they try to unlock nature's secrets, it will be necessary to remember that there must be a range of diets that will support excellent physical performance, there will inevitably be attempts by scientists and laymen alike to distill the diets to some common denominator — a formula for success. The CRC series in *Nutrition in Exercise and Sport* is dedicated to providing a stage upon which to explore these issues. Each volume seeks to provide a detailed and scholarly examination of some aspect of this topic. Ultimately, the series will comprise a set of authoritative volumes for consultation by scientists, physicians, and a broad range of health-care providers and individuals who participate in exercise and sport, whether for recreation or competition.

We welcome the contribution by Luke Bucci to the series.

Editors
Ira Wolinsky, Ph.D.
James F. Hickson, Jr., Ph.D., R.D.

CRC SERIES ON
_____ NUTRITION IN EXERCISE AND SPORT

Editors, Ira Wolinsky and James F. Hickson, Jr.

Published Titles

Luke Bucci
Nutrients as Ergogenic Aids for Sports and Exercise

Ira Wolinsky & James F. Hickson, Jr.
Nutrition in Exercise and Sport, 2/E

Ronald R. Watson & Marianne Eisinger
Exercise and Disease

Luke Bucci
Nutrition Applied to Injury Rehabilitation and Sports Medicine

Forthcoming Titles

Catherine G. R. Jackson
Nutrition for the Recreational Athlete

James F. Hickson, Jr.
Sports Nutrition

Editor, Ira Wolinsky

Forthcoming Titles

Constance V. Kies
Sports Nutrition: Minerals and Electrolytes

Jaime S. Ruud
Nutrition and the Female Athlete

E. R. Buskirk & S. Puhl
Body Fluid Balance: Exercise and Sport

Jana Parizkova
Nutrition, Physical Activity and Health in Early Life

AUTHOR

Luke R. Bucci received his Doctorate in Biomedical Sciences (Biochemistry and Cell Biology) from the University of Texas Health Science Center at Houston, Graduate School of Biomedical Sciences in 1983. The dissertation topic was a characterization of DNA-binding proteins (High-Mobility-Group proteins) during the different cell types in spermatogenesis. A postdoctoral appointment to the Department of Experimental Radiotherapy at M.D. Anderson Hospital and Tumor Institute (University of Texas System Cancer Center) followed, where Dr. Bucci studied the effects of chemotherapy and radiotherapy on normal animal and human tissues. Next, Dr. Bucci was Director of Research for a nutritional supplement company, where he conducted human research and wrote and lectured extensively on a variety of nutritional topics. In 1991, Dr. Bucci formed InnerPath Nutrition, a nutritional consulting and education company. In 1992, Dr. Bucci became Director of Science and Quality for SpectraCell Laboratories, Inc., a clinical laboratory that offers testing for functional nutrient status by lymphocyte growth responses in a series of serum-free media. Dr. Bucci also conducts continuing medical education and relicensing seminars on nutritional applications for physicians and consults for home health care companies. Dr. Bucci authored the CRC Press book *Nutrients as Ergogenic Aids for Sport and Exercise* as part of the Nutrition in Exercise and Sport Series.

FOREWORD

The study of enhancement of healing dates to prerecorded history. Injury is a normal happening in living organisms. The study of healing has progressed both without and with the benefit of scientific design, with the application of scientific method appearing recently within the last 100 years. As with any complex system, the study of human healing has been wrought with difficulties, mostly because the type, severity, and individual responses are highly variable among individuals. Nevertheless, enough suggestive information has been documented to enable the completion of this book. After pulling together many separate lines of research, the concept of using nutrients as therapeutic agents has shown scientific and clinical merit, and deserves to be compiled into one source.

Many excellent books and thousands of articles on surgical healing have appeared in the last 50 years. The obvious impetus is that surgery is intentional wounding, and surgical results are easily visible to both patients and physicians. The impetus to save lives and physical abilities during wartime has made great strides in the knowledge and treatment of traumatic injuries. The epidemics of automobile collisions and criminal violence has supplied a steady stream of research subjects and clinical successes in healing. Thus, a solid basis of biological knowledge has been accumulated, which has parallels to sports injuries.

Modern day warriors are more likely to be professional athletes instead of Roman gladiators or soldiers. Most of the injuries common to athletes and warriors are traumatic in nature. Of special concern to healing in athletes is return to former physical function, rather than merely return to "normal" or acceptable function. This demand to perform drives athletes and nonathletes alike to expect a full recovery from most traumatic injuries, and a return to former physical activities. The pressure to enhance healing, recovery, and rehabilitation may lead to efforts beyond those approved by health care agencies. Some of those efforts may involve nutritional modulation. This book hopes to cast a rational light on nutritional rehabilitation.

Injury is defined as damage to body parts, and trauma is a physical injury or wound caused by external force or violence. Rehabilitation is concerned with restoration to maximum potential from a physical, psychological, social, and vocational standpoint of individuals with disabled musculoskeletal systems. Nutritional rehabilitation is the effort to enhance recovery and return to optimum physical function by modulation of nutrient intakes, including overall dietary changes in selection and amounts of foodstuffs, and/or specific increases in intake of micronutrients as dietary supplements.

This book will focus on the readily available choices of dietary supplements, since no current text has combined the present knowledge on dietary supplements and injury rehabilitation into one source. Since the research is scattered into several nonoverlapping areas of interest, much material in this book may seem new to readers. The goal of this book is to support the rational use of specific nutrients for specific healing conditions, as indicated by research. Whenever possible, guidelines for nutritional programs applied to specific conditions will be given, so that practical application of the enormous amount of research can be practiced.

Luke R. Bucci, Ph.D., C.C.N., C(A.S.C.P.)

ACKNOWLEDGMENTS

William Kaufman, Ph.D., M.D., for graciously supplying information on niacinamide and joint disease. Stanley J. Dudrick, M.D., for supplying key reprints and unpublished data. Forrest Nielsen, Ph.D. and Curtiss Hunt, Ph.D. for their helpful discussions and preprints of papers on boron. Steven Paul, Ph.D., of Metagenics, Inc. for graciously supplying information and discussions on hydroxyapatite. David L. Watts, Ph.D., DC, CCN, for supplying data and references on hair mineral analysis. U.S. Council for Coconut Research/Information, Suite 600, 1629 K Street, N.W., Washington, D.C., 20006, for supplying information and reprints on dietary fatty acids. Ron Overberg, Ph.D., for helpful discussions and reprints on carotenoids and vitamin E. Elizabeth Reilly for computer software expertise. Karen Briggs for manuscript handling. Many other persons deserve mention, and their contributions are remembered warmly.

TABLE OF CONTENTS

Chapter 8

Calcium and Magnesium

Chapter 9

Trace Minerals

Chapter 10
Ultratrace Minerals

This book is dedicated to my wife, Naniece.

Chapter 1

INTRODUCTION AND REVIEW OF
BIOLOGICAL BACKGROUND

I. INTRODUCTION

"More medical manpower is expended in treating musculoskeletal problems than in treating disorders of any other single system."

Rosse and Clawson, *The Musculoskeletal System in Health and Disease.*[1]

The human body is amazingly capable of repairing damage to its supporting structures. Given adequate time, the outcome of almost every injury, trauma, or insult will become resolved so that an individual can survive and continue existing. It seems that humans have the ability to heal themselves under even extremely adverse conditions (starvation, bitter cold temperatures, concurrent infections). The practice of surgery to physically alter biological structures by inducing physical trauma (wounds) in order to correct or ameliorate more significant problems is one example of healing connective tissues. With considerable skill and care, thousands of patients each day are routinely wounded and expected to heal. By far, the vast majority of surgical patients heal quite well. However, after resolution of an injury by healing, seldom is a full return to preinjury status attained. Fear of a degradation in physical performance after an injury has healed is perhaps most important in athletics and sports, where physical skills are paramount for performance. This fear and biological facts have spurred attempts to enhance the healing process by any means possible. This book will consider the nutritional means that have been applied to injury rehabilitation and sports medicine.

A. PURPOSE AND SCOPE

The purpose of this book is to acquaint the reader with scientific evidence on attempts to use nutrients to more fully effect a favorable outcome of healing. Since this endeavor has been practiced since before recorded history, this book will focus on use of specific nutrients or combinations of nutrients taken by mouth and will not focus on intravenous administration of nutrients, except where the data are needed to illustrate a particular concept or hypothesis. An extensive body of literature has been developed to explore and apply nutritional repletion by intravenous means. Several journals and many authoritative books are devoted to the subject of enteral (tube) and intravenous feeding (parenteral alimentation or TPN), which has become standard medical procedure.[2-7] Since nutritional support by TPN is usually reserved for the severely ill, and not commonly practiced on injured athletes, this book will emphasize nutritional practices that are readily available via oral routes.

This book represents the first comprehensive text on the application of a wide range of nutrients and dietary substances to the enhancement of human healing from injuries and other musculoskeletal conditions. The subject of applying nutrients to enhance healing is enormous, and this book will attempt to concentrate on the effects of nutritional therapies. However, because musculoskeletal healing is complicated and somewhat different from healing of other tissues, brief reviews of the musculoskeletal system and the healing process are necessary to provide the requisite background for understanding the results of therapeutic trials with nutrients.

Guidelines for use of nutritional therapies will be given whenever merited. One goal of this book is to distill conclusions into a clinically useful format. Therefore, it is hoped that this book will have practical applications for those health care providers involved with musculoskeletal healing. With an overwhelming amount of information that is increasing daily, helpful advances often become lost or forgotten. This book will help to resurrect some nutritional therapies that are not fully recognized for their utility.

As always, a stimulation of discussion and research is anticipated by the collection of findings found in the following pages. The ultimate goal of this book is to ease human suffering by casting light upon methods to enhance the human healing process.

B. BRIEF PERSPECTIVE ON THERAPEUTIC USE OF NUTRIENTS

The idea of using nutrients as therapeutic agents in medical practice has met with much resistance in recent times. With the current Food, Drug & Cosmetic Act, nutrients are legally considered foodstuffs, and not drugs. Foodstuffs are not legally drugs, which means that any claims for mitigation, cure, prevention, or treatment of illnesses or disorders involving the human body cannot be made in the U.S., regardless of their veracity. Only drugs can have therapeutic claims attached in their marketing and advertisement. This leaves many nutrients in a modern-day limbo. Since nutrients are classified as foodstuffs, and, therefore, not amenable to patent protection as therapeutic agents (like drugs), there is little economic incentive to pursue research into clinical applications of nutrients as therapeutic agents. If a nutrient is patented for a specific purpose (drug claim), and becomes classified as a drug after millions of dollars spent and years of time, then there is still little protection against consumers buying a similar product that is classified as a food at considerable savings over the drug version. Economic suicide awaits any pharmaceutical company foolish enough to engage in converting nutrients into drugs. As a result, few nutrients are patented as drugs, and much research in this country has been nonexistent because of the prevailing legal framework.

However, the legal framework does not prevent research funded by the U.S. government, pharmaceutical companies, and other countries to examine the clinical utility of nutrients applied to clinical settings. Thus, a sizeable body of literature has accumulated which has demonstrated the ability of certain nutrients or foodstuffs to benefit human health in many ways that were unsuspected when the Food, Drug & Cosmetic Act was passed. Almost every one of these nutrients is commercially available, and a modest number of companies has marketed nutrients to fill the gap between drugs and foodstuffs. For example, a recent study found that zinc lozenges could decrease the duration of colds.[8] Zinc supplements have been available for many years as a dietary supplement. However, if someone put the claim that zinc can reduce duration of colds (a drug claim) on a bottle of zinc without having that particular product approved as safe and effective for reducing cold duration by the Food & Drug Administration (FDA), then that product is misbranded and subject to confiscation and punitive measures in the same manner as a bogus cure for cancer. Meanwhile, the zinc product on the shelf next to the misbranded product may be enjoying brisk sales. The legal status of a nutrient does not alter its clinical effectiveness.

Of course, the quality control of foodstuffs is an issue that is not completely resolved, and is a major difference between drugs and food supplements. Even though many nutrients exist as products available to consumers, there is still some question as to the potency and identity of a food supplement as compared to a drug. While some mislabeling has occurred, the large majority of dietary supplement products, especially those manufactured by pharmaceutical companies, meet their label claims for identity and potency (unpublished data). The important point is that almost every nutrient that will be discussed in this book is available to health care providers via pharmacies or specialty companies, and many are available to the general public in grocery stores, pharmacies, health food stores, and health care providers' offices.

Therefore, do not judge the effectiveness of nutrients as therapeutic agents by their lack of common medical usage. Legal, political, and economic factors are often more effective at preventing the clinical application of nutrients as therapeutic agents than their clinical performance. This book will endeavor to present what is known and what is known to be likely about the clinical performance of nutrients applied to healing of musculoskeletal tissues.

II. REVIEW OF CONNECTIVE AND MUSCULOSKELETAL TISSUES

A brief review of the identity of connective and musculoskeletal tissues of the human body is necessary in order to better understand the results and implications of successive chapters on nutrient functions and effects. Many excellent books offer detailed treatises on the anatomy and physiology of musculoskeletal tissues.[9-18] Since healing of sports injuries invariably involves musculoskeletal tissues, the knowledge of basic biology of such tissues cannot be overemphasized. In addition to anatomy, the physiology of musculoskeletal and connective tissues is equally important, especially for insight into the abilities of nutrients to benefit healing. Connective tissues are much different from other tissues in their nutritional supply and mechanical stresses,[19-21] which directly impacts how to use nutrients in clinical settings. Knowledge of the healing process, which includes inflammation and the recent strides in cytokine and eicosanoid metabolism, is also helpful for insight into the effects of nutrients and will be briefly covered.

A. CONNECTIVE AND MUSCULOSKELETAL TISSUES

1. Muscle[22-28]

Many excellent reviews exist on muscle structure, function, and physiology, from which this section is a synopsis. Skeletal muscle tissue, distinct from cardiac and smooth muscle tissues, makes up almost half of human body weight. Muscle is the major musculoskeletal tissue in quantitative terms, but is packaged into several hundred individual muscles. The primary function of skeletal muscles is to provide motion and control motion of body parts. Other functions are to maintain posture, generate body heat, and provide protection (by their mere presence) to other tissues. Both stored and generated chemical energy is converted to mechanical energy by the specialized proteins in muscle tissue (actin, myosin, tropomyosin, and troponins). Muscles are built up from smaller units, much like collagen fibers. Actin, myosin, tropomyosin, and troponins form thick and thin filaments on a subcellular, microscopic scale, which are arranged in myofilaments. Myofibrils (subcellular organelles) are made up of numerous myofilaments, and muscle fibers (muscle cell units) are made up of numerous myofibrils. Muscle fibers are grouped together with endomysium (a connective tissue septa surrounding each muscle fiber) into macroscopic units called fascicles. Perimysium, a collagenous sheath, surrounds each fascicle. Finally, several fascicles are bundled into a discrete muscle (organ), wrapped by the epimysium (deep fascia sheath). Muscles are attached to bones and other structures in two basic manners. First, direct attachment involves fusion of the epimysium to the periosteum of bone or perichondrium of cartilage. Second, indirect attachments involve the muscle fascia becoming a distinct, long tendon or flat aponeurosis anchored to periosteum, perichondrium, or fascia of other muscles. The musculotendinous junctions are frequent sites of injuries. Capillaries and nerves are embedded in the endomysium, after entry from one or two points (neurovascular hila).

2. Connective Tissues

a. *Loose Connective Tissues*[29-32]

Many reviews offer descriptions of loose connective tissues. Three types of loose connective tissues are listed: areolar, adipose, and reticular. Areolar connective tissue is also known as a ground substance and is comprised of a hyaluronic acid gel with several types of collagen fibers. Areolar connective tissue wraps and cushions organs, and holds considerable body fluid (water). Fibroblasts, macrophages, mast cells, isolated fat cells, and transitory immune cells occupy areolar tissue. Distribution in the body is widespread, but especially fills in spaces inside of tissues not occupied by parenchymal cells, lamina propria, under epithelia (skin, mucous membranes, etc.), around organs, and around capillaries. Areolar connective tissue is the predominate tissue type involved in wound healing and inflammation.

Adipose tissue has a matrix very similar to areolar connective tissue, but adipose (fat) cells are densely packaged, with only blood vessels and nerves as accessory components. Adipose tissue is located under the skin, around kidneys, in bone marrow, in the peritoneum (abdomen), and in breasts, where it provides a store of energy, insulation, protection, cushioning, and support of other tissues.

Reticular connective tissues are composed of a network of reticular fibers in ground substance that forms the internal framework for visceral organs, such as liver, spleen, lymph nodes, and bone marrow. Some reticulocytes are fibroblast-like, while others are macrophage-like.

b. Dense Regular Connective Tissues[29-32]

Dense connective tissues are also referred to as fibrous connective tissues, since the predominant component is collagen or elastin fibers. Dense connective tissues comprise the more familiar components of the musculoskeletal system such as cartilage, tendons, ligaments, and bones.

Tendons, Ligaments, and Aponeuroses (Dense Regular Connective Tissue)

Dense regular connective tissues form tendons, aponeuroses, and most ligaments. These tissues are characterized by parallel collagen fibers, with fibroblasts in between. Their chief function is to attach muscles to bones, bones to bones, or muscles to muscles, and are all involved in joint structures and attachments. The primary feature of dense regular connective tissues is their enormous tensile strength (resistance to pulling force in one direction). Microscopically, dense regular connective tissues appear as wavy lines of collagen fibers with fibroblasts sprinkled throughout. Because of their near ubiquitous association with mechanical forces from muscles and bones, dense regular connective tissues are frequent sites of traumatic sports injuries. Loss of function, sometimes severe, is associated with damage to dense regular connective tissues.

Tendons and aponeuroses[29,32-34] — In general, tendons attach muscle to bone. Tendons are longitudinal and rope-like in shape, while aponeuroses are flat sheets, to connect similarly shaped muscles. Type I collagen bundles are interwoven with a reticular network of Type III fibers, along with blood vessels, lymphatics, and fibroblasts. Attachment to bone is accomplished by a gradual merging of collagen fibers to fibrocartilage to mineralized fibrocartilage to bone. Tendon sheaths cover tendons, allowing for smooth gliding of tendons in their traverses. The ratio of collagen to elastin in tendons is 50:1, which makes tendons very tough and resistant to pulling forces. However, this trait also makes tendon injuries pull apart from bones and muscles.

Ligaments[29,32-34] — Ligaments are structurally very similar to tendons, except that ligaments connect bone to bone across joints. Some ligaments are elastic and contain a collagen-to-elastin ratio of 4:1. Thus, ligaments have more flexibility than tendons. Ligaments offer passive stabilization of joints (when little or no load is applied). In fact, some ligaments are seen as extensions of the fibrous joint capsule.

c. Dense Irregular Connective Tissue[29,32]

Irregularly arranged collagen fibers, with some elastic fibers, characterize dense irregular connective tissues. Found in skin (dermis), fibrous capsules of joints and organs, fascia and septae, and submucosa of the digestive tract, the chief function of dense irregular connective tissues is to provide structural strength and resist tension from many angles in joints and organs. The major cell type is the fibroblast.

d. Elastic Connective Tissue[32]

Some authors differentiate certain connective tissue as elastic. The ligamenta flava that connect vertebrae, vocal cords, some parts of trachea and bronchi, and aortic walls are the main sites of elastic tissue. As their name implies, elastic connective tissues provide stretching ability with durability and resistance to tearing. They are associated with body structures that are undergoing almost constant movement. Elastic connective tissues are composed chiefly of elastin, produced by fibroblasts.

e. Cartilage[20,29-51]

Few connective tissues have attracted as much attention as cartilage. As a result, many reviews have explored many facets of cartilage anatomy, structure, physiology, biochemistry, function, aging, repair, and response to trauma. The chief function of cartilage is to provide structural support and shape to tissues. Cartilage is a highly resistant tissue in mechanical terms, and its resilient properties cushion and resist compression. Cartilage offers properties of load distribution and load transmission. Thus, cartilage is present in tissues that receive considerable load forces and require some flexibility and ability to withstand movement. There are three basic types of cartilage: hyaline (cartilage), fibrocartilage, and elastic cartilage. Hyaline cartilage forms the embryonic skeleton and bone growth plates, covers the ends of long bones in joints (articular cartilage), and forms costal rib cartilage, nose, trachea, and larynx. Fibrocartilage is found in invertebral discs, pubic symphysis, and knee menisci. Elastic cartilage is found in the ear (pinna) and epiglottis. All cartilage is distinguished by being avascular, anervic, and alymphatic. Cartilage appears to be a homogeneous, amorphous substance to the unaided eye. Actually, cartilage is a stiff, firm matrix of collagen, proteoglycans, and cells (chondrocytes). Chondrocytes produce the extracellular matrix, and reside in lacunae, which appear because of artifacts during preparation of light microscopic sections. Mature articular cartilage is avascular, with embryonic and bone-forming cartilage possessing canals with blood vessels. Menisci also have a small blood supply in their periphery.

Articular cartilage covers long bones inside joint capsules and provides efficient lubrication, resistance to compression, and resiliency needed to protect bones from the rigors of movements. Articular cartilage exhibits distinct patterns or zones. Zone I has been called the tangential or superficial zone, and faces the joint cavity and synovial fluid. After a very thin surface devoid of cells (lamina splendens) that is high in collagen and low in proteoglycans, chondrocytes are present, flattened along the plane of the surface, for about 10 to 20% of articular cartilage area. Zone II (transitional, middle, or intermediate) comprises 40 to 60% of cartilage area and consists of spherical chondrocytes randomly distributed in complex but ordered layers of collagen sheets and proteoglycans. Zone III (radial or deep) makes up about 30% of articular cartilage area and exhibits chondrocytes and collagen fibers arranged perpendicularly to the cartilage surface. The tidemark is a distinct band, 2 to 5 μm wide, that separates Zone III from Zone IV (calcified cartilage). Zone IV consists of fewer chondrocytes in cartilage that is partly calcified and physically connects and anchors to underlying bone (subchondral bone).

The metabolism of cartilage is very low compared to other tissues. Turnover for large proteoglycan aggregates in articular cartilage in various adult human joints ranges from half-lives of 200 to 800 d. Some smaller proteoglycans exhibit rapid turnover, with half-lives of 5 to 8 d. Collagen fibers exhibit much slower turnover, with half-lives of several years. Thus, cartilage is a living, metabolically active tissue, but with severe restraints on ability to maintain itself or repair damage. A more thorough discussion of cartilage metabolism will be presented later in this book.

Fibrocartilage is similar to hyaline cartilage, but has more thick collagen fibers that resemble ligaments. Thus, fibrocartilage is found in joints where extreme load forces are present, and resistance to shear and tensile strength are also required to absorb shocks. Elastic cartilage has elastin fibers in its matrix, in order to provide flexibility and return to original shape for the external ear and epiglottis.

f. Bones (Osseous Tissue)[29,52-58]

Bone is perhaps the most-studied internal connective tissue. Some recent reviews on bone anatomy, structure, function, physiology, biochemistry, and metabolism have been examined for this section. The major functions of bone are to contribute to body shape and form, support and anchor soft tissues, protect soft tissues, operate as levers for movement, store fat and minerals, and provide a site for hematopoiesis (blood and immune cell formation). Bone should be viewed as separate organs composed of several different tissues, rather than an inert calcified structure. The primary feature of bone is its hardness, which has the tensile strength of cast iron (17.0 gigapascals) with only one third of the weight. In addition, bone is slightly flexible, with bending strength equal to oak (200 to 250 megapascals). To accomplish these engineering marvels, bone is constructed in a laminar (layered) fashion of a composite structure, somewhat like reinforced concrete. The tubular design of long bones, with internal reinforcement from a trabecular mesh, helps to distribute loads in a radial fashion. Bone is 92% solids and 8% water, or 65% mineral and 35% matrix. Two major types of bone are apparent: compact (cortical) bone and spongy (cancellous) bone (composed of trabeculae, hence the name trabecular bone). Bones are long, short, flat, or irregular in shape and range in size from almost microscopic middle ear components to the femur, nearly 2 feet long. The outside of bones is covered by the periosteum, a tough, double-layered membrane to which many tendons and ligaments are physically attached. The inside cavity (medullary cavity) and canals of bones are covered by the endosteum, a thin membrane containing osteoblasts and osteoclasts. Articular cartilage covers the ends of long bones in joints. Spongy bone is present inside of compact bone.

Bone itself is subdivided into contiguous units called osteons (Haversian systems) based on concentric lamellar layers of calcified osteoid matrix surrounding a central Haversian canal. Osteocytes (osteoblasts) occupy interconnected lacunae within each osteon. Thus, each osteocyte is able to remain readily accessible to its blood supply, which makes bone an interactive, metabolically active, hormonally responsive tissue. The usual diameter of osteons corresponds to the limit of diffusion from the central canal of nutrients. Bone receives 10% of cardiac output and is richly endowed with blood vessels and nerves. Lymphatics are located in the periosteum. The blood vessels inside of bone are thin and have frequent anastomoses, sinusoids, and plexi. Venous supply has six to eight times greater capacity than arterial supply, in order to accommodate entry of new blood cells from marrow and facilitate metabolism of mineral ions.

Bone is constantly being remodeled, with 10% of a young adult's skeleton per year regenerated. The remodeling process is influenced by genetics, physical stresses, growth factors, hormones, and nutrition. The well-ordered process of remodeling has three basic steps: activation, resorption, and formation. Activation of osteoclasts by parathyroid hormone (PTH), physical forces, and other means leads to generation of a cutting cone about 400 μm wide and 2 to 10 mm long in around 20 d. Behind the cutting cone, the defect is filled by neovascularization and osteoblasts, which produce a cement line composed mostly of proteoglycans to wall off the cone. Osteoid matrix is synthesized by osteoblasts. Osteoid matrix is mostly Type I collagen, with other proteins and proteoglycans. Mineralization of osteoid matrix starts 8 to 10 d after osteoid formation, and the filling cone is refilled in around 80 d. Mineralization of the filling cone is complete by 300 to 400 d. It is apparent that synthesis of proteoglycans is a seminal event in osteoid formation, followed closely by collagen synthesis. The ability of bone to remodel allows bone to slowly adapt to its physical load forces and strains, as well as quickly respond to and repair damage.

g. *Joints*[32-34,36-38,42,58-61]

Joints, or articulations, are the means by which different musculoskeletal tissues convert their functions into controlled movement by individuals. Joints connect bones together and allow movement of bones by muscles via tendons and ligaments. Three basic types of joints exist in the human body: fibrous synarthroses, cartilaginous amphiarthroses, and synovial diarthroses. Amphiarthroses are represented by the symphysis pubis and invertebral joints. Most joints encountered in injuries and sports medicine are diarthrotic, freely movable joints such as the knee, hip, ankle, elbow, wrist, fingers, thumb, and shoulder. The enthesis is the area of attachment of tendons, ligaments, and joint capsules onto bone, which is frequently injured in trauma. In general a typical joint structure consists of several basic parts: (1) bone; (2) articular cartilage; (3) joint cavity with synovial fluid; (4) synovium; and (5) joint capsule. Menisci, bursae, ligaments, tendons and associated blood vessels, nerves, and lymphatics complete the structures of joints. Joints are the focal point for many traumatic injuries to the human body, especially in sports medicine. In addition, degenerative joint conditions are a major health concern. The components of joints that have not been previously covered will be described briefly.

Synovium[32,33,37,38,42,58,62-64]

Just under the fibrous joint capsule, the dense irregular connective tissue that surrounds most joint structures, the synovium, is found. The synovium is divided into two layers — the subintima and intima.

There is no basement membrane in synovium. The subintima is highly vascular, loose connective tissue and contains nerves and lymphatics. The intima is one to four cells thick and faces the inside of the joint cavity. Two major cell types are present in the subintima. Type A cells are macrophage-like, and Type B cells are fibroblast-like. However, these cells have overlapping functions, which has led some investigators to identify Type C cells (intermediate synovial cells). Both synthetic and phagocytic properties are possessed by synoviocytes. *In vitro*, synovial cells secrete hyaluronan, proteoglycans, collagens (Types I, III), collagenases, neutral metalloproteinases, activators of collagenases and proteases, fibronectin, laminin, and many other unidentified matrix constituents. Importantly, synoviocytes also can be induced to secrete interleukin-1 (IL-1), prostaglandin E_2, and possibly other cytokines and lymphokines.[33,63-65] Thus, synoviocytes are extremely important in regulating the degradation of cartilage, and, thus, joint function.

Synovial Fluid[32,33,38,42,58,62,64]

Synovial fluid is produced by synoviocytes and consists mainly of a plasma filtrate with few or no proteins above 150,000 Da and a protein content (mostly albumin) of 1.5 to 2 g/dl. In addition to lubricin, a glycoprotein that helps lubricate joint surfaces, the major feature of synovial fluid is hyaluronate. Synovial fluid is viscous and slimy from an approximately 0.2% solution of hyaluronate, a long, nonsulfated glycosaminoglycan. Hyaluronate helps to reduce friction in joints, allowing easy movement of joints without excessive wear. The friction coefficient of synovial joints is 0.003 to 0.015, compared to 0.02 for an ice skate on ice, and 1 for automobile tires on the road. Synovial fluid is probably the major route for nutritional supply to cartilage and chondrocytes. As such, the gel-like properties of hyaluronate solutions influence the passage of large molecules and proteins. Small molecules and ions, such as oxygen, glucose, and calcium, are free to diffuse through the hyaluronate gel.

Bursae and Tendon Sheaths[32,33,42,58]

Bursae are closed sacs lined with cells similar to synoviocytes and filled with a form of synovial fluid. Their function is to act as ball bearings and facilitate gliding or movement of tendons, tendon sheaths, ligaments, muscles, skin over bone, and joint structures. New bursae may form during life in response to excessive motion or mechanical stress, and bursae may hypertrophy in response to stress or inflammation. Some deep bursae may attach to other joint structures.

Tendon sheaths are discontinuous sheets of collagen fibers wrapped around tendons, especially those with large ranges of motion. Tendon sheaths are lined by mesenchymal cells resembling vascular synovium, which secrete hyaluronate to aid in lubrication of tendons. Tendon sheaths protect tendons from friction in their movements. Fibrous adhesions often form between tendons and tendon sheaths after inflammation or surgical repair, especially upon immobilization.

Menisci[66]

Menisci are like the washers of the human body. Menisci are fibrocartilage wedges or discs inside of synovial joints, and they cushion cartilage against rotation stress while adding stability to joints. Menisci have long been thought to be almost useless and have been frequently removed when damaged. However, menisci are now known to be complex hybrids of cartilage and fibrous tissues. Menisci in adults have a peripheral vascularized area that is capable of repair and healing. The periphery has lymphatic and nerve supplies. The internal areas more closely resemble articular fibrocartilage and have no vascularity, lymphatics, or nerves. Thus, certain areas of menisci are able to heal. Removal of menisci from joints leads to premature arthritic changes, probably by removal of load distribution properties.[66]

h. Accessory Tissues[29,32]

Throughout musculoskeletal tissues, other tissue types are abundant. Except for articular cartilage, connective tissues and muscles include nerves, blood vessels, and lymphatic vessels with associated neurons, neuronal processes, endothelial cells, epithelial cells, and immune cell components (leukocytes). Lymphocytes, macrophages, and mast cells (histiocytes) are present throughout connective tissues and adherent to blood vessels. Transmission of nutrients and removal of cellular wastes involve diffusion through extracellular matrix and transport through endothelial cells to reach connective tissues. Adipose tissues and cells are also adjacent to loose connective tissue, underneath skin, and inside of muscles. Each of these accessory tissues plays important roles in healing by their responses to and interactions with inflammation. While much attention has been focused on the parenchymal components of connective tissues, the accessory tissues fulfill extremely important roles for nutritional and aerobic status of all tissues.

B. CONNECTIVE TISSUE MACROMOLECULES

The ability of small molecules to form very large polymers that interact to achieve structural shape, rigidity, strength, and motion for biological creatures is a marvel of mechanical engineering that is so often taken for granted. Connective tissues respond to complex signals of mechanical, electrical, biochemical, and genetic origins during growth and development as well as in repair by manufacturing and depositing macromolecular components into cohesive patterns. It is often overlooked that these macromolecules are actually polymers of nutrients or slightly modified nutrients (e.g., amino acids in collagen), and thus it is well within the scope of nutrition to address the physiology and biochemistry of connective tissue macromolecules.

1.   Proteoglycans[29,30,34,41,44,67-83]

Proteoglycans (PGs) are ubiquitous components of all connective tissues. PGs are one of the three major components of connective tissues, the others being collagen and cells. PGs form highly structured gels that occupy large amounts of space, especially in amorphous ground substance. PGs are very large aggregates of proteins and glycosaminoglycans (GAGs) that comprise a small percentage of tissues by weight, but exert an effect far larger than their concentration implies. PGs make up 10% of dry weight in articular cartilage and around 1% of dry weight in bones, tendons, and ligaments. Formerly called mucoproteins, PGs stain intensely with cationic dyes toluidine blue and safranin O due to their high electronegativity. PGs are more than simply structural elements of connective tissues. Smaller PGs serve as cross-linking agents in connective tissues, and others serve as membrane-associated markers involved in cell-cell and cell-matrix interactions. Three types of PGs have been found: (1) aggrecan; (2) small PGs (decorin, biglycan, and fibromodulin); and (3) membrane-associated PGs (glypican, perlecan, serglycin, syndecan).[79,83] All are composed of GAG chains bound to core proteins.

a.   Glycosaminoglycans[67-86]

Several texts review the chemistry and biology of glycosaminoglycans. Glycosaminoglycans (GAGs), formerly known as mucopolysaccharides, are the predominant feature of PGs. GAGs are long-chain polymers of repeating disaccharide units. Except for hyaluronan (HA), GAGs are sulfated, and so possess a very high negative charge density. These charges serve to repel neighboring GAG chains, when bound to PG subunits, causing a space-filling function. The attraction of water to GAGs gives compressive and load-bearing effects to PGs and cartilage. There are six major types of distinct GAGs, identifiable by the difference in sugar residues in the repeating disaccharide subunit. Table 1 lists the major GAGs and their sugar components. It can be seen that each repeating GAG subunit is comprised of an aminosugar (glucosamine or galactosamine to which sulfates are attached) and a sugar or sugar acid. Each subunit is repeated from several dozen to several hundred times per GAG chain, depending upon the type and tissue location.

HA is unsulfated and is the backbone of aggregating PGs found in cartilage (aggrecan). HA is also the major component of synovial fluid and vitreous humor in the eye. HA solutions (around 0.3%) are extremely viscous and slimy, which imparts lubricating properties to synovial joints, and also cushioning properties to joints and eyes. A more detailed description of HA is found in Chapter 12. Chondroitin sulfates (CS) are composed of galactosamine and glucuronate subunits, and are usually the longest GAGs. CS are found in most tissues, but are prominent in cartilage, blood vessels, bone, and skin. Keratan sulfates (KS) are found in close association with CS chains, especially in cartilage and blood

TABLE 1   Identity, Composition, and Tissue Location of Glycosaminoglycans in Human Tissues

Glycosaminoglycan	Molecular Weight	Composition	Predominant Locations
Hyaluronan (HA)	0.4–20 million	*N*-acetylglucosamine D-glucuronic acid	All tissues, synovial fluid, vitreous humor, cartilage
Chondroitin sulfates (CS)	5,000–50,000	*N*-acetylgalactosamine D-glucuronic acid	Cartilage, arterial walls, skin, bone, most tissues
Keratan sulfates (KS)	4,000–19,000	2-acetamidoglucosamine Galactose	Cartilage, arterial walls
Dermatan sulfates (DS)	15,000–40,000	*N*-acetylgalactosamine Iduronic acid	Skin, skeletal tissues (cartilage, bone, invertebral disc, tendons), cornea, blood vessel walls
Heparan sulfates (HS)	5,000–12,000	*N*-acetylglucosamine Iduronic acid	Arteries, lungs, cell membranes (not in skeletal tissues)
Heparin (Hep)	6,000–25,000	*N*-acetylglucosamine Iduronic acid	Mast cells, lungs, liver, intestines

vessel walls. Dermatan sulfates (DS) are found mostly in the skin, but are also present in skeletal tissues and blood vessels. The similar heparan sulfates (HS) are located predominantly in tissues such as lungs, intestines, and blood vessels, but are not major components of skeletal tissues. Heparin is unlike other sulfated GAGs in that it is found as single molecules. Heparin is found in many cell types, where it exhibits regulatory properties such as calcium binding, prevention of blood clotting, and mediation of inflammation. Heparin differs from the almost identical heparan sulfates by being smaller and more heavily sulfated.

The seemingly minor differences in GAG components is very important to the three-dimensional shape and structure of GAG chains. Small changes in identity of aminosugar or sulfation can have large effects on the space-filling shape or flexibility of GAG chains. As can be imagined, very linear chains can be packed more densely than kinked chains. These subtle differences account for the different roles of GAGs in different tissues.

b.   Core and Link Proteins

The two major proteinaceous components of PGs are the core proteins and link proteins. Core proteins are large (210,000 Da) polypeptides to which are bound carbohydrate residues and GAG chains in large numbers. Core proteins make up the spine of the bottlebrush structure of PGs. Link proteins are smaller polypeptides that bind core proteins to HA. Three link proteins have been identified, with molecular weights of 40,000 to 50,000 Da. All are derived from the same polypeptide chain and are modified by glycosylation or degradation. Link proteins stabilize the attachment of PG subunits to HA chains.

Other matrix proteins found in cartilage and connective tissues that are associated with GAGs are anchorin, chondronectin, fibronectin, entactin, fibrillin, integrins, laminins, sparc (osteonectin), tenascin, undulin, and cartilage matrix protein.[79,83] These proteins are believed to help attach and bind chondrocytes and fibroblasts to their extracellular matrices. Roles in cell adhesion and regulation of matrix organization or assembly have been presented for these accessory matrix proteins.[79,83]

c.   Proteoglycan Structures

Aggrecan is the new name for the archetypal PG subunit found in cartilage.[79,83,87] Aggrecans form very large polymers of aggregating PGs (40 to 100 million Da or more) by binding to a very long hyaluronan molecule with link proteins. Aggrecan makes up 10% of the wet weight of cartilage and, by virtue of its high concentration of negative charges, is capable of binding large amounts of water. *In vivo*, aggrecan is underhydrated, which exerts a swelling effect in cartilage. Thus, aggrecan PG is the main contributor of compressive, load-bearing properties in cartilage. Aggrecan is space-filling in three dimensions and is intertwined among collagen fibrils in cartilage. The architecture of aggrecan begins with a single, long-chain hyaluronan molecule of 1 to 20 million Da. To this hyaluronan molecule, about

40 PG subunits are attached. Each PG subunit is composed of a large core protein (210,000 Da) with attached carbohydrates and GAGs. The amino terminus of core proteins is attached to hyaluronan by several specialized link proteins. A region of single or small chains of carbohydrate residues is attached to core protein, followed by a region rich in keratan sulfate GAGs. Finally, a region of chondroitin sulfate GAGs is found on core protein. GAGs are attached to core protein by a linker assembly of sugars bound to asparagine residues. Chondroitin sulfate chains are usually longer than keratan sulfate chains, so that a net effect of longer and longer GAG chains is found on the length of each core protein. Thus, each PG subunit resembles a bottle brush in appearance, well-designed to fill spaces.

Three small PGs have been recently identified.[79,83] Decorin and biglycan consist of one GAG chain (usually chondroitin sulfate or dermatan sulfate) bound to a single protein. Fibromodulin has four keratan sulfate chains and a heavily glycosylated protein chain. These PGs are about 45,000 Da total and comprise about 5% of all PGs in cartilage. Small PGs are found in all connective tissues. Their roles are suspected to be as cross-linking agents between PG subunits, between cells and PGs, or between collagen fibrils and PGs. Thus, small PGs play a key role in the structure of cartilage and other connective tissues.

Membrane-associated PGs are ubiquitous to all cells and come in two basic types.[79,83] One type is a heparan sulfate PG (syndecan, perlecan, glypican); the other is a chondroitin or dermatan sulfate PG (serglycin). These PGs bind to FGF and TGF-β, suggesting a role in cellular responses to cytokines. Cell–cell and cell–matrix interactions have also been proposed as roles for membrane-associated PGs.[79,83] Membrane-associated PGs make up 1% of total cartilage PGs. The membrane-associated PGs will probably become extremely important for connective tissue responses to cytokines, which is of primal importance for inflammation and degenerative conditions, both of paramount interest in healing. The metabolism of membrane-associated PGs remains to be determined.

d. Proteoglycan Synthesis

Synthesis of PGs involves the coordination of both protein and carbohydrate polymer synthesis, along with collagen synthesis. In adult articular cartilage, the half-life of core protein precursor pools is about 30 min.[79] Core proteins are glycosylated inside of cells, and GAG chains are synthesized, sulfated, then added to core protein chains in Golgi apparati of chondrocytes and fibroblasts. The resulting nascent PGs are secreted into the extracellular matrix. Interaction with link proteins and HA then occurs in the matrix to form PG aggregates. Aggregation occurs within 15 min after secretion. Thus, the synthesis of PGs is a rapid event. A final note on the biosynthesis of PGs is the enormous scale of production, compared to outputs of other cell types. Not only are large amounts of very long carbohydrate polymers produced and modified rapidly, but noncollagenous and collagenous proteins are also produced simultaneously in large quantities. In cartilage, these production attributes are accomplished with an anaerobic tissue devoid of blood vessels, lymphatics, and nerves, meaning that supply of nutrient building blocks for PGs and collagen (glucose and amino acids) becomes a limiting factor in connective tissue synthesis.

Precursors for GAGs are mostly glucose itself, which is quickly modified by donation of an amine group from glutamine, and converted into other sugars by epimerases.[88] Preformed components of GAGs can also be incorporated into GAG chains.[88] Sulfate for GAG synthesis is derived from high-energy phosphate compounds and sulfur amino acids or inorganic sulfate. Incorporation of radioactive sulfate into connective tissues is a time-tested marker of GAG synthesis. In Chapter 9, the roles of trace minerals manganese, copper, and zinc for PG synthesis will be discussed in more detail. Vitamin A exhibits some regulatory effects on PG synthesis, mostly by stimulation of degradation.

2. Collagens[29,76,89-103]

The major component, 70 to 90% by weight, of connective tissues is collagen. Collagen is the most abundant protein in the human body, making up about 30% of total proteins. Collagen is 6% of human total body weight. Because of its prevalence and importance, collagen studies have accumulated into many recent reviews. Collagen provides tensile strength and structural rigidity to tissues. Collagen protein is actually a layered buildup of polypeptide chains intertwined and cross-linked in exact manner

TABLE 2 Collagen Types and Predominant Tissue Locations

Collagen Type	Tissue Location
I	Skin, bone, tendons, ligaments, scars, vessel walls, viscera
II	Cartilage, nucleus pulposus
III	Skin, bone, tendons, ligaments, scars, vessel walls, viscera
IV	Basement membranes
V	Basement membranes, endothelial cells
VI	Fetal tissues (lungs), transformed cells
VII	Chorioamniotic membrane, basement membranes
VIII	Endothelial cells
IX	Cartilage
X	Cartilage
XI	Cartilage
XII	Cartilage

to form physically large fibrils and fibers. Collagen is a prime example of using the submicroscopic to form macroscopic structures. At least 15 distinct forms of collagen are known,[100,103] as listed in Table 2. Types I and III are found primarily in skin, bone, tendons, ligaments, and blood vessel walls, whereas Type II is the predominant collagen in cartilage. Types IV and VII are associated with basement membranes. Types V and VI are associated with cell surfaces and other collagen fibers. Types IX to XII are minor types found in cartilage. Collagen exhibits long half-lives in tissues, ranging from weeks to months to years, depending upon the tissue.

a. Collagen Structure[93,94,96,100,103]

Collagen structure begins with synthesis of procollagen chains. Procollagen chains are unique to each type of collagen, but are approximately 1055 amino acids in length. Three procollagen chains form a triple helix, which is the basic unit of collagen. Because of the amino acid sequence of collagen, which is mostly a trimer of glycine, a variable amino acid (usually lysine) and proline, each polypeptide chain forms a left-handed helix which can be intertwined with two other chains to form a right-handed triple superhelix (tropocollagen). Tropocollagen is 300 nm in length and around 285,000 Da. Extensive posttranslational modifications ensue, which are dependent on adequate nutrient status, as will be detailed in subsequent chapters. Collagen is glycosylated, and modified proline and lysine residues provide stabilization of the triple helix structure. Cross-linking with other collagen molecules forms collagen microfibrils. Collagen fibrils are formed from further cross-linking of large numbers of microfibrils. Finally, collagen fibers are formed by aggregation of collagen fibrils, which by now are macroscopic in size. Thus, simple chains of amino acids can be amplified into large physical structures.

b. Collagen Biosynthesis[91,93,94,96,100,103]

The synthesis of collagen is briefly outlined in Table 3. The influences of nutrients have been listed where applicable. It can be seen that energy, amino acids, magnesium, and zinc are needed in general for any protein synthesis. More specific nutrient needs for collagen synthesis include iron, copper, manganese, vitamin C, and, perhaps, vitamin A. Calcium is necessary for enzyme activity of collagenases providing controlled degradation. The synthesis of collagen places enormous demands for energy and amino acids on fibroblasts, chondrocytes, and osteoblasts. Fortunately, synthesis of collagen is given a high priority during healing processes.

3. Elastins[76,94,103-108]

Elastins are very large, highly cross-linked proteins similar to collagens. Elastins form a three-dimensional mesh network in various tissues to give elastic, resilient properties to tissues. The mesh network can be stretched into almost parallel fibers, which return to their original shape. Elastins are rich in ligaments, skin, large blood vessels, and lungs, which are all tissues with the need for expansion and reversion to original shape. Because of the highly cross-linked structure of elastin meshes, turnover is very slow (months to years), and elastins are very resistant to degradation. Unlike collagens, elastins

TABLE 3 Collagen Biosynthesis and Nutrient Requirements

Biosynthetic Event	Nutrient Needs
1. Transcription (mRNA synthesis)	Energy, amino acids, zinc
2. Translation (polypeptide chain elongation)	Energy, amino acids, zinc
3. Hydroxylation of lysine and proline residues	Iron, vitamin C, oxygen, α-ketoglutarate (lysyl and prolyl hydroxylase activity)
4. Helix formation	
5. Limited proteolysis	
6. Glycosylation of hydroxylysine	Manganese, vitamin A? (glycosyltransferase activities)
7. Disulfhydryl bond formation	Redox status (antioxidants, glutathione, protein sulfhydryls)
8. Secretion of procollagen into extracellular space	Zinc, vitamin A
9. Fibril formation (fibronectin-directed)	
10. Conversion of procollagen to tropocollagen	
11. Cross-link formation (collagen maturation)	Copper (lysyl oxidase activity)
12. Controlled degradation	Calcium (collagenase activity)

form desmosine, an amino acid unique to elastin, that forms covalent bonds for cross-links to adjacent elastin polypeptide chains. Some of the synthetic machinery used for collagen synthesis is also duplicated for elastin (such as prolyl hydroxylase), but there is no hydroxylation of lysine in elastin. For nutritional purposes, elastin synthesis relies on many of the same nutrient needs as collagen, but without the specific needs for copper or calcium (see Table 3).

C. MAJOR CELL TYPES INVOLVED IN MUSCULOSKELETAL HEALING

Table 4 lists the major cell types involved in healing of musculoskeletal tissues.[29,30,32,63,109-117] In addition to the obvious cellular components of connective tissues, such as fibroblasts, chondrocytes, and osteoblasts, other cell types found in accessory tissues are of equal importance for healing of connective tissues. Blood cells and immune cells not only provide nutrients to connective tissues, but they are also transitory players in healing processes with key regulatory roles. Endothelial and epithelial cells provide framework for blood vessels and skin, respectively.

1. Fibroblasts[109-118]

Fibroblasts are crucial for proper healing to occur in loose connective tissues, which surround practically every tissue in the body. Under the light microscope, fibroblasts appear as elongated, spindle-shaped cells. However, in electron micrographs, fibroblasts appear as elongated cells with many convoluted processes that look like tentacles. Fibroblasts are responsive to extracellular factors, such as cytokines, growth factors, and inflammatory mediators, which allow fibroblasts to maintain and repair connective tissues. Fibroblasts are capable of prodigious production of collagen, PGs, and extracellular matrix, and are capable of proliferation to repopulate a region. The nutrient needs and demands of fibroblasts during wound healing have been fairly well studied. Fibroblasts produce Types I and III collagen, which form a scar in dermal wounds. In subsequent chapters, the effects of nutrients on fibroblast proliferation and synthetic capabilities will be presented as indicators of nutrient effects.

2. Chondrocytes[119-121]

Cartilage is an underprivileged tissue, and chondrocytes are underprivileged cells from a nutritional supply viewpoint. Without a direct supply of nutrients from blood vessels or lymphatics, and without direct neural support, chondrocytes are destined to an anaerobic metabolism. Chondrocytes manufacture and are immobilized in lacunae in hyaline cartilage, fibrocartilage, elastic cartilage, and epiphyseal cartilage. Chondrocytes are responsible for formation, maintenance, and repair of articular cartilage. Like fibroblasts, chondrocytes have the ability to proliferate, but this ability is much more restricted than fibroblasts. The complex interplay of cytokines on chondrocyte functions is beginning to be unraveled, showing that chondrocytes are much more responsive than previously thought. Chondrocytes are able

TABLE 4   Major Cell Types Involved in Connective Tissue Healing

Fibroblasts
Chondrocytes
Osteoblasts (osteocytes)
Osteoclasts
Macrophages
Mast cells (tissue basophils)
Lymphocytes
Neutrophils (polymorphonuclear, eosinophilic, basophilic)
Platelets
Endothelial cells (vascular and lymphatic vessels)
Epithelial cells (dermis, epidermis)
Synoviocytes

to produce large amounts of collagen and PGs in spite of poor oxygen tension, limited nutrient supply, and anaerobic metabolism. Type II collagen, other minor collagens, reticular fibers, elastin, hyaluronan, proteoglycans, a host of noncollagenous matrix proteins, and even degradative enzymes, cytokines, and eicosanoids are produced by chondrocytes.

3. Osteoblasts (Osteocytes) and Osteoclasts[52-58]

The cells that produce, maintain, and repair bone are known as osteoblasts. Like chondrocytes, osteoblasts have encased themselves in extracellular matrix (bone), but unlike chondrocytes, osteoblasts enjoy a rich blood supply and direct links to adjacent osteocytes in canaliculi. The ability of osteoblasts to respond to trauma enables bone to regenerate and heal completely. Furthermore, bone is constantly being remodeled, which means that osteoblasts are periodically required to produce osseous matrix. Osteoblasts synthesize bone tissue by first depositing osteoid or organic bone matrix. Osteoid is composed of collagen, PGs, and noncollagenous proteins that resemble cartilage. Mineralization of osteoid proceeds with the assistance of specialized proteins and after removal of most PGs. Osteoblasts are hormone-responsive, which greatly affects how these cells convert nutrients into bone. Rapid mobilization of calcium and other minerals (magnesium, phosphate, zinc, copper) from lacunae surfaces is termed osteocytic osteolysis and is vital for maintenance of serum calcium levels.

A cell type probably derived from macrophage lineage, osteoclasts are involved with removal or destruction of bone during normal remodeling. Osteoclasts are gigantic, motile, multinucleated (several hundred per cell), hormone-responsive cells, although usually in a reciprocal manner to osteoblasts. Osteoclasts generate a "cutting cone" of bone removal by generation of organic acids and degradative enzymes *in situ*, forming a cavity which is subsequently filled in with new bone by osteoblasts, along with capillaries.

4. Macrophages (Monocytes)[29-31,109-117,122-125]

Macrophages (in tissue residence) or monocytes (in the bloodstream) are the chief phagocytes of connective tissues. These mononuclear cells literally engulf and digest dead cells, debris, bacteria, and foreign particles. Macrophages also release a host of degradative enzymes (neutral proteases, plasminogen activator, plasmin, collagenases, elastases, acid proteases, and lipases), complement components, protease inhibitors, α_2-macroglobulin, fibronectin, eicosanoids, cytokines, growth factors, and free radicals. Macrophages are essential for normal wound healing to occur.[122,123] Macrophages are involved in all phases of inflammation and serve regulatory roles in addition to structural roles.

5. Lymphocytes and Neutrophils[29-31,109-117,126-130]

A transitory member of connective tissues, lymphocytes are attracted by factors released from macrophages and other cell types during inflammatory processes. Lymphocytes release factors that help to initiate repair of tissues, as well as regulatory factors for macrophage and lymphocyte functions.[126,127]

Neutrophils (segmented neutrophils, polymorphonuclear leukocytes) are another transitory resident of connective tissues called in by inflammatory mediators.[128] Neutrophils are phagocytic and are potent sources of degradative enzymes (cathepsins, elastases, collagenases), free radicals, eicosanoids, and other inflammatory mediators. Neutrophils activate kinin, which produces pain. Neutrophils also release complement, antiproteases, and mast cell-activating factors. Neutrophils are present in initial stages of inflammation in order to prevent bacterial infection.

Mast cells (basophils) residing in tissues release histamine, heparin, and serotonin in response to physical damage, initiating inflammation.[129,130] Eosinophils release basic protein to neutralize heparin. Both cell types interact with macrophages, lymphocytes, and neutrophils to modulate inflammation.

6. Platelets[29-31,109-117,131-133]

During tissue damage, broken blood vessels release platelets, which attempt to form a fibrin clot around the injured area. Platelets also release aggregatory eicosanoids, lytic enzymes, and platelet-derived growth factor (PDGF). The net results of platelet mediators are to attract other immune cells and stimulate fibroblasts to repair.

7. Endothelial and Epithelial Cells[29-31,63,109-117,134-137]

The cells lining small blood vessels are capable of neovascularization during healing to provide a new blood supply to repaired tissues.[135,136] Likewise, epithelial cells manufacture new dermis and epidermis to cover wounds that break the skin.[134] These cell types are essential for proper wound healing to progress. Both are responsive to inflammatory mediators and growth factors.

Synovial cells are thought to be derived from macrophage and fibroblast precursors, and share many of the same attributes as those cells.[63,137] Like their precursors, synoviocytes can be phagocytic and release a wide variety of inflammatory mediators and growth factors. Their involvement in joint inflammation attracts other immune cells, which may exacerbate some conditions, such as rheumatoid arthritis.[137]

D. MAJOR HORMONES AFFECTING CONNECTIVE TISSUES

Although it is beyond the scope of this book to explore the various effects and roles for different hormones on the healing process, it must be kept in mind that hormones are powerful regulatory agents. As such, hormones can influence the utilization or metabolism of available nutrients in either a beneficial or harmful manner to the healing process. The interactions between hormones is complex and can manifest as a delay or acceleration of healing. Table 5 lists some of the major hormones known to play important roles in healing.[111,138-143] Also listed are other mediators with hormone-like effects. Often, nutrients will have effects on synthesis, release, or receptivity to hormones that may have major effects on healing. Where applicable, nutrient effects on hormones that affect healing will be covered in subsequent chapters.

E. REVIEW OF HEALING PROCESS IN CONNECTIVE TISSUES

The process of wound healing has been extensively studied as a model for connective tissue healing. Wound healing is the reparative responses after a surgical incision has been made in the skin and underlying musculoskeletal tissues. Wound healing has been well studied because of the widespread practice of surgery and the desire to enhance healing from surgery. Intense interest in wound healing has aided surgeons to provide increasingly more effective care for their patients. The result has been thousands of intentionally inflicted wounds (surgery) performed routinely each day, with complete or very acceptable healing in almost all cases. The healing response in wound healing is applicable for this book, since surgical repair of connective tissues is common. Many excellent reviews on wound healing have been published, and the reader is referred to those sources for additional information.[111,116,140,143-154] Healing responses of individual connective tissues will follow wound healing.

TABLE 5   Hormones and Other Mediators Affecting Healing

Amines (histamine, serotonin, octopamine)
Androgens (testosterone and derivatives)
Bone hormones (PTH, calcitonin, calciferols, etc.)
Catecholamines (epinephrine, norepinephrine)
Corticosteroids and corticosteroid-releasing factors (ACTH)
Cytokines (interleukins, interferons, TNF, PAF, etc.)
Eicosanoids (prostaglandins, leukotrienes, thromboxanes, etc.)
Estrogens and progestins (oral contraceptives)
Glucagon
Growth factors (PDGF, FGF, TGF-β, etc.)
Heparinoids
Insulin
Nitric oxide
Opioids (endorphins, dynorphins, enkephalins)
Oxygen-derived free radicals and intermediates
Somatomedins
Somatotropin (growth hormone)
Thyroid hormones (thyroxine, etc.)

1. Sequence of Events in Wound Healing

After an injury, a sequence of events is set in motion at cellular and biochemical levels that results in macroscopic resolution. The interaction of tissue systems (nervous, immune, endocrine, cardiovascular, visceral, and muscle) is implied. In general, the healing response can be divided into three major portions or phases: inflammation, repair, and remodeling. These phases will be examined in greater detail, using wound healing as a model.

a. Inflammatory Phase of Wound Healing

An injury can be defined as cell death and disruption. This physical trauma and reduced oxygen supply to cells and blood vessels ruptures intracellular liposomes, which release a variety of lytic enzymes that initiate a cascade of events. Disruption of blood vessels also leads to local cell death via lack of oxygen delivery, with the same effect of lysosomal enzyme release. Lytic enzymes begin to degrade macromolecules from dead cells, but, perhaps more importantly, lytic enzymes release potent chemical mediators: histamines and kinins.

Extravasation of blood initiates platelet functions, forming a clot in the injured area. Proteolytic enzymes released by platelets (triggered by chemical mediators and exposed collagen) include thrombin, which converts fibrinogen present in escaped plasma to fibrin, forming a mesh network, or clot. The injured area enclosed by a clot (or hematoma) is termed the zone of primary injury. Lymphatics become clogged with fibrin, limiting the extent of inflammation. Immediately after injury, acute vasoconstriction lasts for a few minutes until the chemical mediators (especially bradykinins) exert their effects, causing vasodilation and increased permeability of nearby arterioles. Other mediators derived from plasma include activated Hageman Factor (Clotting factor XII), plasmin, kallikrein, and complement. These mediators, along with histamine and serotonin from platelets, and eicosanoids and cytokines from tissue cells and leukocytes, initiate chemotaxis of additional phagocytic leukocytes to the injured area. Leukocytes are designed to debride necrotic tissue and prevent infection. An escalation by leukocytes, which release further proinflammatory mediators, leads to expression of the clinical signs of inflammation. Anaerobic glycolysis from ischemia accumulates lactic acid, with resulting lowered tissue pH. Inflammation may induce further edema and hypoxia, creating a zone of secondary injury. In simple wound healing, the inflammatory phase usually lasts 7 days, but large variations are common.

The classical signs of inflammation were described by Celsus in the 1st century A.D.: "rubor et tumor cum calore et dolore." Redness, swelling, heat, and pain have been the four cardinal signs of inflammation. To these four, a fifth sign has been added — loss of function.

b.   Repair Phase of Wound Healing

The second phase of wound healing is the repair phase. Synonyms have included the proliferative, regenerative, or synthetic phases. Starting approximately 48 h postinjury, and concomitant with the ongoing process of inflammation, reparative processes begin. The repair phase is characterized by cell growth and production of extracellular matrix (collagen and proteoglycans). Hypoxia and cytokines released during inflammation program fibroblasts and vascular endothelial cells to reproduce and form new blood vessels (angiogenesis), respectively. Fibroblasts produce a collagenous matrix rich in Type III collagen, forming granulation tissue. During the repair phase, cell growth occurs on the periphery of a wound and progresses inwards to the zone of first injury, behind an inflammatory front of phagocytic cells. Collagen is gradually cross-linked, increasing tensile strength of granulation tissue. Some fibroblasts differentiate into myofibroblasts and, along with remaining smooth muscle cells, cause wound contracture, or shrinkage. In humans, limited regeneration of epithelium (skin), endothelium (blood vessels), and some components of connective tissues is possible. The repair phase usually lasts 6 to 8 weeks in simple wound healing, but large variations in the time course are common.

c.   Remodeling Phase of Wound Healing

The remodeling (maturation) phase is initiated about 14 days postinjury. Granulation tissue shifts from Type III to Type I collagen, and collagen synthetic activity approaches normal turnover levels. Newly synthesized fibroblasts and blood vessels are reduced in number. Extracellular matrix is further cross-linked, resulting in a plateau of wound tensile strength. Collagen fibers are realigned along lines of mechanical forces and/or electrical fields. During the remodeling phase of simple wound healing, scar formation ensues. Scar tissue usually does not have the tensile strength of original tissue. Remodeling is a relatively slow process in connective tissues and may last up to a year or, quite commonly, even longer.

d.   Wound Healing by Second or Third Intention

The aforementioned wound healing is termed wound healing by first intention and represents uncomplicated, simple healing of wounds that have the cut ends in close contact. Wound healing by second intention occurs when large tissue defects must be filled prior to epithelialization and healing (secondary union). Inflammation is usually more intense and lasts longer, while granulation tissue must grow inwards from margins. Wound contracture is characteristic of healing by second intention. Myofibroblasts deposit actomyosin (not collagen) which contracts to reduce wound size. The repair phase of healing lasts considerably longer, and more scar tissue formation is apparent, along with loss of dermal appendages (sweat glands, etc.).

Wound healing by third intention occurs when healing is delayed by infection or contamination. The wound stays open until leukocytes and macrophages remove bacteria and debris, and granulation tissue then can cover the defect.

2.   Influences on the Healing Response

Table 6 lists some of the factors known to influence wound healing.[111,116,140-154] A very important variable for sports injuries is the type of inflammatory response elicited. Usually, the inflammatory response after an acute injury is resolved in a week and is known as acute inflammation. Subacute inflammation is possible, which lasts longer, and involves different immune system cells. Chronic inflammation is characterized by a less severe intensity of inflammation in vascularized connective tissues, over a prolonged period of time. Neutrophils are replaced by macrophages, lymphocytes, and plasma cells (antibody-producing lymphocytes), which persist at the site of injury and delay repair and remodeling processes.

Inappropriate healing response such as atrophy or degeneration of tissues can occur, which indicates a failure of healing. Immobilization, chronic inflammation, aging, lack of hormonal presence, decreased nutrition, or continued hypoxia are all promoters of healing failures. Atrophy and degeneration weaken mechanical abilities of connective tissues, making additional injuries more likely.

TABLE 6   Factors Affecting Healing of Connective Tissues

Age
Gender
Type of injury
Severity of injury
Underlying disease processes
Hormonal influences
Dietary intake
Nutritional status
Degree of hypoxia (systemic and local)
Type of tissue(s) affected
Electrical fields
Mechanical load forces
Temperature
Pharmacological agents (drugs)
Mobility (local and whole-body)
Type of onset (acute or chronic)
Structural (physical) deformities
Psychological influences (placebo effects and psychoneuroimmunological links)
Metabolic and cell turnover rates of connective tissues
Muscular strength and forces
Blood supply
Overall health status
Timing of return to physical activity
pH and lactate concentration
Growth factors, cytokines, eicosanoids

A primary goal of therapy for injuries has been to reduce inflammation, in order to prevent subacute or chronic situations from occurring, which would delay healing and cause continued patient discomfort and loss of function. Also, a reduction in the length of time of the inflammatory phase has been thought to allow repair and remodeling phases to begin sooner or progress more quickly. However, some inflammation is necessary to promote the repair phase of healing, where tissue repair is enacted. Complete ablation of inflammation (e.g., with massive doses of corticosteroids) can result in delayed or even absent healing.

Of course, the only consistent finding in the study of healing response in connective tissues has been the variability in time course and results among individuals. While each factor listed in Table 6 has a characteristic effect, it is difficult to accurately predict the outcome of healing on an individual basis. For example, aging is associated with increased cross-linking of collagen, resulting in weaker, less compliant connective tissues. Also, water content of proteoglycans decreases, with decreased resilience of connective tissues. Intramuscular bleeding is greater over 30 years of age and also in more highly trained subjects. In general, increasing age is associated with increased time for healing and less closer return to original functions.

The important points to remember when considering the results of studies on nutrient effects on healing to be discussed later in this book are (1) inherent intersubject variability makes enhancement of healing in humans or animals very difficult to "prove" on a rigorous statistical basis; (2) factors affecting healing are usually poorly controlled variables in many studies; and (3) much research was performed before a more detailed understanding of the healing response was known; therefore, some studies did not measure appropriate parameters. Because of the variability of factors affecting healing, the field of healing enhancement has been denied the rigorous scientific proof of cause and effect seen in other medical disciplines (for example, pharmacology). Coupled with an incomplete, but rapidly expanding, knowledge of basic connective tissue physiology and function, scientific rigor has left a gap in application of nutritional therapeutic modalities. However, at this time, there is sufficient research on a number of nutrients to be able to synopsize and collate effects of nutrients as therapy on different types of healing processes. The critical mass of evidence is starting to weigh in favor of beneficial effects for certain nutrients under certain conditions.

TABLE 7   Major Types of Injuries
Affecting Osseous Structures

Fractures
    Acute — compound, simple, comminuted, crush, greenstick, spiral
    Chronic — stress fractures
Osteopenia (bone loss)
    Osteoporosis (senile or involutional, drug-induced, malnutrition-induced)
    Osteomalacia (rickets in children)
Periosteal damage (bone bruise)
Excessive bone growth or deposition
    Soft tissue calcifications
    Osteophyte formation (arthritides)
    Bone spurs
    Acromegaly (hormonally induced)

3.   Healing Responses of Specific Connective Tissues

a.   Bone Healing

Table 7 lists the primary types of injuries affecting osseous structures.[10,11,18,52-57,148,155-159] Bone is one of the few human tissues that can respond to an injury by complete regeneration of original structures. Bones are constantly being remodeled at a slow rate and receive 10% of total blood supply from each heartbeat. Bone is a dynamic, interactive, and responsive tissue despite low cell density. Bone is divided into two major types: cortical or compact bone, and cancellous, trabecular, or spongy bone. Epiphyseal (growth plate) bone is unique to growing young people and exhibits a different healing response.

Acute bone injury (fracture) and resultant healing has been well studied. Five stages of long bone (compact bone) healing have been described:[52-57,116,148,154,158,159]

- Hematoma formation
- Inflammation
- Callus formation (soft callus)
- Consolidation (hard callus)
- Remodeling

In Stage One (hematoma formation), immediately after a fracture injury, bleeding and tissue damage form a hematoma at the fracture site. Broken bone ends die back a few mm. Periosteal and surrounding soft tissues limit the hematoma formation. In Stage Two (inflammation), several hours after fracture, inflammatory cells appear in the hematoma, and proliferation of mesenchymal cells from the periosteum and medullary canal begins. Capillary growth is initiated. Stage Two lasts for several weeks and overlaps Stage Three (soft callus formation). Cell proliferation leads to differentiation into chondrocytes and osteoblasts which deposit organic matrix while the hematoma is absorbed. The organic matrix becomes increasingly mineralized with new bone to form a callus. Dead bone tissue and blood remnants are progressively removed. Usually, within 2 to 3 weeks postfracture, a callus is formed, which roughly replaces the hematoma in size. Stage Four of bone healing (hard callus consolidation) finds replacement of newly deposited woven bone by lamellar bone which firmly and solidly unites the broken bone ends. Size of the callus is gradually reduced. By 4 to 6 weeks for upper limbs, and 8 to 12 weeks for lower limbs, fracture union has occurred. It is not uncommon for full consolidation to take up to 16 weeks. In Stage Five of bone healing (remodeling), the hard callus is further remodeled to eventually return the fracture site to its original appearance (or as close as possible). The time interval for complete healing can be from 8 weeks to several years, depending upon specific factors.

Cancellous bone healing is accomplished by direct repair, since its location is usually inside of compact bone. Hematoma formation occurs, followed by new blood vessel formation and osteoblastic cell migration. Only a small callus, if any, forms, and new osteoid is mineralized and remodeled to resemble the original structures.

Epiphyseal bone is particularly susceptible to acute and chronic injuries, since the newly formed, immature bone is more similar to cartilage at the epiphysis. Fractures may occur on the epiphyseal line, through the epiphysis, or result in a crushed epiphysis. Subsequent bone formation may alter or stop bone growth, resulting in deformities. Chronic injuries to the epiphysis may lead to a slow, gradual degeneration with or without vascular necrosis (osteochondritis). Again, bone growth may be altered or cease, leading to deformity. Epiphyseal bone injury is a significant component in sports injuries of children and adolescents.

Chronic bone injury resulting from overuse results in stress fractures and represents an ongoing adaptive response to stresses on long bones. Microfractures, unraveling of lamellar structures, and increased resorption with bone cavities may be seen. Stress fractures may be asymptomatic or produce pain and heat, indicating bone formation and remodeling is unable to counteract deleterious effects of stress forces. A balance between bone resorption and production is eventually reached, which can be altered towards production (and thus, healing) by removal of stressors.

Osteopenia (bone loss) can manifest as loss of mineral, loss of organic matrix (osteoid), or loss of both. Osteopenia indicates a lack of bone formation relative to bone degradation. Healing of osteopenia occurs by formation of new osteoid by osteoblasts and subsequent mineralization. Formation of osteoid involves collagen and proteoglycan synthesis. Extracellular macromolecule production becomes vital for repair of bone loss syndromes.

b.　Cartilage Healing[37,42,44,49,116,121,158-161]

Cartilage is a unique connective tissue that is avascular, anervic, and alymphatic. Articular (hyaline) cartilage covers bone ends in joints, while fibrocartilage is present in menisci, invertebral discs, glenoid labrum, ears, and larynx. Cartilage is difficult to injure in an acute traumatic manner before other tissues are damaged. Cartilage may split at the tidemark between calcified and noncalcified regions, be depressed into subchondral bone, or be fissured. Fissures or defects that do not involve underlying bone usually heal very poorly, if at all. Some attempts by synovium to repair cartilage may be found in areas adjacent to the joint capsule, and some clonal expansion of chondrocytes near a fissure may be observed, but, usually, the defect remains. No inflammation, bleeding, hematoma formation, fibrin clots, or granulation tissue is formed during healing of cartilage from injuries that do not penetrate the tidemark. Fissures or defects that affect the underlying bone do show repair by hematoma formation, growth of vascular tissue, migration and proliferation of osteogenic cells, and formation of fibrous tissue or fibrocartilage, which is, in essence, scar formation. An impact strain of 10% usually produces no injury and no response; however, an impact strain of 40% leads to chondrocyte death and permanent defects (fissures and surface dents). Continuous passive motion of joints during healing causes more rapid healing with hyaline cartilage instead of fibrocartilage deposition.

Arthritis is by far the more common form of cartilage damage and represents a chronic imbalance in turnover favoring degradation. Healing of arthritic cartilage will be covered in more detail in later chapters. However, contrary to previous beliefs, healing of arthritic cartilage is far from impossible.

c.　Tendon and Ligament Healing[116,148,154,158,162]

Damage to tendons and tendon insertions are common sports injuries. Physical stresses lead to structural defects (tears), which initiate inflammation, similar to wound healing. Tendons are also cut in traumatic accidents. The inflammatory phase of healing peaks at day 4 and continues at least until day 10 postinjury. Granulation tissue, with growth of new capillaries, forms around the injury, and eventually resolves as scar tissue, with decreased mechanical functions. After 6 months, 90% of repair is completed. Antiinflammatory medication can prevent adhesions, but can also delay repair, and result in weaker healed tendons.

An example of tendon healing is after finger flexor tendons are cut. Healing occurs from cut ends and from the surrounding mesotendon by vascular and fibroblastic ingrowth. The epitendon thickens, and fibroblasts proliferate along the tendon surface and at cut ends. Macrophages remove debris (collagen and fibrin) in the cut gap. By 10 to 14 d, a collagenous "tendon callus" forms. Adhesions, which are fibrous bonds connecting the tendon to surrounding soft tissues, are common after healing, but early mobilization reduces their influence. Ischemia is a potent stimulus for adhesion formation.

TABLE 8   Metabolic Changes Postinjury

1. Increased heat production
2. Negative nitrogen, potassium, sulfur, phosphorus balances
3. Water, sodium, chloride retention
4. Increased gluconeogenesis, early hyperglycemia
5. Insulin resistance
6. Increased serum fatty acids and ketosis (altered fat metabolism)
7. Increased adrenal output of catecholamines and glucocorticoids
8. Decreased adrenal cortex levels of vitamin C and cholesterol
9. Increased need for vitamins A, B_1, B_2, B_6, niacin, pantothenate, and C
10. Sequestration of trace minerals iron, zinc, copper
11. Thymic involution and decreased lymphocyte counts
12. Leukocytosis (increased neutrophil counts)

Remodeling occurs during 4 to 16 weeks postinjury. The tensile strength of cut tendons is weakest at day 5 postinjury and is still weak at days 15 to 20 postinjury. Tendon sheaths regenerate rapidly.

Ligaments are usually injured by sprains. Healing of sprained ligaments is similar to wound healing, since ligaments are usually vascularized. Hematoma formation and inflammation are followed by relatively slow repair and remodeling phases. Final outcome may take a year or more and usually does not reach previous strength, with reductions of 30 to 50% in tensile strength common. Immobilization decreases the rate and extent of healing, while careful exposure to loads can accelerate ligament healing. Ligaments differ amongst themselves in metabolic rates and healing capabilities.

An example of ligament healing is after a complete tear of the medial collateral ligament of the knee. After the initial inflammatory phase, collagen is synthesized for up to 6 weeks postinjury. The remodeling phase is slow and gradual and can last 1 year or longer. The healed segment has a higher proportion of Type III collagen, which forms smaller fibrils and deficient cross-linking, resulting in reduced functional capacity. The anatomy, biochemistry, and biomechanics of cut ligaments are never the same as original values.

4. Metabolic Changes After Injury

The changes in metabolism elicited by injury directly affect nutrient needs and utilization of nutrients. Table 8 lists some of the major findings after traumatic injuries.[138,139,163-166] To put these changes in perspective, the absolute change in metabolic rate (caloric expenditure) after elective abdominal surgery is 105 to 110% of normal. Long bone fractures raise metabolic rate to 120%, while massive infections (peritonitis) raise metabolic rate to 130 to 140%. Extensive third-degree burns raise metabolic rate to a maximum, 170 to 250%. Thus, it can be seen that many sports injuries are of minor impact on overall body metabolism. Usually, if an injured subject is not hospitalized, there will be little systemic effects on metabolism. Nevertheless, some of the changes listed in Table 8 may occur acutely or locally at an injured site, which may delay healing in specific individuals. There are still too many variables to consider clinically before a prediction about the metabolic effect of an injury to an individual can be determined. Thus, there are no firm guidelines for nutritional support based on injury severity for nonhospitalized, injured subjects.

Chapter 2

TOTAL CALORIES AND
PROTEIN INTAKE

I. TOTAL CALORIES

A. ROLES AND FUNCTIONS OF CALORIES DURING HEALING

Considerable effort has been expended on determining the caloric needs of humans after injuries, trauma, sepsis, burns, and surgeries, as evidenced by the number of books and book chapters on nutrition in hospitalized patients.[2-7,138,139,163-171] As a result, the roles of calories in healing have been well studied. Calories are derived from metabolic degradation of carbohydrates, fats, and proteins present in foodstuffs, body stores, and body tissues. Calories are defined as the amount of energy needed to raise the temperature of water by one degree Celsius under standardized conditions. Actual caloric units are termed kilocalories (kcal), but common usage has fixed the term calories as equivalent to kilocalories. In theory, carbohydrates and proteins yield 4 kcal/g, and fats yield 9 kcal/g. In actuality, each foodstuff delivers smaller amounts of energy than the theoretical maximum.

Calories provide the raw materials for production of cellular energy. Briefly, foodstuffs are broken down into their respective molecular components of sugars (carbohydrates), acetyl groups (fats), and amino acids (proteins). Conversion of each type of foodstuff allows entry of acetyl groups into the tricarboxylic acid (TCA, Citric Acid, or Krebs) cycle, which produces some ATP and other intermediate compounds which donate energy as electrons into the electron transport chain of oxidative phosphorylation inside mitochondria to produce more ATP and convert oxygen into water. Cellular energy as ATP is used to operate almost every cellular function, including survival. Since tissue repair absolutely requires cellular functions of protein synthesis, macromolecule synthesis, and nucleic acid synthesis, cellular energy is absolutely required for tissue healing, and a steady supply of raw materials is required for cellular energy production. If raw materials in the form of foodstuffs are not available, the body has many means to utilize stored carbohydrates, fats, and amino acids to generate cellular energy. Cellular energy generation is maintained until death of the organism in starvation. Thus, caloric intake is required to prevent excess utilization of body stores during healing.

Glucose in particular is a major energy source for fibroblasts and lymphocytes.[164] Impaired glucose supply (as encountered in diabetes) delays wound healing.[163] Decreased insulin function leads to hyperglycemia, metabolic acidosis, and hyperosmolarity, all of which delay healing. Another illustration of this point is the timing of insulin resistance during the inflammatory phase of wound healing and its return to normal when the repair phase predominates.

Calories also provide the raw materials for building and repairing tissues. Cellular structures are composed of proteins (amino acids), glycoproteins (amino acids and sugars), glycosaminoglycans (sugars), membranes (lipids), and nucleic acids (synthesized from amino acids and acetyl groups). Thus, caloric intake is associated with provision of raw materials needed to manufacture cellular and extracellular components. Calories also trigger hormonal responses, especially insulin, glucagon, somatotropin, and intestinal neuropeptides. These hormones play roles in the healing process as well as homeostasis.

B. EFFECT OF DEFICIENCIES

When caloric intake is deficient, usually protein intake is also deficient, which is why calories and proteins have been included in the same chapter in this book. Thus, many of the effects of caloric deprivation on healing are similar to effects of protein deprivation. Consensus of a vast amount of research has shown that malnutrition (caloric depletion) has a detrimental effect on wound healing.[164,166,170-172] However, delay in healing was significant only in patients with severe malnutrition or extensive trauma (usually not encountered in ambulatory subjects in office settings). Another consensus of research was that the body's resources were mobilized to facilitate wound healing; i.e., healing wounds were given nutritional priority.[172] Also, the subjects with more complications and mortality had problems of intake (gastrointestinal surgery, malignancies) or endocrine abnormalities (insulin-dependent diabetes) that prevented adequate nutrient intake. Thus, while malnutrition of the general surgical population is less than ideal,[173] the usual patient presenting with a sports injury is comparatively well nourished or is able to continue food intake. In routine clinical practice, malnutrition of sufficient severity to significantly impair healing of connective tissues is not common. Nevertheless, it is always difficult to predict nutritional status for each patient without resorting to biochemical or anthropometric measurements.

C. ASSESSMENT OF CALORIC ADEQUACY

In order to determine caloric adequacy, a three-pronged approach should uncover almost every case of nutritional inadequacy. The three prongs are (1) dietary intake surveys and energy expenditure estimates, (2) anthropometric measurements, and (3) biochemical measurements. Dietary intake surveys are relatively simple, inexpensive, and rapid. A nutritionist or dietitian is well trained to estimate the total caloric intake (kcal/d), percentage of protein, carbohydrate and fat, type of fat, adequacy of protein intake, and intake of micronutrients relative to RDA values. Several computer programs available to health care practitioners have enhanced the determination of dietary intakes. In general, dietary records of 3 days are preferable.[170] Estimates of dietary intakes are well known to be imprecise and subject to changes in food selection and amounts during the recording period. However, offsetting these inaccuracies are the facts that dietary intake is easy to apply in outpatient settings, fairly reproducible, and accurate for determination of energy intake. Comparison of the estimated dietary intakes with suggested guidelines involves determination of the energy requirements of each individual. Energy expenditure can be estimated by calculation of the resting energy expenditure (REE), which is also known as the basal metabolic rate (BMR), and then adding activity and injury factors to achieve a total caloric requirement to maintain body weight.[170]

1. Calculation of Energy Expenditure

The estimation of dietary intake and energy expenditure can give an idea of whether an individual is consuming adequate calories to prevent weight loss, and, thus, malnutrition, at the time of estimation. The research methodology for determination of resting energy expenditure involves measurement of oxygen consumption in the morning after awakening, and 12 h after the last meal. This procedure is cumbersome and not practical for routine estimations of energy expenditure. Rather, several other indirect methods involving simple calculations from easily measured anthropometric values can be routinely used in clinical settings. It must be remembered that determination of BMR by calculations is only an estimate that can detect consistent caloric inadequacy (or excess) when compared to dietary intakes. Table 1 lists the simpler methods for estimation of energy expenditure.[169,170] The Harris-Benedict equation is perhaps the most widely used calculation for estimation of energy expenditure or BMR. The Harris-Benedict equation is accurate ±14% and is reported in units of kcal/d. This method underestimates energy expenditure in malnourished patients by about 20% and overestimates BMR in obese patients by the same amount. A newer and more appropriate calculation to determine BMR is the WHO/FAO equation,[170] also listed in Table 1. The WHO/FAO equation calculates units in MJ/d and can be converted to kcal/d by multiplication by 239.2. This method is regarded as being more accurate at the extremes of body composition.

TABLE 1   Methods for Estimation of Energy Expenditure

Harris-Benedict Equation (gender, age, height, weight)

Females: BMR = 655 + (9.6 × W) + (1.8 × H) – (4.7 × A)
Males: BMR = 66 + (13.7 × W) + (5 × H) – (6.8 × A)

WHO/FAO Equation (gender, age, weight)

Age (y)		Males	Females
<3	BMR =	0.249(W) – 0.127	= 0.244(W) – 0.13
3–10		0.095(W) + 2.110	= 0.085(W) + 2.033
10–18		0.074(W) + 2.754	= 0.056(W) + 2.898
18–30		0.063(W) + 2.896	= 0.062(W) + 2.036
30–60		0.048(W) + 3.653	= 0.034(W) + 3.538
>60		0.049(W) + 2.459	= 0.038(W) + 2.755

Multiply result by 239.3 for answer in kcal/d.

Note: W = weight in kg; H = height in cm; A = age in years.

Activity factors are added to the BMR to approximate more closely actual energy expenditure.[169,170] Table 2 lists a crude range of kcal/d to add to the BMR, depending upon each individual's daily activity level. Again, more refinement is available, but for routine clinical practice, an approximation is sufficient to determine whether an individual is ingesting adequate calories or not. Estimation of activity levels for athletes is more difficult, as training intensity varies widely among individuals.

Injury factors are added to the BMR after the activity factor has been added to most closely approximate actual energy expenditure.[169,170] Table 3 lists some injury and metabolic factors in units of change in BMR. Of note is the relatively small changes in BMR associated with soft tissue and osseous injuries (0 to 30%). Thus, for an individual with a BMR of 2000 kcal/d, fracture of the femur would add about 400 kcal/d to energy expenditure. Since many injured persons reduce their activity level, the increase in BMR from an injury process is often canceled by the decrease in activity level. Comparison of the estimated daily energy expenditure to the estimated dietary intake can give information on whether dietary intake is sufficient to provide enough calories for prevention of caloric deficiency during healing. Again, caution in overinterpretation of energy expenditures must be exercised, since these values are estimates and subject to some individual differences as well as inaccuracies in estimating dietary intake, activity level, and injury factors.

TABLE 2   Estimated Energy Expenditures of Activity Levels (kcal/d)

Activity Level	Additional Calories (kcal/d)
Sedentary	400–800
Light (office, clerical, professional	800–1200
Moderate (walking, lifting)	1200–1800
Heavy (construction, athletic)	1800–4500

Activity	Additional Calories (kcal/kg/h)
Sleeping, reclining	0.9–1.0
Very light (sitting, standing, driving, typing, sewing, ironing)	1.1–2.0
Light (walking 2–3 mph, shopping, washing clothes, carpentry, electrical work, golf)	2.1–4.2
Moderate (walking 3–4 mph, gardening, scrubbing floors, biking, tennis)	4.1–6.3
Heavy (running, climbing, swimming, football, handling pick or axe)	6.2–10.3

**TABLE 3   Changes in Basal Metabolic Rate (BMR)
by Injury and Metabolic Factors**

Condition	Change (% BMR)
Normal health	0 ± 12
Fasting	−20–25
Postoperative	−1 ± 16
Soft tissue trauma	+14 ± 17
Fracture	+20–25
Infection, mild	0 ± 20
Infection, moderate	+20–40
Infection, severe	+40–60
Hypothyroidism	−15–40
Hyperthyroidism	+15–80
Malnutrition	−31

2. Anthropometric Measurements

Measurements based on height and weight can estimate whether malnutrition is already present. Like estimations of dietary intake and energy expenditure, anthropometric measurements are not supremely accurate or precise. However, they may be employed to determine or document whether an individual is malnourished compared to a population reference. If malnutrition is evident, more attention can be given to nutritional repletion to prevent delays in healing. Nutritional assessment in hospitalized patients is becoming more common in order to screen for individuals at risk for being malnourished and, therefore, to initiate more aggressive nutritional repletion to avoid complications after surgery.[171] The use of anthropometric measurements in outpatient clinical settings may be used to convince an individual that malnutrition or excess body fat is real. Usually, anthropometric measurements determine body protein mass and body fat mass. Measurements of body weight and skinfolds are frequently used to determine body composition. New techniques to measure body fat, such as bioelectrical impedance, are also available. The creatinine/height index is not suitable for athletes since exercise itself increases excretion of creatinine.

Values obtained are compared to tables found in textbooks to find the percentile value for that individual.[168-170] Values that are 15 to 20% less than usual body weight or muscle mass indicate malnutrition. Usual estimates of body fat and protein stores are accomplished by skinfold thickness measurements made by calipers. Common areas measured are the midarm triceps skinfold and the subscapular skinfold. The triceps skinfold can be combined with midarm circumference to calculate the midarm muscle area. Again, comparisons to tables can find the percentile of the population for an individual. The reader is referred to other texts for detailed instructions on measuring anthropometric values.[174,175]

The most clinically useful parameters to assess caloric adequacy via anthropometric testing are the usual body weight, followed by changes in body weight. Decreases in body weight over the last month of greater than 5%, or greater than 10% decrease in usual body weight over the last 6 months, suggest that malnutrition be considered.

3. Biochemical Measurements

Use of clinical laboratory analysis for determination of malnutrition has been helpful in hospital settings, but is of more dubious value in ambulatory outpatient settings. Measurement of levels of certain plasma proteins can yield information on short-term protein-calorie status. Serum albumin, transferrin, prealbumin, retinol-binding protein, total lymphocyte count, delayed cutaneous hypersensitivity, and maximal respiratory pressure have all been used as indicators of malnutrition and protein status.[170] Since these tests are more specific for protein, further discussion will be found in the next section of this chapter.

D. EFFECT OF REPLETION OR SUPPLEMENTATION

The concept of supplying nutrients to an injured site in order to facilitate healing was tested in rats by Niinikoski and others, from the Departments of Surgery, Medical Chemistry, and Pediatrics at the

University of Turku in Finland.[176] Hollow, cylindrical sponges were implanted subcutaneously into rats, and wound fluid accumulating in the cavity was examined at 7 and 14 d postsurgery. Granulation tissue forms in the sponge, simulating wound repair. One group of rats was injected daily into the sponge cavity with a mixture of amino acids, salts, glucose, B vitamins, and vitamin C. Compared to sham-injected controls, the local hyperalimentation group showed increased PO_2, decreased PCO_2, decreased lactate/pyruvate ratios, decreased fluid hemoglobin, and increased DNA, RNA, and hydroxyproline contents, suggesting an enhancement of the healing process when nutrients were made more abundant at the wound site. Anaerobic metabolism was shifted to aerobic, and more cells with better synthesis of matrix components (collagen) were noted. Thus, in theory, a better supply of essential nutrients directly to the wound site may improve healing.

Likewise, 58 human patients with large open wounds after trauma or third degree burns were treated with viscose cellulose sponges applied to open wound areas.[177] Local application of amino acids, glucose, salts, and B vitamins under the sponge led to enhanced healing and earlier times to skin grafting. Although the concept of supplying additional nutrients to wounds for acceleration of healing was supported, the routine clinical application of local injections of nutrient mixtures had inherent difficulties associated with sterility.

In general, after assessment of nutritional status has found evidence of malnutrition, nutritional repletion by intravenous or enteral means has generally led to decreased morbidity and/or mortality in hospitalized patients.[163-172] For example, hydroxyproline content of healing wound biopsies in patients with abdominal surgery was almost doubled after TPN compared to infusion with glucose (0.302 vs. 0.172 mg hydroxyproline/dl).[167] In another study, 47 malnourished patients exhibited lower levels of wound hydroxyproline than better nourished subjects (0.34 vs. 0.49 µg hydroxyproline/cm Goretex tubing).[178] After TPN, hydroxyproline content increased to 0.88 µg/cm. Other findings were that preoperative nutritional repletion was associated with better healing responses and less complications.[178] Thus, nutritional repletion before or after surgery to malnourished, hospitalized patients appears to improve wound healing and clinical outcome. However, the applicability of these results to sports medicine is unclear. At this time there is insufficient evidence to support indiscriminate application of excess feeding to accelerate healing.

Other areas of interest in injury rehabilitation that are not commonly considered include skeletal muscle function and psychological effects of nutritional repletion for surgical procedures.[178] After 3 weeks of TPN, surgical patients showed a partial restoration of Type II muscle fibers and an increase in phosphofructokinase activity (a key enzyme involved in glucose utilization). Other muscle enzymes (hexokinase, fructose biphosphatase, and oxoglutarate dehydrogenase) were unaffected. Thus, further work on the maintenance of muscle mass and function by nutritional means in injured subjects is warranted.

Another overlooked area of recovery that has a nutritional link is the psychology of the patient. Many injured persons are somewhat depressed due to their circumstances and inactivity, but malnutrition itself leads to inability to concentrate, irritability, and apathy, even though the intellect stays lucid.[178] After 32 patients awaiting major abdominal surgery were given a 2-week course of TPN, objective measurement of psychological scores were significantly improved, with reductions in tension, anxiety, depression, anger, hostility, and fatigue.[178] Vigor and friendliness were increased. Thus, the mood of an injured person may be improved with adequate nutrient intake. The implications for enhanced rehabilitation are obvious since a helpful, committed patient may enjoy a faster recovery than a sullen, depressed, and recalcitrant patient. The need for research into the nutritional link between mood and healing is appealing.

E. SUMMARY

Although the study of caloric requirements and repletion during human healing has centered around hospitalized surgical patients, several findings have been noticed that may be applicable to sports medicine. Malnutrition "need not be overt to be significant physiologically."[164] This means that oftentimes acute nutritional deficiencies or abnormalities at the injured site are not accompanied by systemic signs of nutrient deficiency. The rapidity and timing of metabolic changes during inflammation and repair mean that different nutrients may have deficient status at the injured site at different times during the healing process. This is a difficult phenomenon to explore in humans, especially healthy, ambulatory athletes. Thus, it is not surprising to find that nutritional repletion of malnourished surgical patients results in reduced morbidity and mortality. The improvement in nutritional support coupled with the routine use of antibiotics and advanced surgical procedures means that many operations are successful that just 30 years ago were often very risky. However, the application of results from general hospital patients to sports medicine patients may not be justified because of the likely difference in nutritional states between the two populations. It is clear that if evidence of malnutrition is present, nutritional repletion with calories including protein, carbohydrates, and fats along with vitamins and minerals will result in improved, or "normalized", healing of connective tissues. Reduced morbidity, reduced mortality, reduced nutrient deficiencies, improved nitrogen balance, improved immune function, and, perhaps, improved psychological behavior are all sequelae of adequate caloric intake.

F. GUIDELINES

Guidelines for caloric intake are not different from preinjury time periods, unless severe trauma is encountered. A provision of at least the caloric amounts according to calculations of energy expenditure in Tables 1 to 3 is recommended, taking into account the subject's previous dietary patterns and intakes. For most injured subjects, 35 kcal/kg/d should be sufficient to maintain body weight and muscle mass.[169,170] For extremely severe injuries (usually requiring lengthy hospitalization), increases in total calories may need to be 40 to 50 kcal/kg/d. Protein percentage of about 15 to 25% of total calories appears to be adequate to prevent large losses of muscle mass. Above all else, a decreased food intake is to be avoided, and, if necessary, enteral or even parenteral feeding (TPN) in severely injured subjects should be instituted to prevent decreased caloric intake. Dietary supplements such as Ensure® or Sustacal®, to name only a couple of many enteral products, may be supplied in order to conveniently manipulate a subject's dietary intake and prevent deficiencies. A resulting placebo effect may also be an advantage for the mind-body connection in some persons.

II. PROTEIN, PROTEIN HYDROLYSATES, AMINO ACID MIXTURES

A. INTRODUCTION

Protein appears to be as important as total calories for healing to occur. As previously stated, protein intake and caloric intake are often closely associated, so that malnutrition is frequently termed protein-calorie malnutrition (PCM). In clinical settings, it is unusual to find instances of caloric deprivation without protein deprivation. Many of the effects seen after repletion of total calories may be due to the amino acids present in any type of refeeding (TPN, enteral, solid foods). However, specific effects on protein have been delineated by control of diets fed to animals. Since much of our bodies is constructed of proteins (collagens represents 6% of total body weight), it makes empirical sense that protein nutriture would greatly affect healing, even if our bodies have developed sophisticated homeostatic mechanisms to transfer protein (amino acids) between different organs and tissues.

B. ROLES AND FUNCTIONS DURING HEALING

Dietary protein is eventually converted to its component amino acids by digestion. Amino acids then become protein currency in the body, much as ATP is the energy currency of the body. Thus, dietary protein (or amino acid) intakes equate to serum and cellular amino acid levels or fluxes. Again, since our bodies are mainly constructed of proteins on a cellular level, it is obvious that proteins determine almost every body and cellular function. Amino acids are basic building blocks for construction of proteins, especially collagen, elastin, proteoglycan core proteins, and noncollagenous matrix

TABLE 4   Effects of Protein Deficiency on Healing

Decreased or Delayed	Increased
Fibroplasia (fibroblast proliferation)	Interstitial edema
Neovascularization	Length of inflammatory phase of healing
Collagen synthesis	Length of total time for healing
Proteoglycan synthesis	Catabolism of muscle tissue (protein)
Wound remodeling	Catabolism of visceral tissue (protein)
New lymphatic vessel formation	Catabolism of connective tissues
Immune functions (lymphocyte responses)	Wound dehiscence
Serum, interstitial fluid albumin levels	Wound infections
Skin and granulation tissue wound breaking strength	

proteins (fibronectin, laminin, etc). Other proteins with specific effects on musculoskeletal healing include the hormones made of amino acids (insulin, glucagon, somatotropin, somatomedins, cytokines, lymphokines, neuropeptides) and amino acid neurotransmitters that regulate hormone synthesis and release. Cell receptors, transport proteins for nutrients, and, of course, enzymes are all derived from amino acids. Thus, every aspect of healing is dominated by proteins and their precursor amino acids.

C. EFFECTS OF DEFICIENCIES

Similar to caloric deprivation, protein deficiency has been extremely well studied in terms of healing, especially wound healing and postsurgery. Almost every review on healing covers some aspect of protein deficiency.[138-140,163-172] A simplistic statement is that protein deficiency delays healing. Of course, severity of protein deficiency determines the extent of delay, which can range from imperceptible to complete termination. Table 4 lists the effects of protein deficiency on connective tissue healing (wound healing).[138-140,163-172] Although all phases of healing are delayed by protein deficiency, the major effect is a prolongation of the inflammatory phase, leading to a lag of the repair phase. Proliferation of fibroblasts and endothelial vascular cells is slowed, as is production of proteinaceous matrix components (collagen and proteoglycans). Wound remodeling is also delayed, since remodeling is dependent on collagen synthesis. If protein deficiency is severe enough to depress albumin synthesis, decreased albumin levels in serum and interstitial areas lead to interstitial edema, further hampering fibroplasia. Immune functions, especially those mediated by lymphocytes, may be depressed, leading to lesser amounts of growth factors and increased susceptibility to infections.

During protein deficiency, if dietary protein intake does not meet metabolic demands for amino acids, muscle tissue is catabolized first to maintain a supply of amino acids for other tissues, including healing wounds.[94] If demands for amino acids are still not met, then connective tissues become the primary source of amino acids by catabolism of collagens and noncollagenous matrix proteins.[94] Bone collagens are a primary target of connective tissue catabolism. Not only is collagen synthesis sharply decreased during fasting and starvation, but even food restriction seriously impairs collagen synthesis. Thus, even short-term deprivation or decrease in dietary protein intake, especially when accompanied by the metabolic responses after injury, may seriously affect the ability to heal. Repletion with nonprotein calories does not restore healing to normal in protein-deficient states.[167]

One of the metabolic responses after injury is a net loss of body protein, as discussed above. The duration of protein loss is 3 to 6 weeks when protein intakes are usual (0.8 g/kg/d). The net loss of protein is shown by a negative nitrogen balance (less nitrogen intake than nitrogen excretion in urine and feces). For example, the nonfecal loss of nitrogen (protein) after a simple fracture with immobilization ranges from 16 to 49 g/d.[170]

PCM before major abdominal surgery has been shown to be a risk factor for complications and mortality. For example, although incidence of wound infection and pneumonia were not significantly different in gastric carcinoma patients given TPN before surgery with controls, decreases in major complications (17 vs. 32%) and mortality (5 vs. 19%) clearly illustrated the advantage of repleting protein status via TPN before surgery.[167] Likewise, biochemical indicators of protein deficiency were

TABLE 5   Anthropometric Method for Determination of Long-Term Protein Status: Arm Muscle Circumference

1. Have patient sit with right arm hanging freely at side.
2. Mark the midpoint between the acromion process and the olecranon (from the bone point on top of the shoulder to the elbow bone on the back side of the arm). This is the midarm point.
3. Measure midarm circumference in mm (MAC) with a tape measure.
4. Measure midarm (triceps) skinfold in mm with calipers (TSF).
5. Calculate midarm circumference (MAMC): MAMC (mm) = MAC – (TSF) .
6. Compare the patient's value with tables listing the percentiles for MAMC based on age group and gender.
7. Compare percentile ranking of MAMC with percentile ranking of usual body weight. If percentile rank of MAMC is 15–20% below percentile rank of usual body weight, then significant protein malnutrition is present.

associated with greater incidence of postsurgical complications.[167] For example, surgical patients with serum albumin levels below 3.0 g/dl showed a 55% complication rate compared to 21% for patients with serum albumin levels greater than 3.0 g/dl.[167]

D. ASSESSMENT OF PROTEIN STATUS

The assessment of protein status overlaps with assessment of total caloric malnutrition. Interestingly, "eyeball" assessment of nutritional status by using routine clinical information and empirical observation provided an accurate estimation of protein deficiency in over 70% of hospitalized patients.[170] Nevertheless, if documentation of protein deficiency is required, there are two major ways to assess protein status: anthropometric measurements and biochemical measurements. As with calories, dietary intake assessment may locate a deficient protein intake. Anthropometric measurements of arm muscle circumference or area relate to long-term protein status. Table 5 lists the procedure for determining arm muscle circumference. As with most anthropometric measurements and calculations, there is some imprecision. However, the ease of estimation coupled with the limited sensitivity is sufficient to find individuals with severe protein malnutrition, especially if protein deficiency has been prolonged. Other measurements of protein status, such as creatinine/height ratio, muscle strength testing by hand dynamometer, or maximal respiratory muscle strength, are not recommended due to the wide range of "normal" values and high individual variability.

Biochemical indices of protein status have been useful in hospitalized settings. However, the utility of biochemical measurements in outpatient settings is of considerably less value. Table 6 lists some serum proteins used for assessment of protein status. Usually, decreases in serum levels (signifying protein deficiency) are not seen until protein malnutrition is severe. However, the advantage of serum protein levels is the short-term nature of serum protein half-lives. Thus, rapid changes in protein status may be determined or assessed in a serial manner. Since serum albumin is usually included in chemistry profiles of serum, and lymphocyte counts are now becoming routine for complete blood counts, routine laboratory tests offer two biochemical methods of protein assessment. Thus, screening for protein deficiency is relatively low cost to impractical research methods (nitrogen balance, 3-methylhistidine excretion).

The half-lives of serum proteins used for protein status assessment provide a range of times for protein deficiency assessment. Albumin measures protein deficiency over the last 20 d. Transferrin half-lives are 7 to 10 d, prealbumin 2 to 3 d, and retinol binding protein, 10 to 12 h.[170] Thus, by judicious measurement of certain serum protein levels, one can determine the onset of protein deficiency conditions, as well as their remediation.

Immunological measurements (total lymphocyte counts and delayed cutaneous hypersensitivity [DCH] reactions) are less sensitive than other measures and subject to many interferences, but if the values are decreased below normal limits, then a protein deficiency is strongly indicated. Total lymphocyte count tends to correlate best with visceral protein status. Mild malnutrition is indicated by a count from 1200 to 2000 cells per mm^3, while severe depletion is indicated by counts below 800 cells per mm^3. Of course, other nutrient deficiencies could account for a decreased lymphocyte count, as well

**TABLE 6   Biochemical Measurements Used
for Assessment of Protein Status**

Parameter

Serum albumin level
Serum transferrin level
Serum retinol-binding protein level
Serum prealbumin level
Nitrogen balance
3-Methylhistidine excretion
Amino acid analysis (urine and/or serum)
Total lymphocyte count
Delayed cutaneous hypersensitivity reactions (DCH)

as infections (especially HIV) and immunosuppressant drugs (including corticosteroids). Likewise, the same and additional interferences render the DCH test difficult to interpret correctly.

For ambulatory patients or those with less than severe injuries, routine clinical laboratory measurements should suffice to rule out severe protein deficiency. Methods are simply not precise or sensitive enough at this time to faithfully predict who would benefit from protein supplementation for enhancement of wound healing. If healing appears delayed in an individual, then further measurements of protein status would be justified. Also, if PCM is apparent, then deficiencies of other micronutrients can be expected.

E.   EFFECTS OF REPLETION AND SUPPLEMENTATION

1.   Human Studies

Many studies have verified that correction of PCM by administration of enteral or parenteral feeding results in improved healing.[138,139,163,165-167,176-180] To illustrate this finding, a few human studies will be presented. Haydock and Hill, from the University of Auckland in New Zealand, measured the hydroxyproline content (collagen synthesis) in subcutaneous PTFE tubes in surgical patients given TPN presurgery compared to patients not given TPN.[181] The patients receiving TPN exhibited a faster wound healing response 7 d postsurgery, as evidenced by a greater hydroxyproline content of implants. It is now almost dogma that nutritional repletion (especially protein or amino acid mixtures) to patients with protein-calorie deficiencies will result in fewer complications, quicker return to nutritional adequacy, and improved healing from surgery.

The question of whether apparently healthy persons would benefit from additional protein intake during periods of injury and healing has not been well studied. A series of six studies by Cheraskin and Ringsdorf examined the effect of protein supplementation in humans with periodontal disease.[182-188] No subjects exhibited clinical or biochemical signs of protein deficiency. Studies were conducted with placebos for 4 to 15 d. Both whole proteins of animal and vegetable origin were used, as well as mixtures of amino acids. Total supplemental protein amounts were 10 to 40 g/d. Gingival inflammation, sulcular depth, and tooth mobility were assessed. Protein supplementation was associated with significant favorable effects on reduction of inflammation and tooth mobility. The effect of protein supplementation was greater than standard practice of scaling and prophylaxis. Although these studies have not been replicated, they suggest that even in instances of local healing in persons with presumably adequate protein status, protein supplementation led to improvements in healing.

Tkatch and others, from the World Health Organization Collaborating Center for Osteoporosis and Bone Disease (Geneva, Switzerland) measured the clinical outcome and bone mineral density of elderly patients with hip fractures after receiving two levels of dietary protein, in order to determine whether protein was responsible for clinical improvement seen in other studies of protein supplementation with vitamins and minerals.[189] One group (n = 33) of 62 hospitalized patients (mean age 82) with femoral neck fractures received an oral liquid supplement of 20.4 g milk protein daily for 36 to 38 d. The protein supplement accounted for a 60% increase in daily protein consumption, bringing a low intake into the normal range. Both groups received supplemental calcium (525 mg/d), phosphorus (270 mg/d), magnesium (70 mg/d), vitamin A (750 IU/d), vitamin D (25 IU/d), 29.5 g carbohydrate, and 5.8 g lipids. All patients underwent operations (hip screw placements or cephalic arthroplasty), and bone mineral density was determined by dual photon absorptiometry.

Both groups exhibited low serum albumin levels, indicating protein malnutrition. The group receiving the protein-containing supplement exhibited a significantly shorter hospital stay (69 vs. 102 d), better clinical course (79 vs. 36% favorable), better death and complication rate after 7 months of followup (52 vs. 80%), higher levels of serum osteocalcin (+7 vs. +5 ng/ml), and fewer complications (26 vs. 47) after 7 months. Although the femoral neck bone density was not different between the 2 groups after 7 months, the protein-supplemented group had significantly fewer persons with significant bone loss.

These results suggest that elderly subjects with hip fractures are malnourished, including protein malnutrition, and a protein supplement (meaning normal protein intake) is associated with improved clinical outcome. However, these results do not necessarily extrapolate to fracture healing in young, healthy adults. What is important is that protein deficiency impedes healing of osseous tissues, and protein nutriture must be considered during repair of osseous structures.

F. SUMMARY

The importance of protein (amino acids) for all aspects of healing is unquestioned. The use of protein as amino acids is firmly entrenched in surgical nutrition, enteral feeding, and parenteral feeding.[190] Since many hospitalized patients are malnourished to varying degrees, repletion of protein intake and status has been successful in reducing morbidity and mortality, although it is still difficult to predict clinical outcome on an individual basis. The concept of increasing protein intake during times of connective tissue healing in younger patients that are not hospitalized has not been examined in sufficient detail to make any sound conclusions about effects on healing. Since protein intake of athletes and nonathletes varies considerably among sports and individuals,[191] and nutritional demands of some sports exceed the average needs of the general population, there is a distinct possibility that malnutrition may exist prior to or immediately after an injury. Sports at greatest risk for deficient protein intake are gymnastics, road race cycling, endurance running (marathons, cross-country, triathletes), ultraendurance events, mountain climbing, wrestling, female figure skating, and dance.[191] Persons participating in these sports who have become injured should be carefully checked for dietary protein intake, especially if body weight has decreased recently and muscle mass (arm muscle circumference) is less than ideal.

The form and type of dietary protein seems less important at this time than total intake. A large array of choices to increase protein intake are available, including foods and specific dietary supplements. Food sources rich in protein are preferred, since they contain other essential nutrients. Currently, many protein powders are available that contain vitamins, minerals, and other nutrients, simulating whole foods. The preferred protein choices are listed in Table 7. Their selection is mostly a matter of personal preference.

G. GUIDELINES FOR USE OF PROTEIN

Although the question of whether increased protein intake will enhance musculoskeletal healing, or prevent muscle loss from immobilization, is still unanswered, it is known that "normal" intakes of dietary protein allow healing to progress at "normal" rates. Firm guidelines have been established for protein intake in hospital settings.[169,170] At least 1.0 g protein/kg/d is recommended, with daily intake increasing with general elective surgery (1.5 g/kg/d), multiple trauma (1.5 to 2.0 g/kg/d), and burns or severe sepsis (2.5 g/kg/d). These intakes appear prudent for athletes, as most are consuming these levels as part of their normal diet.[191] Thus, dietary intake analysis is recommended to find a usual daily protein intake. During healing, this amount of protein is recommended to be continued, as long as the daily protein intake is at least 1.0 g/kg/d, and caloric needs are satisfied (no weight loss). Table 7 lists these guidelines for protein intake during musculoskeletal healing.

TABLE 7 Guidelines for Protein Intake During Musculoskeletal Healing

1. Determine each individual's usual dietary protein intake in g/kg/d by dietary analysis from 3-day food records or 24-h recall.
2. Continue protein intake at usual levels, unless usual protein intake is less than 1.0 g/kg/d; if usual protein intake is less than 1.0 g/kg/d, increase protein intake to at least 1.0 g/kg/d, and, preferably, 1.5 g/kg/d; higher protein intakes are acceptable.
3. If increased dietary protein is required, intake of foods rich in protein and low in fat are recommended; these foods include: skim milk; egg whites (including Egg Beaters®); skinless poultry white meat; fish and shellfish; lean beef cuts; lean pork cuts; protein powders (casein, lactalbumin, whey, soy, rice and mixtures); protein hydrolysate powders (same as powders, some may be fortified with amino acids); strict vegetarians can increase soy products, legumes, yeast, and blue-green algae intake.

Chapter 3

SINGLE AMINO ACIDS

I. INTRODUCTION

Proteins are composed of amino acids linked together into discrete chains. Peptides are short chains of amino acids (2 to 20 amino acid residues). Amino acids are the precursors and raw materials for proteins, peptides, nucleotides, and parts of phospholipids. Amino acid metabolism encompasses and directly impacts almost every aspect of cellular function. Pools of individual amino acids exist inside of cells, in plasma, and in other extracellular fluids. Amino acids are ubiquitous in the human body. This chapter will explore the use of individual amino acids for enhancement of musculoskeletal healing. The range of studies is from enhanced absorption of minerals to pharmacological pain control, illustrating the enormous breadth of functions for amino acids. One caveat must be considered about single amino acids, or, for that matter, any single nutrient. The human metabolism and the healing response is a complex, dynamic system with numerous homeostatic controls. Simply adding one ingredient to a complex system may or may not accentuate the desired result, or it may have unforeseen consequences. In other words, adding a single nutrient to metabolism and expecting it to exert measurable effects on the net outcome is an uphill climb. Nevertheless, with the widespread availability of pure, individual amino acids, a considerable literature has accumulated on the effects of single amino acids on musculoskeletal healing.

A comment about the essentiality of amino acids is also in order. Amino acids are referred to as either essential (indispensable) or nonessential (dispensable). This classification has colored amino acid research and understanding of the true roles of amino acids. The notion of essentiality came from experiments in young, growing animals. Thus, the common term of amino acids being essential is for dietary intake to support animal growth. Later research has confirmed the essentiality of the same amino acids (and perhaps others) for human infants. Thus, the term essential amino acid means only that dietary intake of the amino acid is absolutely required to support growth. Unfortunately, the terms essential and nonessential have caused a mindset that dietary dispensable amino acids are not essential. Nothing could be further from the truth. For example, glutamine is widely agreed to be nonessential, and young animals will grow when glutamine is absent from the diet. However, glutamine is not absent from metabolism and protein synthesis. In fact, glutamine is the predominant amino acid, in quantitative amounts, in the human body. If glutamine is absent from cell environments, cells do not grow and frequently die. This simple fact was noticed when cells were first routinely cultured by Eagle in the 1950s.[192] Because glutamine was thought to be less important than other amino acids, understanding of the actual importance of glutamine was severely delayed until only very recently. Thus, every amino acid is essential and indispensable for proper metabolic functions, including healing. Whether the amino acid is derived from dietary or cellular sources is inconsequential on a cellular level.

A new class of amino acids may one day become dogma: conditionally essential. In other words, some amino acids are required during periods of stress to maintain optimum metabolic function. Table 1 lists the known indispensable and dispensable amino acids, with those known to be conditionally essential. All amino acids are indispensable to the body.

TABLE 1 Identification of Amino Acids as Essential From a Dietary Intake Viewpoint

Indispensable	Conditionally Indispensable	Dispensable
Isoleucine	Arginine	Alanine
Leucine	Cysteine, Cystine	Asparagine
Lysine	Glutamine	Aspartic acid
Methionine	Histidine	Citrulline
Phenylalanine	Taurine	Glutamic acid
Threonine	Tyrosine	Glycine
Tryptophan		Ornithine
Valine		Proline
		Serine

Note: Conditionally essential amino acids are synthesized by the body in inadequate amounts to meet requirements during periods of growth or physiological stress. Therefore, an exogenous (dietary) source is required.

II. ARGININE

A. ROLES AND FUNCTIONS

Arginine is one of the basic amino acids, along with lysine, histidine, ornithine, and citrulline. Initial work on arginine found that it was a dietary essential amino acid during periods of growth in rats, but not in stable adults.[193] Table 2 lists some roles of arginine pertinent to connective tissue healing.[138,180,193-196] Arginine is involved with many pathways that influence healing, especially modulation of immune function.

B. ANIMAL STUDIES

Studies in injured rats (postsurgery or postfracture) found that arginine administration enhanced wound healing, ulcer healing, fracture repair rates, nitrogen balance, or protein synthesis.[194,195,197-204] For example, in rats fed by intravenous hyperalimentation after surgical wounding and implantation of sponges, the group receiving a diet with 7.5 g/l of arginine exhibited significantly greater wound breaking strength (376 vs. 252 g) and sponge hydroxyproline content (1698 vs. 1299 µg hydroxyproline per 100 mg sponge wt) than a group fed with 4 g/l of arginine (standard diet).[201] In addition, numerous studies have found that supplemental arginine (either intravenous or in the diet) improved immune function in animals after surgery, cancer, sepsis, burns, or fractures.[194-199,201,205-218] Since immune system cells play important and essential roles in connective tissue healing, the enhancement of immune cell functions after injury by arginine may be helpful to prevent trauma-induced immunosuppression, infections, or sepsis.

C. HUMAN STUDIES
1. Wound Healing and Immune Function After Surgery and Trauma

Similar to controlled studies in animals, arginine administration to humans (either intravenous or oral) after surgery or other injuries was associated with significant improvements in wound healing and nitrogen balance.[138,139,180,194-196,219-222] Elsair and others added 15 g of intravenous arginine·HCl/d for 3 d to patients undergoing routine cholecystectomy.[219] A reduced urinary nitrogen excretion in the arginine group resulted in an improved nitrogen balance after arginine. Daly and others added 25 g/d of arginine to enteral feedings for 16 adult patients with gastrointestinal malignancies undergoing major operations and compared the results to a control group of 14 similar cancer patients given an isonitrogenous amount of glycine (43 g/d).[221] Although mean nitrogen balance over the first 7 d postsurgery were not significantly different between groups (-2.3 ± 6.5 vs. -3.9 ± 7.0), the arginine group achieved positive

TABLE 2   Functions of Arginine Related to Healing

1. Conditionally essential as dietary component during growth and trauma, essential for cell growth *in vitro* (component of newly synthesized protein and peptide chains)
2. Endocrine secretagogue (stimulates somatotropin, insulin, prolactin, glucagon)
3. Precursor for nucleic acid synthesis (cell growth, fibroplasia)
4. Component of polyamine synthesis (cell growth regulator)
5. Source of endogenous nitric and nitrous oxide (vascular dilation, increased oxygen delivery, hepatocyte protein synthesis inhibitor, hepatocyte mitochondria electron transport inhibitor)
6. Improve immune functions posttrauma and postsurgery (increased T lymphocyte numbers, enhanced delayed cutaneous hypersensitivity reactions, increased thymic weight, increased lymphocyte mitogenesis, preservation of lymphocyte functions, increased rejection of allografts, reduction of sepsis)
7. Removal of ammonia produced by increased flux of amino acid catabolism in liver via urea cycle
8. Precursor for ornithine and citrulline at wound site by arginase from dead macrophages (for polyamine synthesis and arginine regeneration)
9. Precursor for proline synthesis (collagen synthesis)
10. Precursor for kyotorphin (L-tyrosinyl-L-arginine), an endogenous analgesic peptide and methionine–enkephalin releaser
11. Precursor for creatine synthesis (high-energy phosphate compound in muscle and nerves for maintenance of muscle bioenergetics)

nitrogen balance after day 5, while the glycine group never reached positive nitrogen balance. Plasma arginine and ornithine levels were increased two to four times by arginine feeding, but were unchanged after glycine feeding. Cerra and others, from the University of Minnesota, compared the protein status of two group of ICU patients (polytrauma, major elective general surgery, or major surgical infection) given total enteral nutrition support as either Osmolite (controls) or Impact (experimental group). Both formulae were nutritionally complete, except that Impact contained additional arginine (12.5 g per 1500 ml), RNA, and menhaden oil (source of omega-3 fatty acids). After 7 d of feeding, the Impact group showed significantly less 3-methylhistidine urinary excretion (a measure of muscle catabolism) (189 to 105 vs. 222 to 224 mg/kg/d), indicating a conservation of muscle mass after trauma or surgical stress. However, a 12-month followup showed no differences between groups in survival, infections, or return to work.

A new model for human wound healing involves the subcutaneous implantation of a polytetrafluoroethylene tubing (5 cm length by 1 mm outside diameter, 90 μm pore size) into the right deltoid area, with subsequent removal and biochemical analysis of granulation tissue.[222] Barbul and others, from the Departments of Surgery at Sinai Hospital and Johns Hopkins Medical Institute in Baltimore, divided 36 healthy volunteers into 3 groups of 12 subjects each.[222] One group was given a placebo, a second group was given 30 g arginine·HCl (25 g arginine), and a third group given 30 g arginine aspartate (17 g arginine) daily for 2 weeks. Arginine·HCl supplementation significantly enhanced collagen deposition as measured by an increase in hydroxyproline content, compared to the placebo group (24 vs. 10 nmol/cm graft). Likewise, arginine aspartate supplementation significantly enhanced hydroxyproline content (18 vs. 10 nmol/cm).

Arginine supplementation to human patients has been associated with improvements in immune functions after surgery, trauma, sepsis, and in normal adults.[138,139,180,194-196,213-215,218,220-226] Daly found large increases in lymphocyte mitogenesis and increased CD4 phenotype (% T helper cells) (43 vs. 29% at day 7 postsurgery) in patients undergoing major abdominal surgery for gastrointestinal cancers.[221] Likewise, there were similar findings in normal subjects[222,224] and ICU patients (trauma, major surgery).[223] One report found that arginine infused as the sole source of nitrogen to postsurgical patients did not improve immune parameters when compared to a mixture of amino acids (Travasol).[226] This study confirms that arginine effect is stimulatory when nitrogen needs are already met or almost met by other amino acids.

2. Hormone Secretion

One documented effect of arginine is induction or release of somatotropin in normal and diseased subjects after intravenous administration of high doses of arginine·HCl (15 to 30 g).[227-231] European research has found that oral administration of arginine·HCl or arginine aspartate can release small but significant amounts of somatotropin at high levels of intake (250 mg/kg/d or 38 g) both short-term and long-term.[232-238] One study, by Isidori, found increases in serum somatotropin and somatomedin in healthy athletes after oral administration of 1.2 g arginine pyroglutamate (L-arginine-2-pyrrolidone-5-carboxylate) plus 1.2 g L-lysine.[231] Either amino acid alone was incapable of stimulating somatotropin after oral administration. Products with this formula are available in some health food stores and mail order companies in the U.S. as dietary supplements. Somatotropin and somatomedins (insulin-like growth factor I) have known enhancement effects on wound healing in humans.[239-241] Therefore, any increase in their serum levels may likely be of benefit for healing processes and overall anabolism.

Other anabolic hormones released by oral arginine supplementation are prolactin,[230,231,233] insulin,[228] glucagon, and somatomedin C.[220,221,231] Thus, arginine may have beneficial multifactorial effects on anabolic hormonal responses to injury, trauma, and healing. Another newly discovered hormone-like compound is nitric oxide (NO). Arginine is the direct precursor for NO production by endothelial cells, macrophages, and many other tissues.[242] NO is a potent vasodilator and is a component of normal immune cell responses. Two reports on oral administration of L-arginine to patients with Raynaud's phenomenon found relief from pain and cyanosis and improvement of circulation in affected extremities.[243,244] If these findings can be extrapolated to other studies of arginine effects on wound healing, then another mechanism of action for arginine may be applicable — increased local vasodilation and oxygen/nutrient supply at wounded or inflamed sites. The increased supply of oxygen and nutrients would theoretically enhance healing, as found by local hyperalimentation of animal wounds.[176,177] The role of arginine as an anabolic hormone secretagogue in humans after oral administration of doses used in human trials has been documented and may represent a major role for arginine supplementation during healing.

3. Pain Control

Kyotorphin, a recently discovered endogenous analgesic opioid peptide and methionine-enkephalin inducer in the human brain, is a dipeptide composed of L-tyrosinyl-L-arginine.[245] Kyotorphin showed relief from chronic pain in animal models.[246] As a direct precursor of kyotorphin, clinical trials of short-term, intravenous L-arginine supplementation (30 g) to 12 patients with persistent pain of at least 6 months duration was described by Harima and others, from Kyoto University in Japan. Significant analgesia compared to saline infusion was measured for 6 to 24 h after arginine infusion. Analgesia was blocked by naloxone administration, an opioid peptide antagonist. Therefore, arginine may also play a role in management of chronic pain if oral doses can be shown to sufficiently affect kyotorphin levels.

4. Exercise (Possible Anabolic Effects)

Elam administered a 5-week resistance training program to 18 untrained adult males (3 workouts per week).[247] While 10 subjects received 1 g each of arginine and ornithine split into 2 daily doses, the other 8 subjects received a placebo. After 5 weeks, body fat decreased significantly more in the arginine/ornithine-supplemented group (–0.85 vs. –0.20%) and body mass decreased significantly more in the supplemented group (–1.3 vs. –0.81 kg), but composite muscle girth changes were not different. Results suggested that modest arginine/ornithine supplementation reduced body fat (and thus body weight) to a greater degree during initial stages of a resistance training program for untrained, sedentary adult males. The evidence is consistent with an anabolic effect mediated by somatotropin and perhaps other anabolic hormones.

III. ASPARTATES

Another dietary dispensable amino acid — aspartate (aspartic acid) — has been studied in relation to fatigue in humans.[248,249] Several studies from the 1950s found subjective improvements in fatigue, which were not replicated. Further studies found mixed results in terms of ergogenic effects during exercise in humans. The research seemed to support hypothetical mechanisms of action for aspartates: (1) transport of minerals to subcellular sites of action; (2) participant in tricarboxylic acid cycle (cellular energy); and (3) part of urea cycle (removal of ammonia). Thus, aspartate shares some mechanisms in common with arginine, and arginine aspartate has been used with clinical success in human wound healing and immune function preservation. However, no specific information on the effect of high doses of aspartates on animal or human connective tissue healing is available.

IV. BRANCHED-CHAIN AMINO ACIDS
(LEUCINE, ISOLEUCINE, VALINE)

The branched-chain amino acids (BCAAs) are indispensable in the diet. During injury, trauma, or severe physiological stress, muscle tissue is progressively catabolized to provide the liver with precursors for glucose. The glucose–alanine cycle, as this loop is termed, has a direct bearing on status of BCAAs.[250-253] Muscle protein contains about one third of its amino acids as BCAA (leucine, isoleucine, and valine). During periods of stress, pyruvate in muscle is transaminated to form alanine, which is then released into circulation to be taken up by liver and converted to glucose, with concomitant removal of the amine group and conversion to urea via the urea cycle. Muscle pyruvate derives its amine group for alanine synthesis mostly from muscle BCAAs. Thus, muscle protein is catabolized into glucose and urinary urea during periods of severe stress, resulting in negative nitrogen balance (net loss of nitrogen from the body). This feature is common during musculoskeletal injuries, and severity of amino acid flux is closely related to severity of injury. In this manner the body conserves integrity of vital organs at the expense of less active tissues (muscle). Muscle catabolism provides amino acids and glucose for other tissues, including healing tissues.

Because of the obvious muscle wasting and negative nitrogen balance during prolonged physiological stress, and the association of protein deficiency with complications and delayed healing, a considerable amount of effort has been directed toward the repletion of critically injured or postsurgical subjects with intravenous amino acid mixtures enriched in BCAAs (35 to 100% of total amino acids).[254-273] A consensus of research has shown that when only amino acids, or amino acids with hypocaloric carbohydrates, are infused, higher proportions of branched chain amino acids led to improved nitrogen retention. However, when caloric needs are met (usually by infusion of lipids and carbohydrates, along with amino acids), there is no difference in metabolic effects between branched chain-enriched amino acid formulas and standard formulas (10 to 20% branched chain amino acids). Also, a greater effect of branched chain amino acids was seen for patients in more severe metabolic stresses. These combined results suggest that oral use of BCAAs would not be advantageous for healing processes in patients normally found in sports medicine settings.

BCAAs have been shown to stimulate release of somatotropin[227,231] and insulin after very high intravenous doses (20 to 30 g). No studies have examined the somatotropin-releasing effects of orally administered BCAAs. Thus, unless further research indicates otherwise, oral use of BCAAs to enhance healing from injuries is not supported.

V. GLUTAMINE

Glutamine had been a forgotten amino acid until recently. Compared to other amino acids, glutamine is relatively unstable in aqueous solutions (such as cell culture media), and, as a result, has not been included in most intravenous amino acid feeding solutions given to animals and humans.[192] Also, since glutamine was originally determined to be a dietary nonessential amino acid for animals and humans, little research interest into the role or importance of glutamine for healing was initiated.[192] In fact, the original studies on essentiality of glutamine did not present details of specific experiments. Thus, the research basis for the nonessentiality of glutamine was grossly inadequate. Nevertheless,

TABLE 3   Roles and Functions of Glutamine Pertinent to Connective Tissue Healing

1. Essential for synthesis of macromolecular cellular components (proteins, glycosaminoglycans [proteoglycans], DNA, RNA, other amino acids)
2. Specific stimulatory effects *in vitro* on production of extracellular matrix by connective tissue cells
3. Primary energy source for gut enterocytes, lymphocytes, myocytes, brain
4. Prevention of intestinal atrophy after injury or total parenteral nutrition
5. Control of serum pH during acidosis and alkalosis
6. Prevention of immunosuppression after stress or surgery
7. Increase in urea flux and removal of ammonia
8. Enhanced host survival after major stress
9. Prevention or reduction in metabolic catabolism after physiological stress
10. Enhancement of protein synthesis and nitrogen retention after major stress
11. Conditionally essential during periods of major physiological stress (surgery, trauma, burns, sepsis)

mostly due to lack of knowledge on specific roles of glutamine (there were so many, researchers could not pinpoint the "major" role of glutamine), the lack of need for glutamine in stressful situations was taken at face value until recently. In spite of the fact that glutamine was shown to be absolutely essential for cell growth in culture systems by Eagle in the 1950s, research interest in glutamine lagged behind interest in other amino acids until the 1980s.[192] Fortunately, much recent research interest has finally determined that glutamine is exceptionally important to metabolism, as exemplified by new texts entirely devoted to glutamine metabolism.[274-276]

A. ROLES AND FUNCTIONS

Table 3 lists some roles and functions of glutamine pertinent to musculoskeletal healing.[192,274-277] It turns out that glutamine is absolutely essential for cell growth and is a major energy source for many cells, especially gut enterocytes, lymphocytes, and brain cells. The list of cellular components synthesized via glutamine is staggering, and includes DNA, RNA, proteins, collagens, glycosaminoglycans, glycoproteins, other amino acids, and their products. Indeed, it is difficult to find cellular components containing nitrogen that do not have a link to glutamine somewhere in their biosynthesis or metabolism. Glutamine is a major interorgan carrier for carbon chains and nitrogen (amine groups) and is the amino acid in highest amounts in cell pools and serum. In fact, the plethora and interconnectivity of glutamine roles and functions has perplexed researchers for decades. Recent research has vindicated the usefulness of glutamine, but inertial resistance to glutamine importance still exists.

Glutamine levels in muscle cells are greatly reduced (50%) after injury, surgery, or sepsis.[277] Serum levels may fall by 20 to 30% after stress. Depressions in glutamine levels are of greater magnitude than for any other amino acid and persist for longer time periods, even after levels of all other amino acids are normal.[277] Synthesis of glutamine is accelerated after injury and during other catabolic states, representing transfer of muscle amino acids to glutamine and alanine for transport to the liver. Corticosteroids accelerate the efflux of glutamine from muscles.[277]

Glutamine has specific stimulatory effects on collagen synthesis and glycosaminoglycan (cartilage) synthesis in connective tissue cells.[278,279] Thus, modulation of extracellular glutamine concentrations by dietary intake, hormonal levels, or pathological changes can greatly influence the anabolic metabolism of connective tissue cells.

B. HUMAN STUDIES

One of the earliest uses of glutamine in human healing was for treatment of peptic ulcers.[279a] Empirical observations of the effectiveness of raw cabbage juice against ulcers led to the search for the "active" ingredient. From this effort, methyl methionine sulfonium chloride (MMSC), later (and erroneously) termed vitamin U, was discovered. MMSC will be considered later in this section. Glutamine was the most potent "active" ingredient in fresh, raw cabbage juice that exhibited antiulcer activity. Placebo-controlled clinical trials of oral L-glutamine (1.6 g/d) to 46 patients with peptic ulcer was compared to 11 controls by Shive et al., from the University of Texas at Austin. Subjects consuming glutamine were all healed in an average of 22 d, compared to half of the placebo group at the same time period. Thus, oral glutamine was shown to enhance peptic ulcer healing in humans.

A large series of human clinical studies found that inclusion of glutamine in parenteral feeding solutions exhibited better improvements than glutamine-free amino acids solutions (even those enriched in BCAAs) for reduction of loss of muscle glutamine, reduction of muscle protein synthesis, reduction in synthesis of muscle polyribosomes, nitrogen loss, nitrogen balance, infection rates, and length of hospital stay in patients undergoing abdominal surgery or bone marrow transplantation.[280-286] However, there is little recent information on the specific oral use of glutamine supplements for enhancement of human healing processes. Nevertheless, the importance of glutamine for healing of any tissues has been demonstrated, setting the stage for further experiments of glutamine supplementation and musculoskeletal healing. Oral glutamine administration is quite safe and bioavailable,[277] and glutamine is widely available as a dietary supplement at relatively low cost. Amelioration of glutamine metabolism after stress by other amino acids has also been demonstrated, as will be covered in the section on ornithine-α-ketoglutarate.

VI. GLYCINE

Although glycine is considered to be dispensable in the diet, it is still an important amino acid in the metabolism.[276] Glycine makes up one third of the amino acids in collagen and a high proportion in elastin. Thus, glycine supply during healing is essential for proper progression of repair. Almost no studies have specifically examined the effects of glycine on injury rehabilitation or connective tissue healing. Glycine supplementation has been used in control groups in studies on arginine effects on human immune function and wound healing after surgery.[221] Although glycine administration was associated with favorable results for nitrogen balance and immune functions, the responses from arginine were even better. Thus, supplementation with large amounts of glycine is not considered to be as effective as other amino acids for postsurgical healing.

Glycine does have a role that may impact healing — release of somatotropin.[287-289] Oral intake of large doses of glycine (6.75 to 30 g) or intravenous infusion of glycine (4, 8, 12 g) led to increases in serum somatotropin levels from 2 to 10 times baseline 2 h after dosing in healthy subjects. Like other amino acids, the role of somatotropin release for possible enhancement of healing is desirable, but the effects of increased anabolism via somatotropin release elicited by oral ingestion of amino acids have not been studied directly.

VII. HISTIDINE AND CARNOSINE

Histidine is a conditionally essential amino acid (dietary intake viewpoint) and carnosine is the dipeptide β-alanyl-L-histidine. As with other amino acids, a dietary deficiency of histidine leads to reduced wound breaking strength and impairment of wound healing in lab animals.[290] Repletion of histidine deficiency by either histidine or carnosine supplementation returned wound healing to normal, but supplemental histidine or carnosine to animals with adequate histidine intake did not enhance wound healing at doses of 1 mg/100 g body weight per day (intraperitoneal injections).[290] However, higher intraperitoneal doses of carnosine (2 mg/100 g body weight per day) given to rats for longer time periods (up to 25 d postsurgery) were associated with accelerated rates of wound healing, as demonstrated by sooner peaks of glycosaminoglycan synthesis and histological development of granulation tissue in rats.[291] Similar results were found after carnosine injections to guinea pigs after experimental lung injury. Acceleration of fibroblast proliferation, connective tissue regeneration, and alveolar reformation was twice that of control groups.[292]

Another aspect of carnosine function is as a scavenger (or protective agent) against hypochlorite and lipid peroxides.[293,294] Hypochlorite is produced by activated immune system cells as a microbicidal agent. Excess hypochlorite is toxic and can delay healing response by prolongation of the inflammatory phase of healing.[294] Carnosine appears to be one effective scavenger of hypochlorite, as demonstrated by significantly reduced serum and brain lipid peroxide levels, increased superoxide scavenging activity in serum and brain, and increased levels of easily oxidized phospholipids in brain lipid extracts in stressed rats.[293]

Along similar lines of evidence, zinc salts of carnosine (zinc carnosinate or Z-103) have been reported to be effective inhibitors of gastric mucosal damage (ulceration) in animal models.[295-298] Additional research on the protective mechanism of action of zinc carnosinate has found scavenging of superoxide radicals, inhibition of superoxide generation from activated neutrophils, inhibition of hydroxyl radical formation by the Fenton reaction, decreased serum, gastric mucosal, liver and brain lipid peroxide levels, and membrane stabilization (preventing release of degradative enzymes).[297-300] Antioxidant effects of zinc carnosinate were not attributable to zinc salts at equivalent doses of zinc; therefore, antioxidant effects were due to the carnosine moiety. Effective doses of oral or injectable zinc carnosinate ranged from 10 to 30 mg/kg. The effect of zinc carnosinate on healing of existing ulcers has not yet been determined, but zinc carnosinate shares properties with other drugs used to treat peptic ulcer disease that have cytoprotective actions.[301] Application of zinc carnosine to human wound or ulcer healing awaits testing.

Another interaction of histidine with human healing is the reproducible finding from over a dozen separate studies of decreased serum histidine levels in rheumatoid arthritis, as reviewed by Gerber from the State University of New York Downstate Medical Center in Brooklyn.[302] Hypohistidinemia was not found in other arthritides or chronic illnesses, and seems to be a specific feature of rheumatoid arthritis. Severity of disease was directly correlated with serum histidine levels. A single-blind trial of oral histidine supplementation to 61 rheumatoid arthritis patients for up to 10 months by Gerber found significant improvements compared to a placebo period in grip strength, walking time, morning stiffness, erythrocyte sedimentation rates, hematocrit, and analgesic drug requirements.[303] A random-ized, placebo-controlled, double-blind study by Gerber and others on the effects of oral histidine supplementation (4.5 g/d for 30 weeks) on rheumatoid arthritis patients found that histidine did not exhibit significant advantages over placebo for most clinical measurements.[304] However, a small decrease in rheumatoid factor titer and small increase in hematocrit were found in the histidine group. In addition, a suggestive benefit for patients with more advanced or prolonged disease was discovered by subjective, double-blind evaluations by physicians and patients. Therefore, histidine is not univer-sally applicable to treatment of rheumatoid arthritis, but may be of some benefit to a subset of patients. However, oral doses of 4.5 g/d of histidine did not raise histidine into normal reference ranges. Perhaps a higher daily dose of histidine is required for normalization of histidine levels (and actions) and for therapeutic benefits to occur more often. Interactions of histidine with copper, zinc, gamma globulin aggregation, gold salts, penicillamine, and sulfhydryl groups may present a possible mechanism of action for histidine. It should be pointed out that histidine is the amino acid residue that binds zinc and copper atoms in superoxide dismutase, and that copper salts of histidine have superoxide dismutase activity *in vitro* (reviewed in References 305 to 307). There are parallels with antioxidant activity of carnosine mentioned earlier in this section.

At this point, there is insufficient evidence to suggest that supplementation with histidine or carnosine can benefit conditions of human connective tissue healing. However, conclusive studies have yet to be performed, and histidine or carnosine therapy at doses over 5 g/d may yet offer some therapeutic benefits as an additional protective antioxidant with mild antiinflammatory effects.

VIII. SULFHYDRYL AMINO ACIDS (METHIONINE, CYSTEINE) AND SULFHYDRYL COMPOUNDS

The sulfhydryl-containing amino acids are linked in metabolism.[252,276] Methionine is absolutely indispensable in terms of dietary intake, but ample cysteine can reduce quantitative requirements for methionine. Other sulfhydryl amino acids present in metabolism or diet are methyl methionine sulfonium chloride, homocysteine, cystathionine, taurine (actually an α-amino sulfonic acid), S-adenosyl methionine, and methyl sulfonyl methane (MSM). The sulfhydryl amino acids function as sources for sulfur (sulfate) in glycosaminoglycan synthesis and sulfate conjugation in detoxification pathways. Sulfhydryl groups in general contribute to redox potentials in cells, and cysteine is a direct precursor for glutathione synthesis. Glutathione is arguably the most important antioxidant in quantitative terms in the body (reviewed by Halliwell[305]). Thus, sulfhydryl amino acids and compounds are considered to be one type of antioxidant.

Studies on wound healing in animals made protein-deficient found that the impairment of healing caused by protein deficiency could be corrected almost to normal by administration of methionine or cysteine.[308-312] Improved fibroblastic proliferation, reversal of prolonged lag phase, and collagen synthesis were found after repletion with methionine or cysteine. Sulfhydryl amino acids were suspected to be integral to collagen synthesis since it was known that cysteine disulfide bridges were critical for proper formation and maturation of newly synthesized procollagen. Now it is known that the important roles of sulfhydryl amino acids as antioxidants and precursors for glutathione may have accounted for some of the observed effects. However, a subsequent study did not find beneficial effects of methionine repletion on wound healing in protein-deficient rats.[313] Additional supplies of methionine or cysteine did not enhance wound healing in animals with adequate intake or status of sulhydryl amino acids. These studies, performed in the 1950s, utilized D,L forms of amino acids (not nature-identical L forms). Thus, the known problems associated with administration of D amino acids may have obscured possible beneficial effects of sulfur-containing amino acids on enhancement of healing. At this point, the use of high doses of sulfur-containing amino acids as single agents to enhance wound healing is not supported, but conclusive research has not been performed.

Another aspect of sulfur-containing amino acids and healing is the effects of S-adenosyl methionine (SAM), a metabolic intermediate of methionine involved in methyl donor metabolism and glutathione synthesis. Oral administration of SAM to animals (20 to 100 mg/kg) showed antiinflammatory and analgesic activities.[314,315] Human trials of oral SAM administration in over 22,000 patients with osteoarthritis have routinely exhibited clinical benefits when compared to placebo or reference NSAIDs.[316-325] A consensus of research has indicated antiinflammatory, analgesic, and antiphlogistic effects along with a stimulation of proteoglycan synthesis by articular chondrocytes.[321] For example, the study by Marcolongo and others from various Rheumatology Institutes in Italy will be described.[320] A randomized, double-blind, multicenter study of oral SAM (400 mg t.i.d. for 30 d) compared to oral ibuprofen (same dose) was conducted with 150 patients with osteoarthritis of the knee and/or hip. SAM showed statistically more significant improvements in active movement pain, night pain, and muscle spasms compared to ibuprofen. Both physician and patient evaluations of effectiveness were equivalent for each treatment. However, side effects were considerably reduced and less severe in the SAM group. SAM also proved as effective as ibuprofen,[322] indomethacin,[323] piroxicam,[324] or naproxen[325] for relief of arthritic symptoms, without side effects seen for the NSAIDs in a series of additional studies. Oral administration of SAM was shown to be effective for elevation of serum levels of SAM, indicating that SAM is bioavailable as an oral nutrient.[326] Thus, SAM has been shown to be equally effective as current analgesic NSAIDs (ketoprofen, ibuprofen) for osteoarthritis management, without gastric side effects.

Very recent research with DL-methionine methyl sulphonium chloride (also known as vitamin U or MMSC) or DL-cysteine in human ulcer healing has exhibited beneficial effects. Topical application of MMSC or DL-cysteine to patients with venous leg ulcers resulted in total healing of 93% of leg ulcers for each sulfhydryl agent, compared to total healing of 70% of leg ulcers in the control group, a significant difference in favor of the sulfhydryl agents.[327] Likewise, oral administration of DL-MMSC (500 mg q.i.d.) or DL-cysteine (200 mg q.i.d.) to 86 or 87 patients with duodenal ulcers was studied.[328] Another 65 patients served as a control group. All groups received equivalent cimetidine treatment, and all subjects smoked and drank coffee, both risk factors for recurrence. After 8 weeks, all patients in the MMSC and cysteine groups exhibited healed ulcers, while the control group (cimetidine alone) exhibited total healing in 74% of subjects, a significant difference. After 1 year of continued treatment, both sulfhydryl agent groups exhibited significantly less recurrence of ulcers (3% each) compared to cimetidine alone (29%). Thus, oral use of sulfur-containing amino acids has improved existing therapy for duodenal ulcer healing in humans. Long-term oral administration of MMSC or cysteine was well tolerated and safe.

MSM is a metabolite of dimethyl sulfoxide (DMSO) and is normally found in foodstuffs.[329] MSM showed clinical benefits at oral doses of 100 to 750 mg/d for a variety of inflammatory diseases in humans, including sensitivity to oral NSAID medications.[329] More research is needed to determine whether MSM would have therapeutic benefits for connective tissue healing.

In summary, consistent evidence has been found to support the use of SAM in management of osteoarthritis. Effects seem to be reductions in pain, but research has not been directed towards modification of osteoarthritis pathophysiology. At this time, there is no firm evidence to support use of sulfur-containing amino acids methionine or cysteine as single agents to enhance connective tissue healing in humans. However, definitive studies have yet to be performed. Later sections of this book concerning antioxidants will address the issue of cysteine supplementation as a precursor for glutathione synthesis and the role of sulfur-containing amino acids as antioxidants, rather than metabolic precursors.

IX. ORNITHINE AND ORNITHINE-α-KETOGLUTARATE (OKG)

Ornithine is a dibasic amino acid derived from arginine that is not incorporated into proteins. Ornithine serves as a metabolic intermediate for production of urea, polyamines, and other amino acids (directly forms citrulline via the urea cycle, and glutamate or proline via Δ-pyrroline-5-carboxylate).[330] Ornithine-α-ketoglutarate (OKG) is a manufactured ionic salt consisting of one molecule of α-ketoglutarate with each carboxy group bound to the end amino group of an ornithine molecule.[330] OKG consists of one α-ketoglutarate per two ornithine molecules. α-Ketoglutarate is the oxo acid corresponding to deaminated glutamine. Since α-ketoglutarate is rapidly absorbed and metabolized and is an efficient precursor for glutamine, and since ornithine levels are elevated whenever arginine levels are elevated, and arginine has shown beneficial properties for the healing process (see previous section in this chapter), the combination of ornithine and α-ketoglutarate was thought to possibly influence protein metabolism in a positive manner. These effects have indeed been observed numerous times for OKG in experimental and clinical studies, and these effects have not been seen when either ornithine or α-ketoglutarate alone has been examined.[330]

A. ROLES AND FUNCTIONS

Ornithine is a key intermediate in the urea cycle, which is involved with conversion of ammonia derived from amino acid (protein) or nitrogen catabolism into urea for safe excretion of nitrogen, since ammonia is a toxic substance in the body.[331-333] Ornithine is also capable of somatotropin release after intravenous administration[334-336] and after oral administration of 170 mg/kg of ornithine hydrochloride to bodybuilders.[337] Lower oral doses of ornithine hydrochloride (40, 100 mg/kg),[337] a 1:1:1 mixture of arginine to ornithine to lysine (2 g each per d for 4 d),[338] a mixture of arginine (1.8 g), ornithine (1.2 g), methionine (0.48 g), and phenylalanine (0.12 g),[339] and a combination of ornithine (1.1 g) and tyrosine (0.75 g)[340] all failed to promote release of somatotropin in athletic subjects. Thus, a threshold of effect for oral induction of somatotropin release appears to exist. An acute dose of at least 10 g or more of a single amino acid known to induce somatotropin release from intravenous studies, such as ornithine, is needed before there is a possibility of somatotropin release. However, at the highest dose tested, 170 mg ornithine per kg, osmotic diarrhea was noted in almost every subject.[337] Therefore, further research is necessary in order to justify the potential use of high-dose amino acids for somatotropin release.

By itself, oral ornithine administration has not been shown to stimulate release of insulin in athletes or healthy persons after acute single doses of 2 to 20 g.[341,342] A small increase in serum glucagon after 6.4 g of oral ornithine was found in healthy subjects.[342] Ornithine has also been shown to enhance polyamine synthesis[343,344] and liver protein synthesis[344] under experimental conditions, although the implications for *in vivo* use are unclear.

OKG has been exceptionally well-studied, mostly by the group of Cynober at Hopital Saint Antoine in Paris, France.[330] Many roles and functions unique to OKG, and not shared by ornithine, α-ketoglutarate, or a mixture of ornithine plus α-ketoglutarate, have been identified.[330,345] Most of these properties have been documented in humans. Oral ingestion of 5 to 20 g of OKG has resulted in significant increases in serum levels of ornithine, α-ketoglutarate, arginine, proline, citrulline, glutamate, somatotropin, insulin, and glucagon.[330,342,345-348] Intravenous administration of OKG has also shown the same results, even in cirrhotic patients.[349-354] Thus, OKG has consistently shown protein-sparing and anabolic effects *in vivo* after oral administration of 5 to 10 g in humans. Single doses of 20 g were associated with osmotic diarrhea, but doses of 5 to 10 g were well tolerated, even 2 to 3 times daily.[330]

B. HUMAN STUDIES

A plethora of human studies has shown that OKG administration (either 5 to 10 g/d per os or OKG infusions) consistently produced beneficial results in a variety of stressed patients.[330] Surgical patients (cholecystectomy, colorectal resection, head and neck surgery, amputations, severe plastic surgery) have exhibited quicker wound healing rates, more satisfactory cicatrization, fewer postsurgical complications, better survival, improved skeletal muscle protein synthesis, prevention of the usual decrease in muscle polyribosomes, improved or normalized nitrogen balance, reduced loss of muscle glutamine levels, and improved changes in muscle amino acid levels.[280,330,345,355-362] Likewise, several human studies have found that 20 to 25 g/d of OKG (enteral or parenteral) improved nitrogen balance and other markers of protein status in patients hospitalized for polytrauma.[363-365] Burn patients given OKG as part of their nutritional support demonstrated better survival, shorter lengths of hospitalization, faster return to normal values for plasma amino acid patterns and protein status markers, lower urea excretion, faster normalization of nitrogen balance, and amelioration of glucose intolerance.[330,347,348,366,367] Intake of OKG in normal and malnourished subjects improved measures of lymphocyte function, such as mitogenesis and antibody production.[368]

X. PROLINE AND HYDROXYPROLINE

Collagen is comprised of almost one third proline residues.[100] It would seem logical to assume that addition of proline to cells synthesizing large amounts of collagen (fibroblasts in granulation tissue) may show enhanced collagen production. However, an early experiment by Peacock found that the addition of 1% DL-proline to the diet of protein-depleted rats did not affect wound healing.[369] Likewise, the addition of 0.5% DL-hydroxyproline to the diets of scorbutic guinea pigs did not affect wound healing. Unfortunately, no further experiments by any investigators have examined the effects of oral intake of nature-identical L-proline, rather than DL-proline (which may exert toxicity), on the healing response. Thus, no evidence suggests that proline supplementation would be beneficial for enhancement of collagen synthesis or healing.

XI. PHENYLALANINE

The D form of phenylalanine (D-phenylalanine, or D,L-phenylalanine) has been identified as inhibiting the enzymes that degrade analgesic enkephalin peptides in the brain. The effect of D-phenylalanine is inhibited by naloxone, suggesting a mechanism on opioid peptides. Several studies in humans with oral D-phenylalanine have found reduced tourniquet-induced pain,[370] enhanced acupuncture analgesia,[371,372] increased pain threshold,[371,372] enhanced analgesia after acupuncture treatment of chronic low back pain,[372] and enhanced analgesia after tooth extractions.[372] Significant pain relief was found in the last 2 weeks of a 4- to 5-week study of D-phenylalanine administration to 43 patients with pain from osteoarthritis.[373] The effectiveness of D-phenylalanine improved as pain severity decreased. In a double-blind, crossover study, 7/21 patients with chronic pain taken off all other pain medications noted over 50% pain relief after D-phenylalanine, but not placebo.[374] Another placebo-controlled study found that all patients who were responsive to acupuncture showed increases in pain tolerance and analgesic persistence after D-phenylalanine administration, compared to placebo.[375] Subjects who were not responsive to acupuncture showed only a response rate of 50% to D-phenylalanine. However, a double-blind, crossover study conducted by Walsh did not find any difference between placebo or D-phenylalanine periods for pain relief in 30 subjects with intractable chronic pain.[376] Also, statistical reevaluation of the studies by Balagot and Budd by Walsh did not find significant changes from D-phenylalanine administration on pain.[377]

Effective oral doses of D-phenylalanine were either 4.0 g 30 min before an event or 500 mg of D-phenylalanine 3 times daily before an event. Thus, D-phenylalanine has shown short-term analgesic effects in human musculoskeletal pain. Further research should clarify the questions that remain. Is D-phenylalanine safe for long-term use, since phenylalanine is an indispensable amino acid, and D amino acids are known to be eventually toxic? Is D-phenylalanine effective for acute or chronic pain or both? Is D-phenylalanine additive or synergistic with other analgesics? Can doses of commonly used analgesic agents be reduced when D-phenylalanine is coadministered? D-Phenylalanine appears to be a promising short-term, nutritional analgesic agent with sufficient merit as a last resort for intractable pain in selected patients.

XII. TRYPTOPHAN

Tryptophan appears to have two major applications for injury rehabilitation. One is in reduction of pain as a mild analgesic, and the other is as a somatotropin-releasing agent. Other uses of tryptophan (hypnotic, antidepressant) will not be covered in this book. Tryptophan is the dietary precursor for the brain neurotransmitter serotonin.[378] When plasma unbound tryptophan levels are increased, either absolutely or in relation to other large, neutral amino acids (BCAAs, methionine, tyrosine, phenylalanine), uptake of tryptophan into the brain is enhanced, and conversion of tryptophan to 5-hydroxytryptophan, and then to serotonin (5-hydroxytryptamine), commences.[378] Serotonin is involved in nociception and behavioral responses to pain.[379] Increased brain serotonin has been associated with analgesia.

Seltzer and others, from Temple University in Philadelphia, conducted a double-blind study of placebo or tryptophan ingestion (2 g/d for 7 d) in healthy volunteers.[380] Pain was measured by electrical stimulation of tooth pulp (onset of pain and unbearable pain). Although threshold perception of pain was not altered by tryptophan, the tolerance to pain was significantly increased by tryptophan, compared to the placebo group (10.5 vs. 2.7 scores). King, from the State University of New York in Syracuse, administered 500 mg of tryptophan 3 to 4 times daily to 5 patients with recurrent intractable pain from previous injuries.[381] Pain was relieved in all cases over a period of several months. Seltzer and others placed 30 subjects with chronic maxillofacial pain on a high carbohydrate, low fat, low protein diet.[382] Half were given placebo, and the other half were given 3 g/d tryptophan for 4 weeks. While both groups showed less anxiety and less depression, the tryptophan group showed a greater increase in pain tolerance threshold. Shpeen and others administered placebo or 3 g tryptophan in 6 divided doses over the first 24 h after root canal procedures.[383] The tryptophan group recorded a lower level of pain at 24 h than the placebo group. However, Stockstill et al. did not find reductions in chronic myofascial pain in a tryptophan-supplemented group compared to a control group.[384] Both groups were instructed to alter their diet to increase carbohydrate intakes. Postoperative pain (cholecystectomy) in 45 females was measured by Ceccherelli et al., from the University of Padova in Italy.[385] No neuroleptics or narcotics were used for anesthesia. Patients were given intravenous doses of either 100 ml of 5% mannitol (control) or 7.5 mg/kg or 15 mg/kg of tryptophan for 30 min, after patients awoke from surgery and asked for analgesics. All patients initially had pain >55 on the Scott-Huskisson visual analog scale. Assessment was continued for 6 h. Both tryptophan doses exhibited significantly less pain compared to placebo, and longer lasting relief from pain was seen at 15 mg/kg tryptophan. Drowsiness was the only side effect reported, which is a typical effect of high tryptophan levels. For pain reduction, tryptophan was rated as better than pentazocine, lidocaine, amidone, pethidine, and electroacupuncture, but not as good as epidural anesthesia. Therefore, intravenous tryptophan was shown to produce effective postoperative pain management.

Broadhurst, from West Suffolk Hospital in England, reported on the use of oral tryptophan in a large number of patients for depression.[386] Some patients had rheumatoid arthritis, and a few of these patients had "dramatic lessening of symptoms" as well as reductions in erythrocyte sedimentation rates. When tryptophan was discontinued, joint pain increased. Whether the effect was on joint pain itself or disease course was unknown. Interestingly, almost all antirheumatic drugs have the ability to displace tryptophan from serum protein binding sites, increasing plasma unbound tryptophan levels. This suggests that one factor for efficacy of antirheumatic drugs is their modulation of the tryptophan/serotonin pathway.

Another application of tryptophan has been in fibromyalgia. The fibromyalgia symptoms of musculoskeletal pain, tender points, fatigue, and disturbed sleep suggested a defect in serotonin, and possibly a tryptophan deficiency. Fibromyalgia patients consistently exhibited decreased plasma tryptophan[387,388] or ratio of plasma tryptophan to large, neutral amino acids (LNAAs).[383] Another study found that although plasma levels of tryptophan were normal, the plasma unbound tryptophan levels were inversely correlated to severity of pain symptoms in fibromyalgia.[389] Ratios of tryptophan to LNAAs were inversely correlated with paresthiasis, headaches, number of tender points, and Hassles score.[388] Puttini and Caruso, from the Rheumatology Unit of L Sacco Hospital in Milan, Italy, conducted a double-blind trial lasting 30 d on 50 patients with fibromyalgia.[390] The patients who received 100 mg of 5-hydroxytryptophan (OHTRP) 3 times daily showed significant reductions in symptoms compared to placebo and initial values. "Good" or "fair" clinical improvement was seen in 50% of OHTRP-treated patients, with reductions in number of tender points, anxiety, pain intensity, fatigue, and improvement of sleep quality. Thus, tryptophan supplementation appeared to ameliorate pain symptoms of some fibromyalgia patients.

Supplementation with 1200 mg of tryptophan 24 h before a treadmill exercise capacity test found a greatly increased total exercise time and total work load performed (49%) compared to unsupplemented tests.[391] Ratings of perceived exertion were lowered, consistent with an analgesic effect of tryptophan.

Several reports have found small but significant increases of serum somatotropin after oral tryptophan administration (5 g or more) to healthy subjects.[392-396] Number of responders averaged 60%, and increases in serum somatotropin reached 10 to 15 ng/ml, which is less than stimulation by other amino acids or other methods. Side effects of drowsiness and mellow feelings were consistently noted, in accordance with known effects of tryptophan.[397]

Tryptophan has substantial evidence for relief of chronic pain from musculoskeletal conditions. Either tryptophan or 5-hydroxytryptophan was able to influence both acute and chronic pain. Effective doses seemed to be 2 to 5 g of tryptophan daily in divided doses on an empty stomach or with sugar, or 300 mg OHTRP daily in divided doses. However, at this time in the U.S., tryptophan sales and distribution have been banned since 1989 by the Food and Drug Administration, except for parenteral feeding solutions and protein fortification. An outbreak of Eosinophilia-Myalgia Syndrome (EMS) was traced to one batch of tryptophan produced by a single Japanese manufacturer.[398-401] The single batch was contaminated with a small amount of a tryptophan dimer produced by a procedural change in tryptophan isolation. The dimer acted as an antagonist of tryptophan, causing tryptophan deficiency symptoms. The single batch was widely dispersed to many manufacturers, hence the widespread incidence of EMS. Over 15,000 cases of EMS have been documented, with 27 associated deaths.[398-401] A novel treatment of contaminated tryptophan-induced EMS with uncontaminated tryptophan led to remissions of EMS.[400] Other companies producing tryptophan have been continuously monitored for tryptophan contamination, but no evidence has been found that past or current tryptophan batches were contaminated, or ever will be, since the isolation procedure used by the single Japanese company was unique among manufacturers. Nevertheless, even though tryptophan is widely used in parenteral intravenous amino acid solutions and fortification of protein and infant formulas, the use of tryptophan as a dietary supplement has not been returned. Thus, until the FDA agrees to allow tryptophan sales, it is unavailable in the U.S. and should not be used. However, research and use of tryptophan continues in other countries.

XIII. AMINO ACID SUMMARY

A final finding on amino acids and connective tissue healing is concerned with L-lysine. A recent study verified the ability of L-lysine supplements (400 to 800 mg/d) to significantly enhance the intestinal absorption of calcium (from 3.0 g of calcium chloride) in 74 osteoporotic women.[402] In addition, lysine supplementation blunted the urinary excretion of calcium normally seen after a calcium load. Thus, ingestion of 400 to 800 mg of L-lysine along with a calcium supplement can positively affect calcium balance, with important implications for prevention and treatment of bone loss disorders.

In summary, an extensive amount of research has found that several amino acids appear to possess benefits for musculoskeletal healing after oral intake in humans. Arginine and ornithine-α-ketoglutarate both have repeated evidence of acceleration of healing from surgery and other trauma, and prevention of catabolic events after injury. Perhaps there is a common mechanism, since arginine loads also increase ornithine levels as well as other amino acids, just as OKG does. The multiplicity of metabolic effects shown by arginine and OKG overlap and include mediation of anabolic hormone response, reduction of potential ammonia toxicity, and improvement of nitrogen retention. Thus, clinical use of large oral doses of arginine and/or OKG to enhance musculoskeletal healing is supported in the literature.

For other amino acids, the evidence of usefulness is less clear. Although glutamine is now essential for healing, the research evidence on effects of oral glutamine supplements is too recent to draw any firm conclusions on effectiveness. Due to the enormous importance of glutamine to metabolism, it is likely that glutamine supplements may exhibit clinical benefits in the near future. BCAAs did not deliver expected improvements in clinical results hypothesized from their roles in injury metabolism. Their oral use has been virtually unstudied, however, and lack of research in less severely injured subjects means that BCAA supplementation may yet become clinically useful. Other amino acids do not seem to be able to affect the course of musculoskeletal healing from injuries, trauma, or surgery.

Possible roles for histidine or carnosine in rheumatoid arthritis need further research to predict responsive patients. However, the amino acids S-adenosyl-L-methionine (SAM), D-phenylalanine (DPA), and tryptophan (or its equivalent, 5-hydroxy-L-tryptophan) have some encouraging evidence as mild analgesics for musculoskeletal pain conditions, including the difficult fibromyalgia syndrome. The majority of studies on each have found decreased pain after short-term treatment periods, especially for intractable pain not corrected by other means. The use of oral amino acids as analgesics deserves further study and application. SAM has generated a substantial database as an effective therapy for osteoarthritis without the side effects associated with NSAID usage. The large number of patients and equivalent results to standard therapies means that long-term treatment of osteoarthritis may be accomplished with fewer problems caused by the treatment. Disease-modifying activity (similar to chondroprotective agents) in the form of aiding synthesis of proteoglycans may allow osteoarthritic cartilage to eventually stabilize or even repair itself, which is less likely with progressive increases in analgesic drug dosages. Thus, SAM represents an underutilized resource for safe therapy of degenerative joint diseases.

The use of large doses of single amino acids or amino acid mixtures to release somatotropin has become popular with some athletes and exercising persons. However, the available data shows that possible induction of somatotropin is only accomplished at very high doses that usually cause unwanted side effects (diarrhea or drowsiness). The chance of being a responder to oral amino acid induction of somatotropin release is up to 60%, meaning that each individual has about an even chance for high-dose

TABLE 4   Guidelines for Use of Single Amino Acids

Amino Acid	Oral Dosage	Conditions
Arginine (L-arginine hydrochloride) or	10–30 g daily in 3–4 divided doses	Surgery Wound healing Fracture repair Immune suppression Burns
Arginine aspartate	Same as for arginine hydrochloride	Prevention of muscle mass loss by immobilization
Ornithine-α-ketoglutarate (OKG, Ornicetil®, Cetornan®)	5–20 g daily in 2-3 doses	Surgery Wound healing Fracture repair Immune suppression Burns Prevention of muscle mass loss by immobilization
S-Adenosyl-L-methionine (SAM)	1200–2400 mg daily in 3 divided doses	Degenerative joint conditions (osteoarthritis, chondromalacia, bursitis, tendinitis, chronic low back pain) Sprains? Tendon and ligament repair?
D-Phenylalanine (DPA)	Acute: 4.0 g 30 min before event Chronic: 1500 mg daily in 3 divided doses	Chronic pain from musculoskeletal conditions or injuries Acute use for postoperative pain Acute use for postinjury pain?
Tryptophan (TRP)[a] or	2–5 g daily in divided doses	Chronic pain from musculoskeletal conditions or injuries Fibromyalgia Syndrome/Fibrositis
5-Hydroxy-L-tryptophan (5OHTRP)	300–600 mg daily in divided doses	Acute use for postoperative pain Acute use for postinjury pain?

Note: All amino acids (except D-phenylalanine) should be in the L-form, not the d- or DL-form. Divided doses should be taken 30 min before each meal and/or before bedtime, preferably with at least 1 large glass of water or sugar-containing beverage (fruit juice, sports electrolyte drinks, lemonade, sweetened iced tea).

[a] Tryptophan is unavailable at the present time in the U.S. and its use is not recommended for legal reasons. 5-Hydroxy-L-tryptophan can legally be considered as tryptophan, even though it has not been associated with Eosinophilia-Myalgia Syndrome.

single amino acids to elicit a somatotropin response. Lower doses are reproducibly useless for inducing somatotropin response, unless the findings of Isidori can be reproduced.[238] Also, the long-term implications of amino acid somatotropin releasing agents is unclear. Does long-term intake of high doses of single amino acids desensitize hormone release? Does catabolism of that amino acid increase to negate the effects? Does the hormone released have physiological benefits that are maintained for long time periods? Many pertinent questions still remain to be answered before use of single amino acids as somatotropin (or other hormone)-releasing agents can be fully condoned. Therefore, at this time, the general application of single amino acids to elicit somatotropin release is impractical.

One final note concerning the use of single agents for enhancement of complex, homeostatically regulated systems is apparent. It is always difficult for any single agent, even a rate-limiting agent, to affect whole body function sufficiently to produce significant results. The results seen in studies to date are therefore clinically applicable for a large portion of potential patients, although not for everyone. The effects of specific combinations of amino acids have not been fully explored, especially when combined with other types of nutrients (such as L-lysine and calcium). Targeted nutrient repletion is starting to combine several nutrients with additive functions, but many potentially beneficial combinations are completely untested. This concept will be discussed further in the chapter covering nutrient combinations.

XIV. GUIDELINES FOR USE

In general, a few guidelines pertain to efficient use of amino acids. First and foremost is the proper dose. Supplemental amounts must be sufficient to safely increase serum and tissue levels of the desired amino acid. In most cases, useful doses have been determined. Second, ingestion of single amino acids should be on an empty stomach about 30 min before a meal. Usually, ingestion of amino acids with a simple carbohydrate (such as fruit juice or sweetened drinks like lemonade, sports electrolyte drinks, or iced tea) does not interfere with absorption of the amino acid and may improve the function of tryptophan and other large, neutral amino acids.

Table 4 lists the potential clinical applications of single amino acids. The listed doses appear to be safe and well tolerated, even for long time periods. The potential for detrimental imbalance of protein metabolism by excess intake of single amino acids has not been demonstrated in humans to date at the doses listed. The clinical application of certain amino acids certainly deserves more widespread use than is currently practiced. At the very least, certain amino acids may be very useful adjuncts to current therapeutic modalities and, possibly, alternatives for persons intolerant of other treatments.

Chapter 4

FATS, FATTY ACIDS, AND LIPIDS

I. INTRODUCTION

Fats have become important to health for more reasons than caloric contributions to diet. Fats will always represent a rich source of food energy for humans and a considerable storage site for bodily caloric reserves. In the last 25 years, entirely new fields of research have sprung forth about the noncaloric roles of fats as fatty acids and membrane phospholipids. Fats now have critical and essential regulatory roles for every facet of metabolism and health. Consideration of fat intake must take into account more than merely calories, for instance, what type of fatty acids are present, their amounts, and relative ratios. Interactions with different body pools of fatty acids (serum, cell membranes, adipose tissues) complicate the ability to quickly modulate fatty acid contents of cells by dietary or pharmacological means. Analogous to amino acids as dietary and metabolic precursors to peptide hormones, fats are dietary and metabolic precursors for steroid hormones and eicosanoids.

One crucial factor about fats and lipids is their inherent insolubility in aqueous systems (cells). Humans have developed elegant and complicated mechanisms to digest, absorb, package, transport, incorporate, metabolize, and utilize fats and their components. Some recent reviews that provide a background on fats and lipids in the human body are recommended for further information on identity, structure, and roles.[403-410] Another very important concern about fats relates directly to their structure. Fats with carbon–carbon double bonds (unsaturated fats) are extremely prone to oxidation reactions from oxygen and oxygen-derived reactive species (free radicals).[305-307] Fats have an inescapable link with antioxidant status.

A. NOMENCLATURE AND BIOCHEMISTRY

A brief review of lipid identities and structures is necessary in order to comprehend the results and implications of studies on fats and healing. Lipids are composed of carbon, hydrogen, and oxygen (same as carbohydrates), but with much less oxygen than carbohydrates. Table 1 lists some basic classifications of lipid types. This chapter will be mainly concerned with fatty acids, which make up over 90% of lipids in our food supply. Fat-soluble vitamins will be covered in Chapter 5.

Triglycerides represent the major storage and transport form of fatty acids. Triglycerides consist of three fatty acids esterified to a glycerol molecule (triacylglycerol). The identities of the three fatty acids can be similar or completely different. Fatty acids are lengths of hydrocarbon chains with a terminal carboxylic acid group. Chain lengths vary from 1 to 32 carbons in frequently occurring foodstuffs. Due to the nature of atomic carbon bonding, fatty acids can be saturated or unsaturated (with respect to hydrogen atoms and available bonds to carbons). A fatty acid with every hydrogen attached to every available carbon bond is a saturated fatty acid. If a hydrogen atom is removed from each of adjacent carbon atoms, a carbon–carbon double bond forms. Carbon–carbon double bonds have a flat, rigid geometry — each bond angle is very close to 120°. Presence of even one carbon–carbon double bond changes the identification of a fatty acid to an unsaturated fatty acid. Fatty acids with one double bond are monounsaturated fatty acids, while fatty acids with two or more double bonds are polyunsaturated fatty acids (PUFAs). The carbon–carbon double bond can have two possible spatial orientations: *cis* and *trans*. Almost all natural PUFAs have double bonds entirely in the *cis* format, which leads to large angles of change in the shape of the usually linear saturated fatty acid chain. *Cis* double bonds have the two hydrogen atoms on double-bonded, adjacent carbons on the same side of the double bond. *Trans* double

TABLE 1   Classifications of Lipids

Fats (triglycerides, triacylglycerols)
Phospholipids
Fatty acids
Sterols and steroids
Fat-soluble vitamins (A, D, E, K)
Quinones (coenzyme Q_{10})
Dolichols
Glycolipids, sphingolipids, ceramides

Note: Fats are almost as diverse in structure and
function as proteins. Each classification
has considerable heterogeneity in size,
modifications, and structures.

bonds signify that the hydrogens are on opposite sides of the double bond. *Trans* fatty acids are naturally occurring in small amounts (mostly from production by microbes in ruminant guts), but have been introduced in large amounts (>2000 times the intakes of 1850) into diets by partial hydrogenation, which chemically adds hydrogens to double bonds in PUFAs. Some double bonds will reform into *trans* configurations, and some will reform into natural *cis* configurations. *Trans* fatty acids can be mono- or polyunsaturated. *Trans* fatty acids have almost the same molecular shape, size, and physical characteristics as saturated fatty acids.

A nomenclature system for fatty acids has been accepted which immediately informs the reader of the chain length, as well as the number and position of double bonds. Fortunately, not all possible combinations of chain lengths and placement of double bonds are encountered in nature. Most fatty acids have an even number of carbon atoms (chain length). Usually, double bonds are found in discrete locations, known as conjugated double bonds. This means that double bonds alternate with single bonds along the carbon chain. Also, double bonds are frequently found in certain positions along fatty acid chains. The locations of the double bonds in a fatty acid chain are commonly denoted by the number of carbon atoms from the noncarboxylic acid end of the fatty acid chain. Table 2 lists some more commonly encountered fatty acids and their abbreviations. For example, oleic acid (*cis*-9-octadecenoic acid), the major monounsaturated fatty acid, is abbreviated as 18:1n9. The first number is the chain length (number of carbon atoms in longest linear chain). The first number after the colon is the number of double bonds in the fatty acid. If no double bonds are present, then no further abbreviations are needed. If one or more double bonds are present, the location of the double bonds is designated by the n number. Numbering of carbon atoms in the systematic method of nomenclature (such as 9-octadecenoic acid) starts from the carboxy terminus. The abbreviated nomenclature numbers carbon atoms from the opposite end, termed the omega end. Thus, the carbon atom on the opposite end of the fatty acid from the carboxy terminus carbon is the omega carbon. Thus, oleic acid is 18 carbons long, with a single double bond at carbon number 9 from the noncarboxy (omega) tail end. The ω denotation is equivalent to n.

Another example is caprylic acid (octanoic acid), a medium-chain fatty acid, which is abbreviated as 8:0, meaning it is 8 carbons long with no double bonds. An example of PUFA nomenclature is linoleic acid (9,12-octadecadienoic acid), the most common vegetable oil, which is abbreviated as 18:2n6. Thus, linoleic acid is 18 carbons long, with 2 double bonds. The "first" double bond is 6 carbons from the tail (12 carbons from the carboxy head) of the molecule, and because of conjugation, the "second" double bond is 3 carbon atoms further along the chain at carbon number 9 (measured from the head). Thus, linoleic acid is an omega-6 fatty acid, because the first carbon–carbon double bond is at position 12, 6 carbons from the omega end. Likewise, 5,8,11,14,17-eicosapentaenoic acid (EPA), the most common fish oil, is abbreviated as 20:5n3, meaning EPA is 20 carbons long with 5 conjugated double bonds starting at the third carbon from the omega end.

Fats and fatty acids differ substantially in physical properties. Long-chain fatty acids and their triglycerides are solids at room temperature, and termed fats. Short-chain saturated fatty acids,

TABLE 2   Nomenclature of Fatty Acids Important for Healing and Health

Trivial Name	Systematic Name	Abbreviation	Family
Acetic acid	Ethanoic acid	2:0	Short-chain saturated
Propionic	Propanoic	3:0	Short-chain saturated
Butyric	Butanoic	4:0	Short-chain saturated
Caprylic	Octanoic	8:0	Medium-chain saturated
Lauric	Dodecanoic	12:0	Long-chain saturated
Myristic	Tetradecanoic	14:0	Long-chain saturated
Palmitic	Hexadecanoic	16:0	Long-chain saturated
Stearic	Octadecanoic	18:0	Long-chain saturated
Arachidic	Eicosanoic	20:0	Long-chain saturated
Palmitoleic	*cis*-9-Hexadecenoic	16:1n7	Monounsaturated ω7
Oleic	*cis*-9-Octadecenoic	18:1n9	Monounsaturated ω9
Erucic	*cis*-13-Docosenoic	22:1n7	Monounsaturated ω7
Linoleic	9,12-Octadecadienoic	18:2n6	Polyunsaturated ω6
γ-Linolenic (GLA)	6,9,12-Octadecatrienoic	18:3n6	Polyunsaturated ω6
Arachidonic (AA)	5,8,11,14-Eicosatetraenoic	20:4n6	Polyunsaturated ω6
α-Linolenic (ALA)	9,12,15-Octadecatrienoic	18:3n3	Polyunsaturated ω3
Stearidonic	6,9,12,15-Octadecatetraenoic	18:4n3	Polyunsaturated ω3
EPA	5,8,11,14,17-Eicosapentaenoic	20:5n3	Polyunsaturated ω3
DHA	4,7,10,13,16,19-Docosahexaenoic	22:6n3	Polyunsaturated ω3

Note: The designation n is equivalent to ω. Both denote the terminal carbon atom opposite the carboxy group end.

medium-chain saturated fatty acids, monounsaturated fatty acids, and polyunsaturated fatty acids (and their resulting triglycerides) are liquids at room temperatures, and termed oils. Long-chain fatty acid and triglycerides yield a heat of combustion of 9 kcal/g, while medium-chain triglycerides yield about 8 kcal/g. This is considerably greater than the 4 kcal/g heat of combustion from carbohydrates or proteins. Because of this discrepancy in caloric density, the concentration of fats in food must be clearly specified as mass (weight percentage) or food energy value (% calories).

Phospholipids are similar to triglycerides, but one end carbon of the glycerol backbone has a phosphate group instead of a fatty acid (phosphatide). The phosphate group is usually bound to one of the following: choline, ethanolamine, serine, or inositol to form a phospholipid. Sterols are hydrocarbon ring structures with varying amounts of unsaturation. Steroids (polyunsaturated sterols) have rigid, planar structures. Many modifications of sterols and steroids are encountered, with esterification, hydroxylation, oxidation, and conjugation being more frequently observed. Common sterols and steroids are cholesterol, β-sitosterol, bile acids, estrogens, progestins, testosterones, corticosteroids, and mineralosteroids. Dolichols are long-chain alcohols used in carbohydrate transport and metabolism in cells. Quinones are exemplified by coenzyme Q_{10}, an extremely important link in the conversion of foodstuffs into cellular energy. Quinones possess substituted rings, usually with hydrocarbon side chains, and are present inside of cell organelle membranes.

Triglycerides are commonly found in foodstuffs (fats and oils), adipose tissue, other tissue storage depots, and in lipoprotein particles in blood plasma. Fatty acids are found in smaller concentrations in foodstuffs, plasma, and intracellularly. Phospholipids are found in cell membranes, plasma lipoproteins, nerve cell sheaths, bile fluid, and foodstuffs (especially lecithin). Sterols and steroids are found in foodstuffs (mostly as cholesterol in animal products and sterols in vegetable products), plasma lipoproteins, cell membranes, and intracellularly. Quinones and dolichols are components of intermediary metabolism and minor components of foodstuffs. Glycolipids, sphingolipids, and ceramides are found in membranes and intermediary metabolism. Fat-soluble vitamins will be discussed in Chapter 5.

B.   ROLES AND FUNCTIONS

Fats offer a diverse range of roles and functions, as summarized in Table 3. The major concern of this chapter will be the roles of fats as calories and as precursors for eicosanoids. The term essential fatty

TABLE 3   Roles and Functions of Fats (Lipids)

1. Source of calories
2. Storage form of calories
3. Insulation and shock-absorbing mechanical qualities
4. Cell and organelle membrane structures
5. Cell membrane signaling and transmission (regulatory roles)
6. Source of acetyl groups for intermediary metabolism and biosynthesis
7. Source of precursors for steroid hormones and bile acids
8. Source of eicosanoid precursors (eicosanoids fulfill a large number of significant physiological functions)
9. Essential for growth, development, and health maintenance (mostly via eicosanoid roles)
10. Transport and uptake of fat-soluble vitamins

acids (EFAs) refers to the combination of linoleate and linolenate PUFAs. There is a dietary requirement for linoleic acid (linoleate) in mammals.[403,404] Linoleate is essential mostly as a precursor for dihomogammalinolenic acid (DHGLA) and arachidonate (which can replace linoleate).[403] DHGLA and arachidonate reside in phospholipids in cell membranes throughout the body and are released by phospholipase A_2 action after stimuli from microenvironmental factors, generating eicosanoids of the one and two series. Eicosanoids are powerful autocrine and paracrine hormones that mediate many cellular and tissue functions.[403-410] Decreased synthesis of eicosanoids after dietary lack of linoleate (or arachidonate) leads to symptoms of infertility, reduced growth, impaired wound healing, scaly dermatoses, eczema, increased permeability of skin and gut, alopecia, kidney damage, liver damage, impaired protein utilization, immune deficiencies (increased susceptibility to infection), irritability, and excess water consumption.[403,411,412]

n3 fatty acids (derived from α-linolenate) are also essential dietary components.[403,411-414] n3 fatty acids are required for proper development of eye and brain tissues during fetal and infant periods. A large proportion of PUFA in developing brain and retina is eicosapentaenoic acid (EPA) and docosahexaenoic acid (DHA), which are formed by elongation and desaturation of α-linolenate (ALA). At this time, absolute deficiencies of n3 fatty acids are thought to be rare. A more pressing problem is relative deficiencies of essential fatty acids and contribution to chronic degenerative diseases.

The conversion of dietary fatty acids to direct eicosanoid precursors occurs in a series of enzymatic steps.[403,404,412,415-417] Table 4 illustrates the fate of major fatty acids and the key enzymes needed to modify fatty acids into eicosanoid precursors. Enzymes for each step work on each fatty acid, although with different affinities. Although Table 4 illustrates that fatty acids derived from palmitic and stearic acids are able to undergo desaturation and elongation, these two pathways do not produce physiologically useful eicosanoids. Rather, excess amounts of these fatty acids compete with essential fatty acids for enzymatic conversions, slowing the formation of direct eicosanoid precursors and, possibly, formation of eicosanoids themselves. Desaturation steps tend to be slow and rate-limiting for each pathway, while elongation steps are rapid.[412] This explains why there are low cellular levels of γ-linoleate and 18:4n3 fatty acids (they are elongated as quickly as they are made by desaturation).

Three types, or series, of eicosanoids are formed from direct fatty acid precursors. Series 1 eicosanoids are produced directly from dihomogammalinolenic acid (DHGLA); series 2 eicosanoids are produced directly from arachidonic acid; and series 3 eicosanoids are produced directly from eicosapentaenoic acid.[412,415-417] In general, eicosanoids are formed on demand almost continuously by almost every tissue and cell. Eicosanoids are short-lived and exert local regulatory effects. Eicosanoids are quickly inactivated or destroyed near their site of production.

After release of target fatty acids by phospholipases in cell membranes, two major types of enzyme systems produce eicosanoids: cyclooxygenase and lipoxygenase.[403,404,408,412,415-417] In general, cyclooxygenase products are termed prostaglandins (PGs) or thromboxanes (TXs), while lipoxygenase products are termed leukotrienes, hydroxy fatty acids (HETEs, HPETEs), or lipoxins.[416] Letters after the abbreviations for each eicosanoid signify specific compounds. A subscript may designate the series of fatty acid derivatives. The naming system has many gaps and deletions as a result of early research finding many artifacts or metabolites of the true eicosanoids. In general, series 1 and 3 eicosanoids exert

TABLE 4 Conversion of Fatty Acids Into Direct Eicosanoid Precursors

Diet ↓	n7 Fatty Acids Diet ↓	n9 Fatty Acids Diet ↓	n6 EFAs Diet ↓	n3 EFAs Diet ↓
Carbohydrate →	Palmitic 16:0 →	Stearic 18:0		
-9-Desaturase →	↓	↓		
	Palmitoleic 16:1n7	Oleic 18:1n9	Linoleic 18:2n6	α-Linolenic 18:3n3
-6-Desaturase →	↓	↓	↓	↓
	16:2n7	18:2n9	γ-Linolenic 18:3n6	18:4n3
Elongase →	↓	↓	↓	↓
	18:2n7	20:2n9	DHGLA 20:3n6	20:4n3
-5-Desaturase →	↓	↓	↓	↓
	18:3n7	20:3n9	Arachidonic 20:4n6	EPA 20:5n3
Elongase →	↓	↓	↓	↓
	20:3n7	22:3n9	Adrenic 22:4n6	22:5n3
-4-Desaturase →	↓	↓	↓	↓
	20:4n7	22:4n9	22:5n6	DHA 22:6n3

Note: DHGLA, arachidonic acid, and EPA are direct precursors of eicosanoids. EFAs = essential fatty acids; DHGLA = dihomogammalinolenic acid; EPA = eicosapentaenoic acid; DHA = docosahexaenoic acid.

antiinflammatory actions, and series 2 eicosanoids exert proinflammatory actions. Both actions are necessary to maintain balance and homeostasis, including during wound healing. However, when one series predominates (by predominance of target fatty acid precursor levels in membrane phospholipids), disorders can occur. Therefore, inhibitors of cyclooxygenase (aspirin, NSAIDs) will reduce formation of all series of prostaglandins and thromboxanes. Therapeutic manipulation of cyclooxygenase and lipoxygenase activities has been a cornerstone of analgesic and antiinflammatory therapies for decades.

II. OMEGA-3 FATTY ACIDS

A. BACKGROUND

An explosion of research into the health effects of EFAs and n3 fatty acids has occurred since 1980. This section will be concerned mostly with human trials of fatty acids on conditions of musculoskeletal healing. The rationale for use of fatty acids (oils or fats) is to modulate membrane phospholipid levels of direct precursors for eicosanoid synthesis in such a manner as to enhance production of antiinflammatory eicosanoids and reduce production of proinflammatory eicosanoids. Because of the interaction of many variables, this rationale has not been reproducibly attained. Nevertheless, sufficient studies have accumulated to deduce that modulation of eicosanoid production by dietary intake of fatty acids is reasonable. Table 5 lists some specific actions attributed to EPA and DHA *in vivo* and *in vitro*.[138,139,418] A large amount of animal and human research has found that provision of dietary n3 fatty acids will increase cell membrane levels of ALA, EPA, and DHA, and lead to enhanced production of series 3 eicosanoids. In addition, n3 fatty acids have lower affinity for cyclooxygenase and lipoxygenases, thus reducing the total amount of eicosanoids formed when n3 fatty acids predominate. Extremely high levels of n3 fatty acids can antagonize n6 fatty acid-derived eicosanoid production and function; therefore, absolute ablation of arachidonic acid function is not recommended. Rather, a balance between series 1, 2, and 3 eicosanoids is suggested to maintain reparative processes with the least amount of inflammation.

B. HUMAN STUDIES
1. Antiinflammatory Effects

Since interleukin-1 (IL1) and TNF are major mediators of inflammation, it has been postulated that reduced production of these cytokines may reduce inflammation and ameliorate inflammatory

**TABLE 5   Specific Actions of EPA and
DHA Fatty Acids**

↓ Melting point
↑ Fluidity of membranes
↓ Production of phosphatidyl inositol
↓ Dienoic eicosanoid release
↓ Interleukin-1 and TNF release
↓ N6 PUFA levels in membranes
↑ Production of antiinflamatory eicosanoids

Note: EPA = 5,8,11,14,17-eicosapentaenoic acid;
DHA = 4,7,10,13,16,19-docosahexaenoic acid;
TNF = tumor necrosis factor; PUFA =
polyunsaturated fatty acids.

symptoms.[138,139,180,216] Clinical evidence of antiinflammatory effects of n3 fatty acids is mounting, as evidenced by effects on inflammatory conditions such as psoriasis, eczema, cardiovascular diseases, ulcerative colitis, and other conditions.[439] Increasing status of n3 fatty acids has been associated with significant changes in eicosanoids and other regulatory agents mediated by eicosanoids.

In a study, 9 healthy volunteers ingested 18 g/d of fish-oil concentrate (MaxEPA) to their usual diets for 6 weeks.[419,420] Levels of IL-1β production by peripheral blood mononuclear cells were reduced significantly after the 6-week diet period from a baseline value of 7.3 to 4.3 ng/ml. The depression was continued for 10 weeks after cessation of the diet, but returned to baseline levels 20 weeks after cessation of the fish oil diet. Surprisingly, oral aspirin and ibuprofen (200 mg/d) increased IL-1β and TNF levels 2- to 3-fold. Thus, dietary supplementation with n3 fatty acids (as fish oil) showed the potential to reduce inflammation by reduction of inflammatory mediators IL-1 and TNF in normal volunteers.

Similarly, incubation of isolated human neutrophils or monocytes with arachidonate, EPA, or DHA found that arachidonate enhanced production of proinflammatory leukotrienes (5-HETE, LTB_4) and platelet-activating factor (PAF), while EPA decreased leukotriene and PAF production, and DHA had no effect.[421] When 7 healthy volunteers ingested 18 g/d of fish oil (MaxEPA) for 6 weeks, a 50% inhibition of neutrophil leukotriene production was found, with only very small amounts of EPA-derived leukotrienes produced.[421] These changes were seen after 6 weeks of dietary fish oil supplementation, and not after 3 weeks, although neutrophil EPA contents were similar at both 3 and 6 weeks. Similar reductions in production of leukotrienes and PAF were observed in monocytes.[421] A large decrease in neutrophil chemotactic response to leukotrienes was observed (71% decrease). Thus, fish oil supplementation is able to impair neutrophil adherence, margination, and diapedesis into inflammatory sites (in response to leukotrienes). In studies with specific fatty acids, EPA, and not DHA, accounted for the observed effects.[421,422] Again, n3 fatty acids showed the ability to modulate inflammatory mediators in humans.

Another possible effect of n3 fatty acids is to reduce pain.[423] For 30 d, 13 normal males received either 5 g/d of fish oil (Promega) or 5 g/d of wheat germ oil placebo, followed by a washout period and crossover to the other oil. The time to peak pain for a cold pressor test (immersion of a hand in water at 4°C for 5 min) was significantly prolonged during the fish oil period, compared to the placebo period. Peak pain scores were not different. Thus, enhancement of n3 fatty acid intake and status may improve pain tolerance.

2.   Rheumatoid Arthritis

Rheumatoid arthritis (RA) is a common autoimmune disease resulting in joint inflammation and severe joint damage to the point of disability.[424] Although RA is not an injury directly related to sports or physical activity, for the purposes of this book, RA is a model of human inflammation with a considerable amount of research and clinical trials, including effect of nutrients. Thus, the effect of n3 fatty acids on rheumatoid arthritis in humans will be briefly reviewed.

At least ten original studies on the effects of fish oil supplementation on human RA have appeared.[421,425-437] Three additional studies have examined the clinical effects of n6 fatty acid supplementation on human RA.[431,437,438] Kremer et al., from the Division of Rheumatology at Albany Medical College in New York, reported on clinical results of a pilot study of 17 RA patients switched to a diet high in PUFA and low in saturated fat, with a daily supplement of 1.8 g EPA and 0.9 g DHA in 10 fish oil capsules (MaxEPA).[425] A control group of 20 RA patients consumed a diet high in saturated fat (PUFA/saturated fat ratio of 1/4) along with paraffin placebos. The study was double-blind, randomized, and placebo-controlled, and lasted for 12 weeks, with a 1- to 2-month followup. Significant differences between groups in favor of the fish oil group were an improvement in morning stiffness, number of tender joints, hemoglobin, and prolongation of bleeding time. However, the significant results could be attributed to worsening in placebo group subjects with no change found in supplemented subjects. Also, both groups continued aspirin or NSAID therapy throughout the study.

Another study by Kremer and colleagues compared the effects of fish oil supplements (15 capsules per d for 2.8 g EPA and 1.8 g DHA) in a 14-week double-blind crossover trial with a 4-week washout period in 33 subjects.[426] Diets and medications were unchanged during the study periods. The fish oil period resulted in the following improvements over placebo: longer time to fatigue, decreased number of tender joints, and decreased neutrophil production of leukotriene LTB_4. Other measurements tended to improve in the fish oil group, but did not reach statistical significance. The fish oil group exhibited significant improvements from baseline values, and residual effects of fish oil were seen to be greater than 4 weeks. Thus, the placebo group may have benefitted from insufficient washout of fish oil effects. Thus, crossover studies are not an adequate experimental design for studying the effects of fish oils (n3 fatty acids). Sperling and associates, from the Harvard Medical School, administered 20 g/d of fish oil (MaxEPA) to 12 RA patients for 6 weeks.[427] Findings included large increases in cell membrane EPA, decreased cell membrane arachidonate levels, reduced production of leukotriene LTB_4 by neutrophils, increased neutrophil chemotaxis *ex vivo*, reduced monocyte production of PAF, and appearance of leukotrienes derived from EPA, which were previously undetectable. Thus, high-dose fish oil resulted in biochemical changes congruent with antiinflammatory actions.

Magaro and colleagues divided 12 female RA patients into 2 dietary groups: 1 group received a diet high in saturated fats and low in PUFAs, while the other group consumed a diet high in PUFA and 9 capsules per d of MaxEPA for 30 d.[428] All subjects continued on NSAID therapy. Compared to baseline values, the fish oil group showed improvements in Ritchie Index, grip strength, morning stiffness, and reduction of neutrophil chemiluminescence. The improvements in the fish oil group were also significantly different from the control group. Cleland and colleagues, from the Rheumatology Unit of the Royal Adelaide Hospital in Adelaide, South Australia, studied the effects of fish oil supplementation (18 capsules per d MaxEPA), or an equivalent amount of olive oil, for a total of 60 g of dietary fat daily in 46 RA patients for 12 weeks.[430] All patients continued antirheumatic medications (NSAIDs, prednisone, long-acting agents). Improvements in grip strength and number of tender joints was found for the fish oil group. Neutrophil leukotriene production was reduced 30% by fish oil, similar to other studies. Belch and others, from the Center for Rheumatic Diseases in Glasgow, Scotland, compared the effects of placebo (paraffin), evening primrose oil (EPO, a source of γ-linolenic acid, a DHGLA precursor), and EPO plus fish oil on drug requirements in 49 RA patients.[431] Doses of γ-linolenic acid were 540 mg/d, and EPA doses were 240 mg/d. Oils were given for 12 months, followed by a 3-month crossover to placebo (paraffin without vitamin E) in all groups (subjects remained blinded throughout the study). All subjects also took 120 mg/d of vitamin E, which is a substantial dose that may have its own antirheumatic effects, as will be discussed in the section of this book on vitamin E. Significant subjective improvements were noted for both EPO and EPO plus fish oil groups at 12 months, along with significant reductions in NSAID medication levels. Measures of disease activity did not worsen despite a decrease in NSAID dosage. After 3 months of placebo, all subjects relapsed. Beneficial changes were significant after 6 months. Therefore, low supplemental doses of both γ-linolenate (GLA) or GLA/EPA + DHA for long time periods were associated with reductions in analgesic medication doses and improvements in clinical symptoms. However, the contribution of vitamin E cannot be ignored.

Table 6   Significant Findings After n3 Fatty Acid Supplementation in Subjects with Rheumatoid Arthritis

Decreased Parameters	Increased Parameters
Number of tender joints	Grip strength
Ritchie Index	Bleeding time
Morning stiffness	Time to fatigue
NSAID dosage and usage	Neutrophil chemotaxis
Production of arachidonate-derived eicosanoids (leukotrienes LTB_4, 5HETE)	Cell membrane levels of EPA, DHA
Production of monocyte PAF	Production of EPA-derived leukotrienes
Cell membrane levels of arachidonate	
Neutrophil chemiluminescence	

Kremer and colleagues administered high-dose (54 mg/kg/d EPA and 36 mg/kg/d DHA) or low-dose (27 mg/kg/d EPA and 18 mg/kg/d DHA) EPA + DHA supplementation (as ethyl esters of EPA and DHA) or olive oil to 49 RA patients for 6 months in a randomized, prospective parallel, double-blind, placebo-controlled study.[434] No changes in diet or medications were attempted. The EPA group showed numerous clinical improvements (21/45 measurements) from baseline values between 6 to 24 weeks in the high-dose group. Low-dose supplementation produced 8/45 improvements, and placebo produced 5/45 improvements, compared to baseline values. However, when the high-dose group was compared to low-dose or placebo groups, only the grip strength remained significantly improved in clinical parameters. All groups showed improvements in immune functions (decreased IL-1 production, lymphocyte mitogenesis, decreased IgG production), but improvements were more significant in the high-dose group. This study is important for several reasons. It confirms that long treatment periods (>6 to 14 weeks) are necessary for beneficial effects to be seen for n3 fatty acids, and that more beneficial effects accrue over time. A dose response may exist, with larger doses providing greater responses. Low-dose EPA + DHA supplementation was no better than olive oil supplementation (6.8 g oleate per d). Oleic acid may have its own immunostimulatory properties, which could have masked differences between the high-dose and placebo groups.[435] More dropouts were encountered in the placebo group, due to need for increases in analgesic medications (which indicates that placebo treatment resulted in clinical worsening of symptoms).

Other studies also found various degrees of clinical benefits after fish oil supplementation to patients with RA.[429,432,433] Thus, a consensus of research strongly indicates that supplementation with large doses of EPA + DHA (as fish oil or ethyl esters) possesses some benefits as adjuncts for RA therapy (see Table 6). Results are slow to appear, but suggest a reduction of inflammatory processes and their symptoms, rather than a disease-modifying activity. Possibly, fish oils may offer an alternative to patients with gastric intolerance to standard NSAIDs, since almost no toxicity was found in n3 fatty acid-supplemented groups. Some areas of future research to make application of fish oils more practical include a low fat diet without NSAIDs, since mixed diets or diets high in PUFAs (which were used in all studies) have considerable linoleate and arachidonate contents, which suppress n3 fatty acid conversions to eicosanoids. Likewise, NSAIDs reduce eicosanoid synthesis as their major mechanism of action. The use of flaxseed (linseed) oil, which is almost 50% α-linolenate (the dietary precursor for EPA and DHA), as a source of n3 fatty acids has not been studied in human inflammatory conditions.

A preliminary pilot study by Carmichael administered 6 capsules of Efamol (evening primrose oil) containing 2.2 g linoleate and 270 mg γ-linolenate (GLA) and Efavit containing additional calcium ascorbate, niacin, vitamin B_6, and zinc to 18 patients with severe RA for at least 2 months.[437] Of 18 patients, 10 showed reductions in pain scores and articular index of between 50 to 100% without concurrent NSAID or other medications. However, Hansen et al. did not find significant changes in biochemical or clinical measurements in 20 RA patients after 12 weeks of similar supplementation.[438] However, NSAIDs and other medications were stopped 4 d prior to supplementation, which may have influenced results. From the results of Belch, it appears that 12 weeks is insufficient to determine whether GLA has benefits for RA patients. Thus, GLA, as a precursor for series 1 eicosanoids via DHGLA, deserves further study as an antiinflammatory adjunct in humans.

It appears that increased dietary intake of n3 fatty acids is associated with mild to moderate antiinflammatory effects in humans with severe inflammatory diseases. Antiinflammatory effects from n3 fatty acid supplementation are also apparent in healthy subjects, meaning that application to sports injuries and sports medicine is practical.

3. Trauma

Use of n3 fatty acids has attracted much recent attention in parenteral and enteral feeding.[3-7,138,139,170,171,180,216] Hospital-based use of lipids as major caloric sources has enjoyed a rebirth with the use of structured lipids and combinations of different oil types, including n3 fatty acid sources. A few recent studies that included n3 fatty acids will be examined to further emphasize the point that n3 fatty acids (and GLA) are well tolerated and have beneficial clinical effects in severe inflammation of trauma.

Phospholipids in erythrocyte membranes after enteral feeding of three different types of fatty acids by Diboune and others from Strasbourg, France and Vevey, Switzerland were determined to monitor ability of different fat supplements to deliver certain fatty acids thought to be important for inflammatory processes.[440] Each of 32 patients with severe head trauma or cerebral stroke were given 150 g/d of fat consisting of one of the following three types: (1) soybean oil (54% linoleic acid, 9% α-linolenic acid); (2) 50/50 soybean oil/medium-chain triglycerides; or (3) 50% soybean oil/42.5% medium-chain triglycerides/7.5% black-currant seed oil (27% linoleic acid, 14% γ-linolenic acid, and 4% stearidonic acid). The black-currant oil diet supplied approximately 3.5 g of omega-3 fatty acids. Before administration of fats, each patient exhibited a normal fatty acid profile, compared to healthy controls. There was no difference between groups in the tolerability of each type of fat, which was well tolerated.

Soybean oil greatly increased linoleic acid levels and decreased dihomogammalinolenic acid (DHGLA) levels slightly and briefly, indicating a minor inhibition of delta-6-desaturase. However, the MCT oil diet caused a rapid increase in DHGLA production, while the black-currant oil diet produced an even larger increase in DHGLA production. Arachidonic acid levels did not change at any time with any diet. The only diet that increased levels of the omega-3 eicosapentaenoic acid (EPA) was the black-currant oil diet. Increases of 32% over baseline were measured after 3 weeks of supplementation. The ratio of DHGLA + EPA/arachidonic acid was constant after soybean oil, but increased after the MCT-enriched or black-currant oil diets, with the latter producing an increase of 50% by 3 weeks.

This study clearly shows that feeding black-currant oil with medium-chain triglycerides and soybean oil supplies not only adequate essential fatty acids (linoleate and linolenate), but also supplies medium-chain triglycerides for readily available energy and omega-3 fatty acids. A relatively short time period of 3 weeks for results to be apparent was achieved by feeding large amounts of total fat (150 g/d). The omega-3 fatty acids were present in sufficient amount to significantly alter the ratio of precursor fatty acids used in production of eicosanoids. Thus, supplying GLA from black-currant oil appears to be more favorable at reducing production of arachidonic acid and its subsequent 2-series eicosanoids, and increasing formation of EPA and its subsequent 3-series of antiinflammatory eicosanoids. The implications of less inflammation, less platelet aggregation, and less release of shock mediators which may follow black-currant oil supplementation would have obvious benefits for recovery from major trauma.

Gottschlich and others evaluated the effects of three enteral diets in burn patients in a randomized, prospective trial.[441] A diet containing fish oil and just enough n6 fatty acids to prevent EFA deficiency, with restricted total fat intake, was compared to two commercial formulas modified to more closely reflect the experimental diet, with no limits on fat intake. The fish oil group exhibited reductions in wound infections and ratio of length of stay to percentage of body burned. More deaths (70%) occurred in the two modified commercial formulas, which contained much more linoleate and total fat. Thus, fish oil intake and reduction of competitive fat intake may have significant effects on the outcome of major trauma patients.

Cerra and colleagues compared the effects of an enteral diet supplemented with n3 fatty acids (menhaden oil), arginine, and RNA with another commercially available complete enteral formula on the outcome of ICU patients with polytrauma or major elective surgery.[223] Although both formulas improved nitrogen retention and improved visceral protein status to a similar degree, the fish oil formula was associated with a significant reduction in 3-methylhistidine excretion and stimulation of *ex vivo* lymphocyte proliferative responses, indicating amelioration of suppressed immune function commonly encountered in these patients. Thus, recent evidence is supporting the concept that improvement of n3 fatty acid status plays a beneficial role in recovery from inflammatory conditions and trauma.

At this time, there are no specific studies on the effects on n3 fatty acids (or GLA) on healing sports injuries, trauma, or even surgery. Thus, evidence in other inflammatory conditions must be considered when applicability of n3 fatty acids to sports medicine is called into question.

III. MEDIUM-CHAIN TRIGLYCERIDES (MCTs)

Medium-chain triglycerides (MCTs) are a class of lipids made of saturated fatty acids from 6 to 12 carbons in length (see Table 1).[403,404,442,443] MCTs are found in coconut, palm kernel, babassu, cohune, and tucum oils, and in human milk. MCTs have been purified from these sources and are commercially available as mixed MCTs (6 to 12 carbons long) or pure tricaprylic (C8) triglycerides.[170] Increasing use of MCTs as an energy source for enteral and parenteral feeding is based on years of clinical use when safe, additional calories are needed.[3-7,170,443] MCTs possess different physiological and chemical properties than other lipids and fatty acids. MCT oils are less viscous than their long-chain triglyceride counterparts and are about the only saturated fats that are liquid at room temperature. Medium-chain fatty acids are slightly soluble in water and aqueous solutions, compared to almost total insolubility for long-chain fatty acids. Since MCTs are completely saturated, they do not have the instability to oxidation and storage well-known for unsaturated fats. No eicosanoids are produced directly from medium-chain fatty acids or their possible elongation and desaturation products. Thus, the major influence of MCTs is as a source of calories.

Several properties make MCTs attractive as efficient energy sources. When ingested, MCTs are rapidly and completely absorbed into the portal blood system, not the lymphatic system like other fats. Medium-chain fatty acids are not reesterified and repackaged into chylomicrons. The liver readily takes up medium-chain fatty acids from the portal blood supply. Albumin is the chief carrier of medium-chain fatty acids, although some are dissolved in plasma. In the liver, medium-chain fatty acids do not need carnitine for transport into mitochondria. Medium-chain fatty acids are transported directly to oxidative sites in mitochondria.[403,404,442,443] Medium-chain fatty acids are rapidly and, it seems, preferably oxidized to produce cellular energy and ketone bodies, which may be further oxidized or sent to peripheral tissues.[442] Metabolism of medium-chain fatty acids resembles carbohydrate metabolism in some ways, rather than fat metabolism. Caloric yield of medium-chain fatty acids is 8 kcal/g, rather than 9 kcal/g usually associated with fats.[170]

MCTs have the ability to increase resting metabolic rate to a greater degree than isocaloric amounts of long-chain triglycerides in healthy or obese subjects.[444-447] MCTs are not easily stored as body fat[443,447,448] and assist in mobilization of body fat stores.[447-449] Furthermore, by provision of extra calories, MCTs are able to spare lean muscle mass.[450] Both purified MCTs and coconut oil are nonatherogenic.[451] Coupled with many years of clinical safety,[170,442,443] MCTs represent an excellent source of additional calories when calorie needs are increased, such as after trauma, surgery, or infections. A working hypothesis for sports medicine is that provision of MCTs during recovery from injury can add additional calories that spare lean muscle mass and do not become body fat if excess is ingested. This may be important for athletes desiring to return to peak performance as soon as possible after injury. As with n3 fatty acids, no clinical trials on MCTs and recovery from sports injuries have been attempted. The availability, safety, and known effects of MCTs suggests that they may be of some benefit to recovery from injuries.

IV. COENZYME Q$_{10}$ (UBIQUINONE)

Coenzyme Q$_{10}$ (ubiquinone) is a highly lipophilic compound occupying a key role in production of cellular energy. Coenzyme Q$_{10}$ transfers electrons from food energy converted into NADH, NADPH, FADH$_2$, FMNH, and other substrates into the electron transport chain of oxidative phosphorylation in mitochondria.[452] Coenzyme Q$_{10}$ is the single most important metabolic component of ATP production. Of interest for practical applications is the finding that normal levels of coenzyme Q$_{10}$ do not saturate the respiratory chain and, thus, energy production,[453] thereby leading to a working hypothesis that additional coenzyme Q$_{10}$ may lead to increased cellular energy output, tissue function, organ function, and clinical benefits for healing.

Coenzyme Q$_{10}$ supplementation to humans with periodontal disease has been assessed in a series of studies.[454-462] A deficiency of coenzyme Q$_{10}$ levels and functions in gingival tissues of periodontitis patients has been found.[454-458] Administration of various forms of coenzyme Q (mostly as coenzyme Q$_{10}$) has consistently resulted in significant, but small improvements in tooth mobility, pocket depth, and gingival index.[457-462] Both serum and gingival tissue levels of coenzyme Q$_{10}$ were doubled or tripled after oral supplementation with 60 to 100 mg/d for 8 to 12 weeks. Results were usually not significant until 8 weeks or later. Thus, some evidence suggests that coenzyme Q$_{10}$ enhances healing of gingival tissues by an increase in deficient bioenergetics. This concept should be applicable to other tissues, and extensive worldwide research on the effects of coenzyme Q$_{10}$ supplementation for cardiovascular diseases, immune system disorders, muscular dystrophy, and exercise performance has consistently shown significant and practical clinical improvements (reviewed by Folkers and others[452,463-469]). Thus, sufficient rationale and clinical experience in other conditions argue in favor of conducting clinical trials of coenzyme Q$_{10}$ supplementation and recovery from injury.

V. SUMMARY AND GUIDELINES

Fats and lipids are emerging from the shadow of unwanted caloric intake into potent and useful modulators of physiological functions of great importance for healing. The recent surge in research on eicosanoid effects of PUFAs and clinical uses of MCTs promise to spill over into effects on healing in ambulatory situations. Although few direct studies on healing of musculoskeletal injuries have examined the effects of dietary fat modulation, the number of studies in closely allied fields (rheumatology) is increasing, and results are possibly of clinical value. However, in order to successfully apply n3 fatty acids for enhancement of healing, several conditions must be met. Since turnover of cell membrane phospholipid fatty acids is slow (compared to effects of aspirin and NSAIDs), results may not be immediately apparent. Thus, modulation of inflammation by dietary fat intake may not appear clinically useful in short-lived or acute situations. However, long-term or chronic conditions of inflammation have the most potential for showing clinical responses. Table 7 lists some dietary manipulations necessary to derive optimum effect from n3 fatty acids and their effect.

It can be seen that simply taking fish oil supplements is not a guarantee of success. Intake of other competitive fats must be simultaneously reduced to observe the greatest relative effects from n3 fatty acids. An increase in the ratio of n3/arachidonate in the diet and cells is the goal of enhanced status of lipids for healing. Care must be taken to prevent a complete deficit in linoleate, which is essential for healing. Also, the combination of n3 fatty acids with GLA (the precursor for DHGLA and series 1 eicosanoids) may exert additive or synergistic effects with n3 fatty acids.[407,410,470]

Another major consideration given almost no research attention is the issue of oxidation and rancidity. n3 Fatty acids are highly susceptible to attack by oxygen and free radicals and, as a result, have limited shelf lives, unless protected by lipid-soluble antioxidants (vitamin E).[470,471] It is entirely possible that oxidized n3 fatty acids can cause more harm than good, as shown by early studies that did not take oxidation and rancidity into account.[471] Therefore, it is usually recommended to increase vitamin E intake to protect n3 fatty acids in cellular membranes when consuming increased quantitities of PUFAs.

TABLE 7   Dietary Manipulations to Increase N3 Fatty Acid Status

1. Decrease total dietary fat intake to 10% of calories or less.
2. Decrease intake of foods rich in long-chain saturated fats (red meats; dairy products including whole milk, 2% milk, ice cream, butter, cheeses; margarines; shortenings; lard; tallow; fried foods); no intake of these foods is preferred.
3. Limit intake of vegetable oils rich in linoleate (vegetable cooking oils, especially corn, safflower, sunflower, soybean, sesame); nuts; seeds; peanuts; peanut butter. Ideal intake is 1 TBS daily; do not continue to limit linoleate intake for more than two months.
4. Increase fish consumption, especially fish with colored flesh (salmon, mackerel, sardines, herrings, anchovies, tuna, eel); in general, deep-sea cold-water fish have higher n3 fatty acid contents; shellfish and blue-green algae are also significant n3 fatty acid sources; fish may be consumed at each meal if desired, or at least daily.
5. Optional: add supplements of fish body oil (not fish liver oil); usually, each capsule contains 1 g of fish oil with 20 to 50% n3 content; therefore, 3 to 18 capsules per day in divided doses are a major source of dietary n3 fatty acids (EPA and DHA).
6. Add flax seeds, flaxseed (edible linseed) oil, or flaxseed oil capsules (1 g each) to the diet as an alternative to fish or fish oil supplements; flax seeds contain α-linolenate (ALA), an essential n3 fatty acid and precursor for EPA and DHA. Taking 1 cup of flax seeds, 1 to 4 TBS of flaxseed oil, or 1 to 12 capsules of flaxseed oil daily will significantly affect ALA levels in cells; green leafy vegetables are also significant sources of dietary ALA and should be consumed in large amounts.
7. Add *d*-α-tocopherol (vitamin E) supplement (100 to 400 IU daily).
8. Optional: addition of dietary sources rich in γ-linoleic acid (GLA) may provide a synergistic effect to n3 fatty acids by enhancing production of series 1 eicosanoids, which are similar in effect to series 3 eicosanoids; richest sources are capsules with evening primrose oil, black-currant seed oil, or borage oil; 2–12 capsules daily have increased tissue levels of GLA.

TABLE 8   Speculative Conditions for Application of Dietary Modification of Lipid Intake for Injury Rehabilitation and Sports Medicine

Rheumatoid arthritis
Chronic inflammatory conditions (especially skin and joints)
Autoimmune disorders
Degenerative joint conditions (osteoarthritis, invertebral disc disease)
Bursitis, tendinitis, tenosynovitis
Major trauma (fractures) or major surgery
Delayed healing
Prevention of muscle wasting or catabolism
Adjunct to long-term therapy with aspirin, NSAIDs, or corticosteroids
Alternative when intolerant to long-term aspirin or NSAID therapy
Depressed immune function or resistance to infections

The use of dietary sources of α-linolenate (ALA) to augment n3 fatty acid intake has been virtually ignored.[472] ALA is the precursor for endogenous formation of EPA and DHA by desaturation and elongation. There is insufficient research to determine whether ALA intake can replace EPA and DHA intakes. The addition of ALA with fish oils has not been studied.

Table 8 lists conditions pertaining to injury rehabilitation and sports medicine that may have clinical benefits by modulation of dietary lipids to enhance effects of series 1 and 3 eicosanoids. It must be stressed that specific studies are not available (except for rheumatoid arthritis), and so application of dietary lipid modulation must be considered speculative at this time, even though the basic physiological mechanisms and sources are known.[473-475]

In general, reports on human subjects of high n3 fatty acid intake are reproducibly safe. Although bleeding times have been lengthened, the values were still in normal ranges. Thus, there is little or no evidence to endow n3 fatty acids with ability to prevent adequate blood clotting. Commercial sources of fish oils, flaxseed oils, GLA oils, and MCT oils are all available in grocery stores, pharmacies, health food stores, or mail order companies. Lipid modulation to counter inflammatory processes appears promising at this time, but firm guidelines for use are nascent and not conclusive.

Chapter 5

FAT-SOLUBLE VITAMINS

I. VITAMIN A (RETINOLS) AND β-CAROTENE

"If we consider the role of vitamin A on the widest possible basis, therefore, we may say that it is necessary for the formation of large molecules containing glucosamine."

T. Moore, 1957[476]

This quote is presented to illustrate just one of the many essential roles vitamin A plays in the musculoskeletal system. Vitamin A was probably the first vitamin discovered, by McCollum and Davis, in 1915.[477] Several recent reviews give a substantial amount of background information on the many vital roles and functions of the first vitamin.[170,476-481] Confusion over the identity of vitamin A is common, due to the multiplicity of forms found in nature with vitamin A activity. In this chapter, vitamin A is retinol, with commercially available forms including all-*trans*-retinyl palmitate, all-*trans*-retinyl acetate, and retinol. Retinol and its derivatives are referred to as preformed vitamin A to distinguish retinoids from carotenoids. Over 500 carotenoids are known to exist,[477-479] but by far the most important is β-carotene, which is actually two retinols combined with the alcohol groups removed.[477-481] By itself, β-carotene is primarily an antioxidant, by virtue of its scavenging effects against singlet oxygen.[482,483] However, upon demand, β-carotene is cleaved into two retinol molecules. Thus, β-carotene can supply retinol equivalents when preformed vitamin A is not available or insufficient to meet needs. This book will make a distinction between retinols and carotenoids, since their actions differ, although recognizing that some β-carotene can convert into retinol.

A. ROLES AND FUNCTIONS

Table 1 lists the most important roles for retinol.[476-481] This section will be concerned with the somatic roles of retinol on epithelial tissues, since these retinol-responsive tissues (skin, bone, cartilage, loose connective tissues) are involved in musculoskeletal healing. Retinol functions as a regulatory hormone with effects on specific genes in epithelial cell nuclei.[477-481] Retinol is also converted inside of target cells to retinoic acid, an extremely potent regulator of specific genes.[477-481] Retinol is also converted to retinyl β-glucuronide and retinyl phosphate, with additional regulatory roles for cell differentiation. Thus, retinol metabolism for cell differentiation is a complex and intricate set of regulatory capabilities with profound effects on connective tissue cells. Retinyl phosphate exhibits coenzymatic roles for sugar transport in glycosylation reactions for glycoprotein, and perhaps glycosaminoglycan, synthesis. Possible roles as an electron transfer coenzyme interacting with membrane enzymes and altered membrane stability are additional somatic roles for retinol.

B. DEFICIENCY SYMPTOMS

Table 2 lists some of the more important deficiency symptoms pertinent to healing.[477-481] Deficiency symptoms can occur with lowered dietary intake but normal liver stores of retinol. Rapidly proliferating tissues are very sensitive to retinol deficiency, especially fibroblasts during the proliferative phase of wound healing. Deficiency symptoms of retinol may relate to lack of dietary intake and depletion of tissue stores in the liver, or to deficiency of other nutrients needed to assist in the transport and metabolism of retinol. After trauma, sequestration of zinc may reduce liver synthesis of retinol-binding

TABLE 1   Retinol Roles

1. Somatic (differentiation and maintenance of epithelial tissues)
2. Reproductive
3. Visual
4. Anticarcinogenic
5. Immune function

TABLE 2   Deficiency Symptoms of Retinol Pertinent to Connective Tissues

1. Dedifferentiation of epithelial tissues
2. Less glycoprotein synthesis
3. Lowered immunoresponsiveness and resistance to stress
4. Decreased sulfate uptake into cartilage
5. Increased turnover of chondroitin sulfates in cartilage
6. Reduced adhesion of chondrocytes and fibroblasts to extracellular matrix
7. Decreased collagen quantity and quality
8. Increased urine excretion of sulfate and chondroitin sulfates
9. Decreased binding of cytokines (e.g., Epidermal growth factor)
10. Decreased wound strength
11. Decreased serum and tissue ascorbate levels
12. Decreased appetite
13. Bone loss
14. Skin follicular hyperkeratosis
15. Night blindness

protein (RBP), which has a short half-life of 11 to 16 h.[170,477] Each RBP molecule binds one retinol molecule for transport in plasma to other tissues. Dietary retinol is transported to the liver in lipoproteins, in which form retinol is unavailable to other tissues.[477] RBP-retinol binds to transthyretin (prealbumin) in plasma.[170,477] Both transthyretin and RBP have been used as markers for protein status, since serum levels of RBP and transthyretin are reduced by about 50% in protein deficiency states.[170,477] Thus, deficiencies of protein and/or zinc can adversely affect retinol status independent of the amount of retinol stores. Since retinol is stored in the liver, and sent to peripheral tissues in a highly regulated manner on RBP and transthyretin, functional retinol deficiencies can occur with normal retinol intakes and stores.

Wound healing in rats made deficient in retinol by dietary lack was decreased to 63% of normal at 14 d postsurgery.[484] Wound hydroxyproline content was 67% of normal. These large differences signify the importance of maintaining adequate retinol status and plasma levels during healing. The following parameters of wound healing were decreased: epithelialization; rate of open wound closure; collagen synthesis; collagen cross-links; proteoglycan synthesis; and rate of epithelial cell differentiation.[93,164,485] Corticosteroids in particular antagonize retinol effects, resulting in retinol-responsive impairment of healing.[164,485-487]

C. ASSESSMENT

Retinol status assessment has progressed to include a number of useful measurements. Table 3 lists some of the assessments for retinol status in practical use.[170,477-481] Clinical symptoms center around the eye and are apparent in frank deficiencies of retinol. Night blindness, time to dark adaptation, xerophthalmia, and Bitot's spots signify a deficient retinol state. Conjunctival impression cytology involves collecting an imprint of the conjunctiva and, after staining, histological examination of goblet cells and epithelial cell numbers and morphology. This noninvasive procedure is capable of detecting marginal states of retinol status, before clinical symptoms appear in eyes. The relative dose response test measures the ratio of plasma retinol levels before and 5 h after a standardized oral dose of retinyl

TABLE 3   Methods of Assessment for Retinol Status

1. Serum (plasma) retinol levels
2. Relative dose response or modified relative dose response test
3. Conjunctival impression cytology
4. Xerophthalmia, Bitot's spots, night blindness
5. Tear retinol levels
6. Dietary intakes of retinol equivalents

palmitate (450 µg). An increase in plasma retinol of >20% indicates a marginal status, and an increase of >50% indicates a frank deficiency of retinol. Plasma retinol levels <0.7 µmol/l (<20 µg/dl) are indicative of marginal status, but plasma retinol levels are subject to misinterpretation during liver or kidney failure. Plasma retinol levels are decreased in retinol deficiency, protein-calorie malnutrition, infections, parasitic infestations, and liver disease. Plasma retinol levels are artificially elevated by pregnancy, oral contraceptives, and kidney disease. Plasma retinol levels are also indicative of retinol toxicity when >100 µg/dl. Dietary intakes are generally less useful than clinical or biochemical assessments, but may be of use in frank deficiencies or excess consumption.

D. INTAKES

Two major surveys of nutritional intake in the U.S., NHANES I and NHANES II, found that >20% of the population was ingesting <70% of the RDA at the time for vitamin A (both preformed and precursor).[488] Dietary intake surveys of vitamin A have difficulty in estimating actual intakes, owing to the large day-to-day variability in retinol or carotenoid intakes and storage of retinol. However, other investigators have expressed vitamin A intake in retinol equivalents (RE) and have found average intakes to be about 1000 µg RE per d, and median intakes to be about 620 µg RE per d, which would mean that the majority of the U.S. population is adequately nourished in vitamin A.[477]

Dietary requirements for vitamin A have been very confusing. The Recommended Daily Allowances for vitamin A were originally expressed as International Units (IU), with an assumption of a 1:1 ratio of intake for preformed vitamin A (retinols) and precursor vitamin A (carotenoids).[478] However, refinements in techniques have resulted in changes in estimation of relative contributions from retinoids and carotenoids, and the units for vitamin A requirements have changed. Currently, Table 4 lists the preferred units and amounts for vitamin A intake and conversion factors for interpreting older data expressed in IU.

**TABLE 4   Dietary Requirements of
Vitamin A in Current Units**

Definitions

1 retinol equivalent (RE) = 1 µg all-*trans*-retinol
6 µg β-carotene = 1 RE
12 µg mixed provitamin A carotenoids = 1 RE
1.8 µg retinyl palmitate = 1 RE
1.2 µg retinyl acetate = 1 RE

Group	Age (years)	RE/d
Infants	0–1	375
Children	1–10	400–700
Adult males	>10	1000
Adult females	>10	800
Pregnancy		800
Lactation		1200

Note: Based on 1989 National Research
Council recommendations.[477]

Those at greatest risk for retinol deficiency include those with severe injuries (trauma, burns, fractures), chronic low food intake (anorexics, dieters, elderly), deficiencies of zinc or vitamin E, protein-calorie malnutrition, liver damage, long-term TPN, and chronic fat malabsorption syndromes (cholestasis, cystic fibrosis, sprue, chronic diarrhea, pancreatic insufficiency, biliary cirrhosis), as well as Third World preschool children and alcoholics.[479]

E. DIETARY SOURCES AND INFLUENCES

Preformed vitamin A (retinol) is found only in foods of animal origin.[477-481] Richest food sources include fish liver oils, shark liver oils, liver, vitamin A-fortified milk and dairy products (butter, cream, cheese, etc.), fish (especially sardines, herring, tuna), nonfortified dairy products, egg yolks, and meats. Precursor vitamin A (β-carotene) sources include dietary supplements, carrots, squashes and pumpkins, dark green leafy vegetables, tomatoes, papayas, oranges, cantaloupes, peaches, apricots, corn, and *Dunaliella salina* algae.[477-481] Therefore, by consuming a diet rich in fresh vegetables and fruits, it is possible to consume sufficient β-carotene to prevent deficient vitamin A status, even on low fat diets. Addition of animal foodstuffs, especially fortified milk products, can easily prevent deficient status without leading to toxicity.

F. ANIMAL STUDIES

Much research has focused on the ability of retinol supplements to restore wound healing inhibited by corticosteroids and on the ability of retinol to accelerate normal wound healing. Oral, parenteral, and topical retinol has repeatedly restored healing of skin wounds and corneal wounds to normal or towards normal, as demonstrated in at least a dozen studies reviewed by Hunt.[487] Retinol prevented wound contracture, allowing skin healing to progress strictly by granulation tissue formation and reepithelialization.[487] This finding has the potential to make skin wounds more cosmetic.

Again, many animal studies have found that supplemental retinol (local or systemic) accelerated wound healing (reviewed by Hunt[487]). A typical example was enhancement of wound strength (129%) 14 d postsurgery by combined oral and topical administration (1 mg/d p.o. and 2 mg/d topical) of vitamin A to rats with adequate vitamin A status. Another typical example is data from Hunt and others, who administered 2000 IU retinol intramuscularly on days 7, 9, and 11 to wounded rabbits.[486] Time to wound closure was measured and was 14 d for vitamin A-treated animals, 16 d for control animals, 19 d for vitamin A + cortisone treated animals, and >30 d for cortisone treated animals.[486] The difference between 14 and 16 d for wound closure was not statistically significant, but other studies found significant differences of similar magnitudes.[487] Gerber and Erdmann found that a diet containing 5 times the dietary allowance for rats led to a small but significant increase in wound strength (135%) at 5 d postsurgery.[489] Thus, high-dose vitamin therapy for short time periods during wound healing may have the ability to hasten healing in a positive manner. Likewise, retinol was shown to enhance healing retarded by stress, aspirin, radiation, or diabetes, including healing of femoral fractures and stress ulcers.[487] Vitamin A administration also reversed thymic atrophy and adrenal hypertrophy after injury.[487]

The effects of β-carotene on healing of rat surgical wounds were studied by Gerber.[489] Diets containing 1.2 RE of β-carotene resulted in an increase of 191% in wound strength at 5 d postsurgery, compared to 100% RDA levels for rats (1.2 RE of retinyl acetate). Addition of 4.8 RE of β-carotene to the 100% RDA diet for vitamin A (1.2 RE retinyl acetate) led to a 171% increase in wound strength at 5 d postsurgery. Thus, β-carotene seems to have effects on wound healing that substitute for retinol and appear to be additive to retinol. Perhaps the antioxidant functions of β-carotene play a role in preventing deleterious effects of wound ischemia. The issue of apparent β-carotene enhancement of surgical wound healing (skin healing) is worthy of further research attention.

G. HUMAN STUDIES

Major trauma or burns was associated with large decreases of serum retinol levels to deficient ranges after 1 to 2 d postinjury.[490-492] Incidence of gastric stress ulcers was associated with lowest serum vitamin A levels. As described previously, severe inflammation with corticosteroid release disturbs RBP synthesis, leading to decreased transport of retinol in plasma, and decreased plasma retinol levels with adequate liver stores. Massive parenteral doses of vitamin A (100,000 to 200,000 IU daily) were needed to bring plasma retinol levels into normal ranges.[490,491] Prophylactic administration of high dose vitamin A decreased incidence of stress ulcers in two studies of severe trauma and burn patients by Chernov.[490,491] Combined results from both studies found that 34/52 (65%) control patients developed stress ulcers, while 6/35 (17%) patients treated with retinol developed stress ulcers. Historical controls showed a 62% incidence of stress ulcers. However, soon after these findings were published, it became apparent that nutritional repletion with protein, zinc, and other nutrients (TPN) resulted in a smaller decrease in plasma retinol levels and prevented stress ulcers. Thus, administration of large doses of retinol were not necessary to correct a functional vitamin A deficiency in plasma.

Reductions in gastric ulcer size were found in gastric patients given 150,000 IU vitamin A daily for 4 weeks.[493] Complete healing was significantly greater with vitamin A administration (39 vs. 19%). Thus, retinol may have the ability to enhance current treatments of gastric ulcers, which involves mucosal healing.

A report by Honkanen provided evidence that plasma levels of retinol were decreased in rheumatoid arthritis patients, compared to healthy controls.[494] The decreased levels may have more relevance to corticosteroid and other drug therapy for this subset of patients than a specific disease process.

Cohen and co-workers, from the University of Oxford, administered 300,000 to 450,000 IU of retinyl acetate daily per os for 7 d to an unspecified number of patients scheduled for extensive operations.[495] Measurements of immune function showed that oral vitamin A restored or stimulated lymphocyte and monocyte counts and responses that were depressed by surgery. No toxicity was observed. Thus, short-term, high-dose retinol therapy postsurgery was associated with improvements in immune function. Although this study has not been replicated, the well-known immunostimulatory effects of vitamin A (retinol)[477-481] may provide the ability to reduce incidence of infections and complications in surgical settings. This concept remains to be tested directly.

Hunt and colleagues presented two case reports where vitamin A therapy healed skin ulcers that were otherwise nonresponsive.[486] An 18-year-old girl with lupus erythematosus on prednisone and Imuran therapy bumped her leg and developed a large bruise that progressed to an ulcer (3×5 cm) 18 d postinjury. Topical application of 7500 IU vitamin A ester in anhydrous ointment base 3 times daily was associated with complete healing 28 d after vitamin A application. The other case report was a 5-year-old girl taking prednisone after renal nephrectomy and transplant for Wilm's tumor who developed a nonhealing foot ulcer after extravasation of actinomycin D. The ulcer did not show any signs of healing for 45 d, when healing suddenly began simultaneously with oral ingestion of a multiple vitamin product containing 5000 IU vitamin A (retinol). When the vitamins were stopped, healing stopped. Topical vitamin A application led to rapid and complete healing in 10 d. Both of these cases mirrored animal study results of reversal of impaired wound healing during corticosteroid therapy. As of this date, no controlled trials of oral supplemental vitamin A on wound or ulcer healing have been presented. No direct studies on effects of β-carotene as a single agent on human healing are apparent.

H. SAFETY

Preformed vitamin A (retinol) is the most toxic vitamin. Over 600 cases of hypervitaminosis A toxicity have been reported.[477] Much attention has been focused on the safety and toxicity of retinol (retinyl ester) administration, and ranges of toxic daily doses have been found.[477,488] Table 5 lists some toxicity symptoms of hypervitaminosis A. Toxicity is dose dependent, with longer intakes of higher doses leading to more severe toxicity. Acute doses of vitamin A that cause toxicity in adults range from 1,000,000 to 30,000,000 IU. Acute toxic doses of vitamin A in children are 200,000 to 600,000 IU. Chronic toxicity has been seen at doses as low as 50,000 IU daily when taken for many years (over 20). Chronic toxicity has been seen with doses between 50,000 and 1,000,000 IU daily in adults. Adolescents showed toxicity at chronic intakes of 50,000 to 300,000 IU daily (associated with acne treatments). Vitamin A is known to be a teratogen and cause birth defects in animals (after ingestion of very large

**TABLE 5   Toxicity Symptoms of Acute or
Chronic Vitamin A Overdose**

Alopecia
Anemia
Anorexia
Bone and joint pain
Brittle nails
Cheilitis
Conjunctivitis
Dermatitis
Diarrhea
Edema and papilledema
Fatigue
Fever
Fontanelle bulging
Headache
Hepatomegaly
Insomnia
Irritability
Mucosal membrane dryness
Muscular pain
Nausea
Premature epiphyseal closure
Skin rash, scaliness, desquamation
Vomiting
Weight loss

Note: These symptoms describe toxicity from preformed
vitamin A (retinol and retinol esters) only and are
not associated with even massive doses of
β-carotene.

doses — 100,000 IU/kg body weight). Case reports have yielded a range of 25,000 to 500,000 IU daily as being associated with birth defects in humans. If a woman of child-bearing age wants to consume greater than 25,000 IU daily of preformed vitamin A, a pregnancy test is justified. Thus, a bottom line on vitamin A (retinol) toxicity is that for absolute safety do not exceed administration of 25,000 IU (7500 μg retinol, 9000 μg retinyl acetate, or 13500 μg retinyl palmitate) daily of preformed vitamin A. Pregnant or lactating women should not exceed 10,000 IU daily of supplemental preformed vitamin A. Supplemental doses of 25,000 IU daily or less appear to be safe for long-term ingestion in adults.

On the other hand, β-carotene appears to be almost completely safe at any dosage (aside from oily diarrhea at ridiculously high and impractical doses).[477-481,488,496] Thus, there is no practical concern over β-carotene toxicity. Ingestion of over 25,000 IU β-carotene will lead to yellow or orange coloration of subcutaneous fat (carotenemia) that may resemble jaundice, except that sclera of eyes are not colored. The coloration is harmless, does not exhibit any toxicity, and may have protective roles against ultraviolet radiation. The addition of β-carotene to high doses of retinol vitamin A does not cause additive or synergistic toxicity since conversion of β-carotene to vitamin A is carefully controlled. Thus, high doses of β-carotene will not affect vitamin A status adversely.

I.   SUMMARY AND GUIDELINES FOR USE

The term vitamin A now needs to be split into two types of compounds: retinoids and carotenoids. Carotenoids can be converted to retinoids when intake of retinoids is low. Otherwise, carotenoids possess unique antioxidant capabilities not seen for retinoids. Thus, β-carotene and other carotenoids can be considered to have different effects and actions in the body from retinoids. Carotenoids are part of body antioxidant defense systems. Retinoids have many complex roles in cell differentiation and regulation. Derivatives of retinol, such as retinoic acid and isotretinoin, are becoming used more frequently for medical uses, but since they are not true nutrients, they have not been considered in this book. Although vitamin A was the first vitamin named, it has eluded complete elucidation of its roles and functions, especially for connective tissues. Some animal evidence suggests that retinol may enhance healing of skin wounds when adequate status is present. This interesting concept has not been examined in humans, perhaps because of the legal and ethical fears associated with toxicity of high doses of vitamin A.

Retinol appears to be useful to reverse corticosteroid-induced delays in healing of skin wounds or ulcers, but numbers of subjects studied are exceedingly small. Topical application appears to be quite safe and may accelerate healing when healing is impaired by corticosteroids. Thus, one application of vitamin A (retinol) to connective tissue healing would be administration of 25,000 IU daily in cases of delayed healing of surgical wounds, skin ulcers, or other skin damage.

The immunostimulatory effects of vitamin A and β-carotene are beyond the scope of this book, but another potential application would be in injured subjects who display increased incidence of infections. Again, 25,000 IU per day appears safe and a large enough dose to exert effects. The effects of vitamin A on cartilage and bone are still obscure, and it is not known if moderate doses (25,000 IU/d) would have any effect on those tissues. It is known that vitamin A deficiency and hypervitaminosis A are deleterious to bones and joints, and both conditions must be avoided to maintain health of connective tissues.

II. VITAMIN D (CALCIFEROLS)

Vitamin D is actually a series of lipid-soluble steroid-like hormones with far-ranging regulatory effects, rather than a true vitamin in the coenzymatic sense of the word. The vitamin D family was similar to compounds that possessed antirachitic activity. Since rickets could be caused by removal of certain dietary component in young animals, the antirachitic factors were named vitamin D by McCollum (the discoverer of vitamin A) in 1922.[497] Since the biochemistry of vitamin D has progressed significantly in recent years, including clinical usage of penultimate active agents, the use of vitamin D as a nutrient has been slowly replaced by vitamin D as a prescription item. Therefore, only the basic nutritional facts on vitamin D will be covered in this section.

In the past, the chemistry of vitamin D metabolism has been complicated by technical difficulties in measuring the extremely small amounts of activated metabolites and inactivated metabolites of calciferol. Further compounding calciferol confusion is the multiplicity of analogs with vitamin D activity. Furthermore, synthesis of vitamin D by the human body is a normal event, which is another reason that vitamin D does not fit the definition of a vitamin. However, the entrenchment over many years of food, clinical, and legal uses for calciferols has become too commonplace to change.

A. ROLES AND FUNCTIONS[497-503]

Vitamin D metabolism starts with cholesterol and sunlight. Ultraviolet radiation from the sun penetrates the skin sufficiently to produce cholecalciferol (vitamin D_3) from 7-dehydrocholesterol in the integument. Ergocalciferol (vitamin D_2) is produced commercially from irradiated ergosterol and is commonly added to foods, especially dairy products. Cholecalciferol is hydroxylated in the liver to 25-hydroxycholecalciferol (calcidiol or 25OHD). 25OHD is then hydroxylated in the kidney to form the penultimate active form of vitamin D, 1,25-dihydroxycholecalciferol (calcitriol or 1,25OHD). 24,25-Dihydroxycholecalciferol (24,25OHD) is also produced in the kidney and has some activity. Normal blood levels of 1,25OHD are approximately 20 to 76 pg/ml, depending upon specific methodology. 1,25OHD synthesis is controlled by activity of renal hydroxylases, which are influenced by factors that affect bone, phosphorus, and calcium metabolism (PTH, hypophosphatemia, acidosis, calcitonin, and hyperphosphatemia). 1,25OHD functions as a steroid hormone and has receptor sites on target tissue cell membranes, cellular binding proteins, translocation to the nucleus, and activation of specific genes. The major target organs are the intestine and bone. Intestinal cells respond to 1,25OHD by increasing mRNA for calcium-binding proteins, which facilitate active transport of calcium from the gut lumen through enterocytes and into plasma. In bone, 1,25OHD is an obligatory cofactor with PTH for bone resorption (transport of calcium from mineralized osteoid through osteocytes into plasma). The resultant increase in serum calcium levels caused by vitamin D facilitates mineralization of bone osteoid, which prevents rickets and osteomalacia (adult rickets). Almost every tissue studied possesses receptors for 1,25OHD. Recently, other tissues have proven to be targets for 1,25OHD, such as immune system cells. However, these findings are only now finding potential clinical application.

B. DEFICIENCY SYMPTOMS[497-503]

Vitamin D deficiency results in impaired intestinal absorption of calcium and impaired renal reabsorption of calcium and phosphate. Serum calcium (5 to 7 mg/dl) and phosphate levels are decreased, and serum alkaline phosphatase activity is increased. Hyperparathyroidism in response to lowered serum calcium levels ensues, and PTH and remaining 1,25OHD produce bone demineralization. Rickets occurs in growing humans (children and infants) and osteomalacia in adults. Osteomalacia is characterized by loss of bone mineral, with preservation of osteoid (unlike osteoporosis, which has decreased bone mineral and osteoid). Clinical symptoms include bone pain, muscle weakness, and bone tenderness. Usually, in adults, muscle pain (myopathy) is the foremost or only sign of vitamin D deficiency. Serum levels of CPK or aldolase are normal in vitamin D deficiency with muscle pain. Left untreated, rickets can lead to bone disfigurement, with characteristic bowing of legs and arms. Knock-knees, spinal curvature, and joint enlargement occur. Extreme symptoms of convulsions and tetany may occur.

Vitamin D deficiencies have been associated with changes in collagen cross-linking, proteoglycan abnormalities, increased collagen catabolism, and increased collagenase activity.[93,94] These changes are deleterious to health of all connective tissues, although research interest has focused mostly on bone. Thus, it may be surmised that vitamin D deficiency is harmful to other musculoskeletal tissues.

C. INTAKES AND DIETARY SOURCES[497-503]

Intakes of vitamin D are not absolutely essential if adequate skin exposure to sunlight is available. However, more than 2 h of exposure of the face to the sun in wintertime in northern latitudes is needed to meet body requirements. Thus, people in urban areas or living indoors have difficulty in deriving sufficient vitamin D synthesis from sunlight, and a dietary source is required.

Vitamin D (cholecalciferol) is present only in animal foods and fortified foods. Small and variable amounts of vitamin D are found in food supplies. Fish liver oil and saltwater fish (herring, sardines, salmon) are the richest nonfortified food sources. Other meats, animal livers, dairy products, and egg yolks have small amounts of vitamin D which are significant if eaten in any quantity. Fortified foods (milk, evaporated milk, butter, margarine, cereals, chocolate mixes) contain substantial amounts of vitamin D_2 or D_3. If these foods are part of daily diets, then an individual is probably at little risk for deficient vitamin D intake. However, individuals living in northern latitudes and not receiving sunlight and eating restricted diets may require supplemental vitamin D.

Those at risk for vitamin D deficiency include the elderly and those with chronic fat malabsorption syndromes (sprue, regional enteritis, jejunal diverticulosis, gastric resections, bypass surgery), liver disorders (alcoholism, cirrhosis, primary biliary cirrhosis, obstructive jaundice), renal diseases (renal failure), hypoparathyroidism, genetic variants of hypophosphatemic rickets (vitamin D resistant), anticonvulsant medications (phenobarbital, diphenylhydantoin), and reduced exposure to sunlight at northern latitudes.

The requirement for vitamin D in adults is not precisely known, but the RDA for vitamin D is 400 IU (1 IU = 0.025 µg cholecalciferol). This may represent an upper limit of requirements for both children and adults.

D. ANIMAL AND HUMAN STUDIES

Vitamin D therapy is in use for osteomalacia and rickets. Large doses of 10,000 to 300,000 IU daily of cholecalciferol have been used.[497] However, increasing use is being made of 1,25OHD at small oral doses with equivalent results. Prevention of steroid-induced osteopenia may be prevented by large doses of vitamin D_2, but results have not been replicated.[502] A link between vitamin D metabolism and osteoporosis is still being explored. This has ramifications for amenorrheic female athletes with bone loss. At this time, it is unknown if vitamin D supplements would aid in repletion of bone mass in amenorrheic athletes. Likewise, the effects of vitamin D supplements on fracture healing in humans are not fully known. Topical application of 5 ng per wound per day of 1,25OHD to skin punch biopsies in rats led to significant acceleration of wound closure, accomplished in the first 2 d postwounding.[504]

The role of vitamin D and its metabolites as therapy for postmenopausal osteoporosis is outside the scope of this book. Recent research is reviewed by Norman et al.[503] Usually, vitamin D therapy is administered along with calcium supplementation, which further clouds the specific effects of vitamin D alone. It may become apparent that vitamin D alone will not result in full clinical responses without additional calcium intakes. The field of vitamin D research is quite large, but almost none has been focused on sports medicine or injury rehabilitation, including fractures.

E. SAFETY

Vitamin D is the second-most toxic vitamin, behind retinoids. Excess intakes of cholecalciferol (over 250 µg or 10,000 IU daily) cause hypercalcemia.[500] However, toxicity symptoms are not seen until consumption of over 50,000 IU/d for long time periods (several months).[499] Clinical symptoms of weakness, nausea, anorexia, headaches, abdominal pains, cramps, and diarrhea are associated with vitamin D toxicity.[500] Osteopenia and soft tissue calcifications (including arteries) become apparent.[499] Excess vitamin D metabolites decrease collagen synthesis and cross-linking.[93,94] Thus, excess vitamin D may lead to increased susceptibility of musculoskeletal injuries for athletes. For these reasons, and the greatly increased potency of 1,25OHD, vitamin D metabolites are prescription items. Thus, excess vitamin D intake is harmful when continued.

F. SUMMARY AND GUIDELINES FOR USE

At this time, there are no specific guidelines for use of vitamin D (cholecalciferol) in sports medicine as applied to injury rehabilitation and healing. Since massive doses of cholecalciferol are needed to raise 1,25OHD levels or activity only slightly, the threshold between toxicity and therapeutic benefits is slim for nutrient forms of vitamin D. The introduction of 1,25OHD instead of cholecalciferol for treatment of osteomalacia and other vitamin D-dependent conditions has largely replaced the need for cholecalciferol use. Therefore, guidelines are to ensure adequate vitamin D status by providing exposure to sunlight (or ultraviolet radiation) in normal amounts and monitoring diet for adequate intake of cholecalciferol (100 to 400 IU/d).

III. VITAMIN E (TOCOPHEROLS)

Several specific reviews present background information on vitamin E.[505-512] Vitamin E is another series of compounds of similar structure and properties. Vitamin E is the term used to describe the group of tocopherols and tocotrienols that were found to be essential for reproduction in the rat by Evans and Bishop in the early 1920s.[506] The name tocopherol was derived from the Greek words *tokos,* for childbirth, and *pherein*, to bring forth. Thus, the term vitamin E is a generic term describing compounds with vitamin activity needed for reproduction in lab animals. It turned out that animals exhibited a wide variety of specific disorders from vitamin E deficiency, whereas identification of vitamin E deficiency in humans was not accomplished until recently. However, the mechanism of action for vitamin E differs from every other vitamin, as it is so nonspecific that it is no wonder that a specific condition has been difficult to identify. In fact, vitamin E affects almost every aspect of health to some degree, especially chronic degenerative conditions. Thus, while vitamin E may not be essential for development of a specific deficiency disease, it is essential for life.

A. ROLES AND FUNCTIONS

The role and function of vitamin E is simple: scavenge free radicals in all tissues.[505-512] Vitamin E effectively scavenges several types of free radicals and other reactive species in lipid bilayer membranes and other lipid concentrations.[512] Extensive evidence that vitamin E functions as a free radical scavenger is based on ability to inhibit lipid peroxidation in many experimental systems; replacement of most vitamin E biological activity by synthetic antioxidants with known scavenging activities; protective effects against conditions known to induce free radicals and lipid peroxidation; presence of vitamin E metabolites *in vivo* that are only formed by reactions with free radicals; and increased free radical and lipid peroxidation levels in animals deficient in vitamin E.[512]

A very short review of free radical formation and metabolism is necessary to understand the terminology of studies concerned with vitamin E and other antioxidants to be covered in this book. Many excellent reviews exist, and the reader is referred to a few for further reading.[305-307,509,512] Briefly, free radicals are molecules or atoms with an unpaired electron that exhibit high reactivity. Free radicals can easily attack and physically denature all types of biological macromolecules, especially polyunsaturated lipids. Free radicals are deleterious to biological systems mainly because free radicals initiate chain reactions, where one free radical forms another, and another, and so on, leaving a wake of damaged molecules (after rearrangement or further reactions of the free radicals). Transition metals iron and copper, when present in certain unbound ionic forms, are able to catalyze formation of even more potent reactive species termed hydroxyl radicals. Molecular oxygen (which is omnipresent in biological tissues) usually ends up attaching to the free radicals formed, forming peroxyl radicals, and eventually, peroxides (by removing the hydrogen atom from another atom or molecule, resulting in a new free radical). Often, fatty acid chains are cleaved by free radical reactions (which can become quite complex) into malondialdehyde (MDA), ethane, or pentane, which have become convenient markers for free radical damage and lipid peroxidation. Antioxidants are molecules described as chain-breakers; that is, they are modified by a free radical into a stable radical or compound that does not attack other molecules. The antioxidant is then safely disposed or regenerated by various mechanisms. In this way, a low level of antioxidants is able to prevent large amounts of biological damage by limiting free radical-mediated damage.

Vitamin E has a molecular structure that allows formation of a stable vitamin E radical (chromanoxyl radical), which is then metabolized into safer products that can be safely disposed.[512] Ascorbate, glutathione, dihydrolipoate, coenzyme Q_{10}, and superoxide anion can all "recharge" oxidized vitamin E back to its original reduced form.[512] Enzymatic systems involving NADH, NADPH, and succinate electron transport enzymes can also recharge vitamin E.[512] This explains the interactions of other antioxidants with each other as a networked system of free radical scavenging and antioxidant recycling, which has only recently begun to be understood.

The scavenging ability of vitamin E stabilizes membranes. However, vitamin E prevents membrane damage from phospholipase activity by formation of complexes with phospholipids and phospholipid hydrolysis products.[506,512] Thus, by several mechanisms, vitamin E is vital for membrane integrity, fluidity, and functions. The functions of vitamin E are numerous and vital for proper function of all cells and tissues.

B. DEFICIENCY SYMPTOMS

Frank deficiency of vitamin E is rare in humans.[505-512] Severe deficiencies are found in preterm infants, fat malabsorption syndromes, abetalipoproteinemia, protein-calorie malnutrition, cirrhosis, and biliary atresia.[505-512] Retinopathy, neuropathy, hemolytic anemia, muscular dystrophy, accumulation of ceroid pigments (lipofuscin), thrombocytosis, and other neuromuscular defects have been identified as

TABLE 6 Methods of Vitamin E Assessment

Test	Deficient Status	Adequate Status
Plasma (serum) vitamin E		
(µmol/l)	<12	12–37
(mg/dl)	<0.7	>0.7
Plasma (serum) vitamin E per total plasma lipid		
(µmol vitamin E per g total plasma lipid)	<1.86	>1.86
(mg vitamin E per g total lipid)	<0.8	>0.8
Plasma vitamin E per total cholesterol		
(mmol vitamin E per mol cholesterol)	<2.2	>2.2
(mg vitamin E per g cholesterol)	<2.5	>2.5
Erythrocyte H_2O_2 hemolysis (%)	>10	<10
Erythrocyte malondialdehyde release (%)	>6.0	<6.0
Breath pentane and/or ethane		

frank vitamin E-deficiency symptoms in humans.[505-511] However, functional or relative vitamin E deficiencies are believed to play a role in incidence and onset of a wide variety of conditions related to free radicals.[505-512] Cardiovascular diseases, cancer, arthritis, immune function, senile dementia, Alzheimer's disease, and a long list of other conditions may be influenced by antioxidant status in general. Since vitamin E is a major antioxidant, its functionality will affect ability to handle free radicals and associated adverse health effects. Again, this topic has been covered by many texts.[305-307]

Specific findings pertaining to connective tissues in vitamin E deficiency of animals have found increased soluble collagen in skin, decreased aldehyde content of collagen, and increased susceptibility of collagen to proteases, all signs of defective collagen production.[93,94] Deficiency effects specific to connective tissues in humans are not clear at this time.

C. ASSESSMENT

At present, determination of plasma levels of vitamin E (tocopherol) is the most widely used indicator of vitamin E status.[505-511] Table 6 lists some tests for vitamin E status and their values. Serum or plasma tocopherol is frequently expressed in terms of blood lipid or cholesterol content, since vitamin E is intimately associated with lipids, and tocopherol levels are directly linked to lipoprotein levels. Newer tests that reveal more information on the functional status of vitamin E are measurements of breath pentane or ethane, adipose vitamin E levels (for long-term status), platelet tocopherol levels, and erythrocyte tocopherol levels.[506,509]

D. INTAKES

Determination of vitamin E intakes in humans is hampered by lack of accurate data in listings of food contents of vitamin E. The variable nature of storage and food processing means that tabulated values are frequently incorrect. However, intakes of vitamin E for the general population seems to be around 7 to 10 mg α-tocopherol equivalents.[505-507,512] These values are close to estimated requirements of 8 mg for females and 10 mg for males.[505-507] However, even in adults ingesting 3 to 5 mg α-tocopherol equivalents daily, biochemical evidence of frank deficiency is not normally seen. This does not mean that tocopherol requirements for prevention of chronic degenerative diseases are equal to the RDA of 8 to 10 mg. A small percentage of individuals in developed countries (about 5%) exhibit low levels of plasma vitamin E. Thus, intakes appear to be adequate for the vast majority of persons to prevent frank deficiencies of vitamin E, but there is still concern that current intakes are inadequate to prevent degenerative diseases.

The vitamin E requirements for humans are expressed as tocopherol equivalents (TE). Table 7 lists the various forms of vitamin E vitamers with their relative biological activity (TE). 1 TE = 1 mg RRR-α-d-tocopherol. Whenever possible, units of vitamin E amounts should be expressed as mg or TE (or µmol for specific vitamers), rather than IU. There has been a good deal of confusion and ambiguity in

TABLE 7   Relative Potencies and Biological Activities of Vitamin E Vitamers

Vitamer	IU/mg	Tocopherol Equivalents
RRR-*d*-α-tocopherol	1.49	1.00
RRR-*d*-β-tocopherol	0.75	0.49
RRR-*d*-γ-tocopherol	0.15	0.10
RRR-*d*-δ-tocopherol	0.05	0.03
RRR-*d*-α-tocopheryl acetate	1.36	1.03
RRR-*d*-α-tocopheryl succinate	1.21	1.03
all-RAC-*dl*-α-tocopheryl acetate	1.00	0.76
L-α-tocopherol (seven vitamers)	0.31–1.34	0.21–0.90
d-tocotrienol (four vitamers — α, β, γ, δ)	0.00–0.45	0.00–0.29

Note: 1 mg RR-*d*-α-tocopherol = 1 tocopherol equivalent (TE). Preferred expression of vitamin E is mg or TE instead of traditional IU. RAC = racemic; IU = International Unit.

the literature concerning what type of vitamin E was used in studies. The differences between vitamers is not trivial and may have affected numerous conclusions of numerous studies.

E.   DIETARY SOURCES AND INFLUENCES

Vitamin E activity is found in a series of closely related vitamers and also from synthetic tocopherol.[505-512] The reference vitamer, RRR-*d*-α-tocopherol, is the predominant form in human tissues and the diet. RRR-*d*-α-tocopherol has been assigned a biological activity of 1.0 and has 1.49 IU/mg activity. The original definition of IU for vitamin E was based on a single synthetic preparation (all-RAC-*dl*-α-tocopherol acetate) with an unknown composition of stereoisomers that is no longer available.[508] However, the relative ratios of biological activity for vitamin E vitamers are still applicable. Table 7 lists the vitamers of vitamin E and their relative potencies. Naturally occurring vitamers are all *d* forms, and when synthesized, *dl*-α-tocopherol consists of a mixture of seven possible L stereoisomers with *d*-α-tocopherol. As can be seen from the relative potencies listed in Table 7, all vitamin E sources are not equal. Natural form vitamin E (RRR-*d*-α-tocopherol) has exhibited better absorption, tissue retention, and biological activities than its synthetic and less expensive counterpart.[505-512] Thus, the synthetic all-racemic- (all-RAC)-*dl*-α-tocopherol, which has been used more frequently in studies on vitamin E both *in vitro* and *in vivo*, is not equivalent to *d*-α-tocopherols.

Major dietary sources for vitamin E are wheat germ oil, rice bran oil, wheat germ, vegetable oils, nuts, seeds, cereals, and green leafy vegetables.[505,509] The two oils most consumed in the U.S., soybean and corn oils, have very little *d*-α-tocopherol content, but rather have mostly *d*-δ-tocopherol content. With increasing usage of vitamin E as a food preservative and additive, vitamin E contents of prepared foods can vary widely. Some foods show seasonal variation of vitamin E contents. Many processes can destroy vitamin E in foods. The list includes exposure to air (oxidation), drying in presence of air and sunlight, addition of organic acids, milling, refining of grains and oils, irradiation, canning, and exposure to peroxidized (rancid) lipids.[509] Natural sources of tocopherols are always unesterified, while natural sources of tocotrienols are sometimes esterified. Since plants, but not animals, synthesize vitamin E, animal foodstuffs have very low levels of vitamin E.

Other nutrients that influence vitamin E status are PUFAs, which increase the physiological demand for vitamin E and reduce its intestinal uptake,[506] and medium-chain triglycerides, which improve the uptake of vitamin E.[509] Other antioxidants, especially selenium, cysteine, glutathione, and methionine, have sparing effects on vitamin E requirements to a degree.[506,508] Zinc deficiency can decrease vitamin E levels. Simultaneous presence of ferric ions (Fe^{+3}) with vitamin E will oxidize vitamin E, making it unavailable for absorption. Ferrous ions (Fe^{+2}, the form found in supplements) do not damage vitamin E.

Absorption of vitamin E is low and variable, with 30 to 50% uptake usually encountered.[506] At dietary intake levels (around 10 mg/d), esterified forms of vitamin E are hydrolyzed and absorbed completely, but at higher doses (>400 mg/d), the unesterified forms are absorbed better than esterified forms.[506] Detergents (bile salts, monoglycerides, surfactants) can improve uptake of vitamin E by facilitation of micellar formation. Vitamin E is absorbed as unesterified tocopherol forms and transported via the lymphatic chylomicrons to the bloodstream. Tissue uptake is from lipoprotein particles. Attention has been given to the absorption and dietary influences of vitamin E, since it is now clear that the "natural" form, RRR-*d*-α-tocopherol, possesses several advantages over other forms of vitamin E products available in the marketplace.

F. ANIMAL STUDIES

Antiinflammatory effects of vitamin E in animal models have been reported.[513-516] Free radicals are known to play a role in the inflammatory response, which argues that as an antioxidant, vitamin E should have some effect. Both macrophages and neutrophils produce oxyradicals during inflammation, and production of eicosanoids also generates oxyradicals. Feeding 1000 ppm of *dl*-α-tocopheryl acetate in the diet to rats was associated with decreased production of platelet thromboxane B_2 and platelet malondialdehyde (MDA).[515] Prostacyclin production was increased, suggesting that vitamin E may modulate inflammation via eicosanoid synthesis. Protection of lysosome membranes by vitamin E led to decreased release of histamine and serotonin from mast cells during inflammatory events.[514] If sufficient vitamin E is existent before inflammation starts, then inflammation can be shortened and prevented from expanding. However, adding vitamin E after inflammation has started did not affect the progress of inflammation. Similarly, large oral doses of vitamin E to rats did not affect paw edema or peritonitis models of inflammation.[517]

A close model of rheumatoid arthritis in humans is adjuvant arthritis induced in rats. Oral administration of large doses of vitamin E to rats did not exhibit effects on adjuvant arthritis in one study.[517] Another report did find antiinflammatory effects of synthetic vitamin E at doses of 250 mg/kg in rat models of adjuvant arthritis.[518] Having 7 d of pretreatment with daily oral doses of 147 mg/kg *dl*-α-tocopheryl acetate before induction of adjuvant arthritis in rats increased the depressed serum sulfhydryl levels, increased serum levels of α_2-macroglobulin, and increased the lowered albumin/globulin ratios caused by inflammation.[519] Changes in blood glutathione levels, erythrocyte superoxide dismutase activity, and serum ceruloplasmin levels were unchanged. Administration of vitamin E 21 d after adjuvant arthritis induction did not lead to significant differences, unlike pretreatment. Two other studies found protective benefits from vitamin E administration on rat adjuvant arthritis.[520,521] In cartilage cultures of guinea pigs made osteoarthritic, vitamin E at 200 μg/ml significantly reduced degradative enzyme activities and improved proteoglycan deposition.[522] Thus, vitamin E in large doses tended to have mild protective actions against the inflammation of adjuvant arthritis in rats, a close model of rheumatoid arthritis in humans.

In animal models of wound healing, vitamin E has exerted differing effects. In normal rats, high doses of vitamin E inhibited wound healing by decreasing collagen synthesis and wound breaking strength.[523] This study has been interpreted by other authors as offering evidence that vitamin E may inhibit excess scar or keloid formation after surgery. Subsequent studies of vitamin E administration and capsule contraction after subcutaneous implants in rats found either no effects on wound contraction[524] or very small effects on prevention of wound capsule contraction.[525] Vitamin E decreased adhesions after abdominal surgery in mice (58 vs. 97% of animals with adhesions) at oral intakes of 300 IU/kg diet.[526] Four oral daily doses of 1000 IU/kg vitamin E to rats before abdominal skin flap surgery found an increase in skin flap survival (area of live tissue) of 84% compared to 67% for controls.[527] Likewise, vitamin E led to partial return to normal healing of surgical wounds that were irradiated.[528] Animal models of trauma (spinal cord injury) also showed that prefeeding with vitamin E resulted in less cord damage and improved neurological function.[529,530] Dietary vitamin E levels were 25 times rat daily allowances.

In animal models of thermal burns, vitamin E levels were decreased and lipid peroxide levels were increased at the burn site and systemically in blood and tissues.[531-534] Administration of vitamin E by oral or injectable routes to rats and guinea pigs reduced the anemia, intravascular hemolysis, lipid peroxide levels, and restored intestinal weight and protein content in burned rats and guinea pigs.[533-535]

Most results on vitamin E and healing in animals are very recent and represent initial attempts at determining the ability of vitamin E as an antioxidant to affect the outcome of healing. Almost every study showed significant benefits in outcome after vitamin E supplementation at doses that are practical in humans, suggesting that vitamin E may possess some protective benefits for inflammatory conditions.

G. HUMAN STUDIES
1. Antiinflammatory Effects

Oral administration of vitamin E to humans decreased inflammatory reactions to irritants injected under the skin.[514] Administration of 1600 IU vitamin E to 6 subjects for 7 d led to decreased platelet thromboxane production and decreased arachidonate-induced platelet aggregation, while maintaining prostacyclin synthesis.[536] Administration of 1600 IU of vitamin E for 2 to 3 weeks to 4 subjects doubled serum levels of vitamin E and significantly reduced peroxide production by neutrophils, reduced bacterial killing by neutrophils, increased phagocytosis of neutrophils, and enhanced membrane release of arachidonate.[537] The changes were minimal, and not expected to change susceptibility to infections. Nevertheless, the data indicate that oral vitamin E can modulate inflammatory responses of platelets and immune cells.

2. Wound Healing and Skin Repair

A preliminary report by Baker on the ability of vitamin E supplements to influence contracture around breast implants found that vitamin E was beneficial for preventing contracture.[538] However, the study was open with no control group and thus subject to investigator bias. Similar results were found by Lovas.[539] The administration of vitamin E, along with vitamins A and C, to 95/197 gastric cancer surgery patients found lowered serum lipid peroxide levels and a large reduction in complication rates (from 30.9 to 1.9%).[540] Thus, preliminary studies indicate that vitamin E may possess protective properties after major surgery (along with other antioxidants). The use of vitamin E to reduce visible scarring and improve surgical scar aesthetics needs further confirmation in more carefully controlled studies with objective measurements before conclusions can be drawn for expanded usage.

Ramasastry, from the Department of Plastic Surgery at the University of Pittsburgh, compared venous leg ulcer healing in 10 controls and in 10 subjects given 400 IU vitamin E daily for over 18 months.[541] All ulcers were long standing (over 5 years) and resistant to other therapies. Skin grafts were placed on each ulcer of each patient. MDA levels of skin grafts showed higher MDA levels than adjacent normal skin, indicating free radical damage was increased in venous leg ulcer skin grafts. In the control group, all grafts took at three weeks, but 10/10 (100%) had breakdown within 6 months. The vitamin E-treated group showed complete takes that were stable in 9/10 subjects after 18 months, a highly significant difference ($p < 0.001$) from the control group. These results mirrored the ability of vitamin E to enhance survival of skin graft flaps in rats.[527]

3. Arthritis

In rheumatoid arthritis patients, one report found a decreased serum level of vitamin E,[494] while two others did not.[542,543] However, all studies found increased levels (3×) of serum lipid peroxides in rheumatoid arthritis patients, as well as in other rheumatoid diseases.[494,542,543] A case study of a 70-year-old woman with polymyositis that was refractory to high doses of azathioprine, cyclophosphamide, and corticosteroids was presented.[544] After progression to helplessness, the immunosuppressive drugs were removed, and 800 IU vitamin E daily was given. After 10 d, 1600 IU/d was taken. After 3 weeks, noticeable improvements were seen in daily functions, and after 3 months, the patient was well enough to be discharged from the hospital and take care of herself. Continued intake of 1600 IU vitamin E daily maintained remission. Thus, there is precedent for vitamin E therapy against rheumatic diseases. However, due to lack of information, the possible effects of vitamin E on rheumatoid arthritis is unknown.

Subjects with osteoarthritis were shown to have increased levels of serum lipid peroxides in two studies.[543,545] In one study, after administration of 100 mg vitamin E daily, a decrease in lipid peroxide products was seen.[545] Again, a single case report by Kienholz noticed that supplementation with 68 mg *d*-α-tocopheryl succinate daily plus 1000 µg daily of selenium as sodium selenite for 9 months prevented knee pain after mountain climbing and hiking which had previously proven unbearable.[546] The knee was diagnosed as ligament irritation on lateral and front parts of the knee joint, and the subject was told there was no accepted therapy. Machtey and Ouaknine, from the Rheumatology Clinic at Hasharon Hospital in Petah-Tiqva, Israel, measured the effects of vitamin E administration (600 mg/d for 10 d) or placebo in 29 subjects with osteoarthritis in a single-blind, placebo-controlled, crossover study.[547] Subjects were allowed to take paracetamol and propoxyphene analgesic tablets (Algolysin) as needed for pain. During the placebo period, 1/29 (4%) of subjects noted marked relief of pain, while 15/29 subjects noted marked relief of pain during the vitamin E period, a highly significant difference ($p < 0.01$). The results are remarkable for the short duration of the study. Blankenhorn administered either placebo or 400 IU *d*-α-tocopheryl acetate daily for 6 weeks to 50 patients with osteoarthritis.[548] After 6 weeks, the vitamin E group showed significant differences compared to the placebo group for pain relief at rest, pain relief during movement, and pain induced by pressure. Analgesic usage was reduced in the vitamin E group. Improvement of mobility tended to improve in the vitamin E group. Thus, several studies in humans have seen significant benefits in pain relief and possibly in joint function, after short treatment times with vitamin E as an adjunct to analgesic therapies. The significance of the results and the lack of toxicity seen for vitamin E argue strongly for additional studies with larger numbers of osteoarthritic patients. The data at hand showed that elevated indicators of free radical damage were reduced at the same time analgesic use was reduced and pain relief was apparent in the majority of subjects. Why no additional studies have been conducted on the effects of a simple and inexpensive therapy with evidence of efficacy for osteoarthritis is a mystery. Free radicals are known to be an important part of the osteoarthritic condition, with deleterious effects on cartilage.[549]

4. Miscellaneous Uses of Vitamin E for Healing of Human Connective Tissues

Vitamin E supplementation has shown clinical benefits of varying magnitudes for the following conditions: capillary fragility,[550] periodontal disease,[551-555] leg muscle cramps, and restless legs syndromes.[556-558] Twelve human burn patients showed increased levels of serum and erythrocyte lipid peroxides and decreased levels of serum vitamin E.[559] Plasma lipid peroxide levels were inversely correlated with serum vitamin E levels, and magnitude of changes were greater with increasing severity of burns. A close correlation between injury and lipid peroxidation was found, providing a rationale for vitamin E therapy after burns in humans. These additional studies further reinforce the clinical impact of vitamin E on human conditions of musculoskeletal healing.

H. SAFETY

Oral administration of vitamin E (any form) in doses up to 1600 mg/d has been associated with almost no toxicity or side effects, aside from a very few hypersensitive individuals.[505-509,560] In large population studies of vitamin E supplementation (10,000 subjects consuming 200 to 3,000 mg/d), incidence of nonspecific side effects was 0.8%, a level expected in untreated populations.[561] Oral supplementation with doses of vitamin E ranging from 100 to 400 mg/d for extended time periods (years) appears to be very safe. Higher doses (>800 mg/d) may have a slight chance of side effects, but clinical efficacy and tissue levels are not much different (after long time periods) than with lower doses. Vitamin E does not interfere significantly with coagulation in terms of bleeding risk. However, high doses of vitamin E (>1600 mg/d) may exacerbate vitamin K deficiency by competitive inhibition of uptake in the intestine.[560] Early reports suggested that vitamin E may decrease insulin requirements; so, insulin-dependent diabetics should initiate doses of 100 mg/d of vitamin E and titrate upwards slowly if necessary. Since many vitamin E products are dissolved in oil, very high doses may increase oil intake sufficiently to develop gastrointestinal symptoms of excess fat intake (nausea, flatulence, diarrhea), but these effects were not attributable to vitamin E per se. One consistent finding in all studies of vitamin E in humans has been lack of side effects. Thus, oral doses of vitamin E from 100 to 400 mg/d are extremely safe, while higher doses (up to 3000 mg/d) have a very high order of safety.

I. SUMMARY

Vitamin E is a major antioxidant in humans. As such, vitamin E has the ability to decrease the effects of free radical damage on tissues, regardless of cause. Free radicals are involved in the progression of arthritis, inflammation, injuries, ischemia, autoimmune disorders, and healing processes. Free radical effects are almost always harmful to some degree. Therefore, the rationale for vitamin E supplementation is to depress the deleterious effects of free radical damage. This concept has been verified repeatedly in human studies on healing, in addition to a very large database on other human conditions (cardiovascular disease, cancer, premenstrual syndrome, pregnancy, autoimmune diseases) that has not been mentioned in this section.[439,505-511] Vitamin E supplementation is safe and appears to be compatible with other treatment modalities, including pharmaceutical interventions.

What are the clinical implications of vitamin E and healing? First and foremost is the suppression of excess inflammation during traumatic injuries or arthritis. Vitamin E effects on inflammation are mild and do not have the same clinical impact as aspirin or NSAIDs for relief of pain and other cardinal signs of inflammation. Rather, vitamin E functions as a protective nutrient to prevent free radical damage from delaying or preventing adequate healing. Vitamin E can be thought of as insuring the normal progression of healing, rather than stimulating a normal response. Since the presence of free radicals is pervasive and significant during almost any healing condition, the effects of vitamin E are usually noticeable, even if mild, for almost any condition where free radicals are present.

One important point about the use of vitamin E is garnered from a review of existing studies. Almost every study observed subjects who increased their daily intake of vitamin E from about 5 to 10 mg/d to 400 to 800 mg/d, an increase of 40 to 80 times normal amounts. Thus, effects were seen in "vitamin E-naive" subjects. Since many persons are currently taking vitamin E supplements of 100 to 400 mg/d, the results of studies in this section may not apply to this group. Instead, these persons may have to increase their vitamin E intake to 800 to 1600 mg/d for short time periods (4 to 12 weeks) to enhance vitamin E status.

Another aspect of vitamin E is its protective abilities, rather than its therapeutic nature. Enhanced vitamin E status was definitely more effective at preventing full effects of damage from injuries or free radicals, as opposed to initiating vitamin E intake after damage has already occurred. Thus, vitamin E prophylaxis in populations prone to injuries or arthritis may offer benefits over administration only during times of stress. The protective effects of vitamin E for prevention of chronic degenerative diseases certainly argue for increased intakes of vitamin E in all adult population groups.

The difference between commercially available vitamin E products needs to be addressed. Nature-identical forms of vitamin E (d-α-tocopherol, mixed tocopherols [β, γ, δ forms], tocotrienols, and d-α-tocopheryl acetate and d-α-tocopheryl succinate) have been documented to have increased absorption, uptake, tissue level maintenance, and biological effects compared to the synthetic all-RAC-dl-α-tocopherol or tocopheryl esters. Therefore, long-term supplementation of vitamin E should be with "natural" or nature-identical forms. Ideally, vitamin E in the form of mixed tocopherols (as vitamin E is found in foodstuffs) is a preferred form of vitamin E supplementation.

J. GUIDELINES FOR USE

Table 8 lists conditions of human healing for which enhancement of vitamin E status has proven beneficial in clinical settings. The primary uses of vitamin E are as prophylaxis to reduce adverse effects of inflammation and for degenerative joint conditions.Other specific uses include treatment of restless

TABLE 8 Guidelines for Use of Vitamin E Supplementation in Musculoskeletal Conditions

Dosage

400–800 mg daily of mixed tocopherols, *d*-α-tocopherol, *d*-α-tocopheryl succinate, or *d*-α-tocopheryl acetate. Synthetic vitamin E (*dl*-α-tocopherol forms) is clinically useful, but not suggested for long-term usage. Dosage may be reduced after healing has occurred to 100–400 mg/d for long time periods, which is consistent with suggestions to prevent chronic degenerative conditions.

Conditions for Use

Osteoarthritis
Rheumatoid arthritis
Ankylosing spondylitis
Degenerative joint conditions
Traumatic injuries, burns, or fractures
Periodontal diseases
Night leg cramps and restless leg syndrome
Chronic inflammation
Surgical interventions
Hematomas, contusions

leg syndrome, night muscle cramps, capillary fragility (purpura), and periodontal conditions. The chondroprotective abilities of vitamin E represent an exciting new application that deserves further clinical application.

Vitamin E and wound contracture (prevention of excess scar formation) deserves singular attention. Vitamin E has a popular image of being able to reduce size of existing scars or even to reduce stretch marks after topical application of vitamin E oil. These attributes are not supported by human research. The two studies in humans on this topic have examined breast implant capsule contractures for cosmetic results, with apparent benefits, but studies were not controlled and guidelines for use would be premature until confirmation or denial by other studies. Extremely high doses in animals were needed before an inhibition of wound healing (and perhaps scar formation) was found. These results are almost impossible to achieve in humans with oral supplementation. However, the concept of prevention of excess scar formation by normalization of inflammation following surgery is still valid. The clinical outcomes of vitamin E supplementation after surgery are not fully known, but do not appear to be harmful. Whether benefits of vitamin E supplementation are practical for enhancing cosmesis of surgical wounds in humans is not yet clear.

Expected results for vitamin E supplementation are difficult to predict for individual cases. Usually effects of vitamin E are mild by pharmacological standards, which may be apparent in some individuals, and may not be sufficient for effect in others. The results with degenerative joint conditions appear to be the most impressive at this time.

IV. VITAMIN K

Like other fat-soluble vitamins, vitamin K exists as a series of compounds with the same biological activity.[562-566] Vitamin K is the generic term for menadione, menaquinone, and phylloquinone. As 1,4-naphthoquinone ring compounds, vitamin K vitamers are lipophilic (fat-soluble) and subject to oxidation–reduction (redox) reactions in tissues. The chief role of vitamin K is as a cofactor for enzymes that convert protein-bound glutamyl residues to γ-carboxyglutamyl residues.[562-566] Prothrombin activity is dependent upon gamma carboxylation of glutamyl residues, and, thus, vitamin K is associated with antihemorrhagic and blood clotting properties. Recently, vitamin K-dependent gamma carboxylation of bone-associated proteins (osteocalcin and others) has been confirmed, and another role of vitamin K has been added: regulation of bone mineral formation.[562-566] All gamma carboxylated proteins bind calcium ions in a specific manner that allows for specific functions for each protein.

Deficiency symptoms that are frank enough to affect clotting ability are difficult to produce in humans.[562-566] Groups at risk for severe deficiency of vitamin K are neonates, chronic fat malabsorption syndromes, coumarin (warfarin) treatment or poisoning, antibiotic therapy that destroys gut microbial flora, extended TPN, and possibly salicylate therapy. Usually, several of these factors need to be combined before vitamin K deficiency is elaborated. In healthy populations not taking antibiotics, frank vitamin K deficiency is extremely rare, since about 2 µg/kg of vitamin K is absorbed after production from gut microflora. Thus, dietary requirements are not firm and range from 0.5 to 1.0 µg/kg daily in adults.[562-566] Green leafy vegetables are the richest dietary source of vitamin K, with lesser amounts in fruits, cereals, and grains. Animal foodstuffs have little vitamin K.

Potential clinical uses of vitamin K pertaining to connective tissues focus mostly on bone health. A preliminary study on animals given experimental fractures found better healing after administration of vitamin K supplements, but no experimental details were given.[567] No other studies on use of vitamin K supplements to possibly enhance healing of fractures in young adults are available. Another link between bone health and vitamin K concerns postmenopausal osteoporosis. Decreased circulating levels of vitamin K have been identified in osteoporotic patients with hip fractures or vertebral crush fractures.[568] In addition, urinary excretion of gamma carboxyglutamate residues was increased somewhat by vitamin K supplements.[569] Also, vitamin K supplements decreased urinary calcium excretion in postmenopausal women.[570] Oral administration of phylloquinones or menaquinones are not associated with toxicity; however, menadione has some toxicity and its clinical use is not recommended. Thus, there is sufficient rationale to explore in more detail the link between vitamin K supplementation and bone health. At this time, there are no specific recommendations for vitamin K supplements as an aid to musculoskeletal healing.

Chapter 6

B VITAMINS

I. INTRODUCTION

B vitamins are a group of diverse, structurally different compounds utilized as cofactors for cellular energy production in human intermediary metabolism. Since the discovery of B vitamins, many clinical uses have been studied, but many early reports (before the 1960s) were hampered by lack of knowledge on other nutrient roles and deficiencies, poor experimental design, and, sometimes, inadequate dosages. Conquering classical deficiency diseases such as pellagra, beriberi, and pernicious anemia resolved the importance of frank B vitamin deficiencies, but conditions where B vitamins may have pharmacological significance aside from correcting deficiency states have been less well studied. Assessment of B vitamin status still is not worthy of routine clinical use for a wide variety of reasons. Thus, clinical research using B vitamins as therapeutic agents has fallen out of favor. Nevertheless, sufficient reports on B vitamins indicate that clinical usefulness may be applied to human healing processes. In this chapter, in order to focus on the scope of this book, background information on B vitamins will be pooled and not broken down into individual vitamins until the section on clinical trials is reached.

II. ROLES AND FUNCTIONS

Table 1 lists some of the more important roles and functions of B vitamins that pertain to connective tissue healing. Many excellent reviews on background information on B vitamins are available if further information is desired.[170,571-576] The primary role of B vitamins is in bioenergetics. B vitamins are involved in most of the many biochemical steps in the breakdown of food components (sugars, fatty acids, amino acids) into smaller molecules that enter cellular respiration. Many B vitamins transfer or carry electrons to other components of cellular respiration, aiding in production of ATP, the major energy source for cells. Cellular energy is used to fulfill cellular functions. Any deficit in cellular energy production may have adverse effects on cellular functions. Thus, fibroblasts would be less able to respond to an injury by decreases in proliferation, production of proteoglycans and collagens, and resistance to ischemia and free radicals. Thus, B vitamin deficiencies can indirectly affect healing by affecting cellular function.

In addition, specific enzymes activated by B vitamins participate more directly in healing. For example, lysyl oxidase, involved in collagen and elastin maturation by formation of cross-links, utilizes vitamin B_6 as a cofactor.[93,94,577-585] B vitamins can have very indirect consequences on connective tissues by virtue of their roles in intermediary metabolism. One example is the production and metabolism of homocysteine, which is dependent upon function of vitamins B_6, B_{12}, and folate, in enzyme activities in the pathway of sulfur amino acid metabolism.[93,94,581,586,587] Since homocysteine can interfere with collagen maturation, and thus production, one symptom of homocysteine excess is osteopenia.[93,94]

III. DEFICIENCY SYMPTOMS

B vitamins are found together in foodstuffs and are commonly deficient as a group when total food intake is inadequate. B vitamin-deficiency symptoms often overlap or are difficult to distinguish unless cardinal symptoms specific to a single B vitamin are encountered. Table 2 lists some deficiency

TABLE 1　Roles and Functions of B Vitamins Related to Healing

Vitamin B_1 (Thiamin)

Roles	Energy production from foodstuffs, especially carbohydrates
Functions	Coenzyme for transketolase (pentose phosphate pathway); pyruvate dehydrogenase and α-ketoglutarate dehydrogenases (entry of acetyl groups and α-ketoglutarate into tricarboxylic acid cycle)
Dietary Needs	0.5 mg per 1000 kcal

Vitamin B_2 (Riboflavin)

Roles	Energy production and cellular respiration
Functions	Unique component of coenzymes flavin adenine dinucleotide (FAD) and flavin mononucleotide (FMN), essential for large number of redox reactions, releasing energy from carbohydrates, fats, and amino acids (proteins)
Dietary Needs	0.6 mg per 1000 kcal

Niacin, Niacinamide (Vitamin B_3, Nicotinic Acid, Nicotinamide)

Roles	Energy production, cellular respiration, fat synthesis
Functions	Unique component of coenzymes nicotinamide adenine dinucleotide (NAD) and nicotinamide adenine dinucleotide phosphate (NADP), essential for many redox reactions, releasing energy from breakdown of carbohydrates, fats, and amino acids (proteins); glycogen synthesis
Dietary Needs	6.6 niacin equivalents (NE) per 1000 kcal (1 NE = 1 mg niacin)

Vitamin B_6 (Pyridoxine, Pyridoxal, Pyridoxamine)

Roles	Amino acid metabolism and energy production
Functions	Unique component of coenzyme pyridoxal phosphate, essential for numerous reactions involving transamination (transfer of amino groups), deamination (removal of amino groups), desulfuration (transfer of sulfhydryl groups), decarboxylation (removal of organic acid group), cofactor for lysyl oxidase (collagen and elastin maturation), heme formation, conversion of tryptophan to niacin, glycogen breakdown, eicosanoid synthesis, one-carbon metabolism, hormone modulation, gluconeogenesis, neurotransmitter synthesis
Dietary Needs	2.0–2.2 mg per day

Vitamin B_{12} (Cobalamins, Cyanocobalamin, Hydroxocobalamin, Cobamamide)

Roles	Prevention of anemia and neuropathy, cell division (DNA synthesis)
Functions	Essential for one carbon metabolism and recycling of folate, breakdown of odd-chain fatty acids and branched chain amino acids
Dietary Needs	3.0 µg per day

Folic Acid (Folate, Folacin, Folinic Acid, Pteroylglutamates)

Roles	Blood cell formation and cell division (DNA synthesis)
Functions	Primary carrier of one carbon unit used for numerous biosynthetic events
Dietary Needs	0.4 mg per day

Pantothenic Acid (Pantothenate)

Roles	Energy production from carbohydrates, fats, amino acids (proteins)
Functions	Unique component of coenzyme A, essential for entry of carbohydrates, fats, and amino acids (proteins) into tricarboxylic acid cycle; coenzyme A used in many biosynthetic pathways
Dietary Needs	4–7 mg per day (estimated)

Biotin

Roles	Energy production and fat metabolism
Functions	Biosynthesis of fatty acids; replenishment of tricarboxylic acid cycle; gluconeogenesis
Dietary Needs	100–300 µg per day

TABLE 2   B Vitamin Deficiency Symptoms Pertinent to Connective Tissue Healing

Vitamin B$_1$ (Thiamin) Deficiency Symptoms

General

Early: Fatigue, loss of appetite, nausea, constipation, irritability, mental depression, peripheral neuropathy
Moderate = Wernicke-Korsakoff Syndrome: Ataxia, loss of fine motor control, mental confusion, loss of eye coordination, sonophobia
Severe = beriberi: Muscular weakness, muscular atrophy, edema, heart failure

Specific

↓ Wound strength (55% of normal)
↓ Lysyl oxidase activity in skin and wound (78% of normal)
↓ Hydroxyproline content in collagen
Abnormal maturation of collagen fibers
↓ Collagen accumulation in wounds
↓ Type III collagen in wounds (1st collagen type synthesized in wounds)
↓ Differentiation of fibroblasts
Derangement in macrophage ultrastructure and phagocytosis
↓ Wound healing

Vitamin B$_2$ (Riboflavin)

General

Scaly dermatitis, glossitis, angular cheilitis (fissures at corner of mouth), alopecia, cataracts, depression, photophobia

Specific

↑ Collagen solubility in rat skin (by 150%)
↑ Ratio of α/β chains in collagen
↓ Content of total collagen (by 28%)
↓ Aldehyde content of collagen (by 26%)
↓ Elastin and elastin cross-links (by 50-60%)
↓ Wound healing
Granulation tissue much less dense, more vascular, more cellular
↓ Serum pyridoxal phosphate levels (by 22%)

Vitamin B$_3$ (Niacin, Niacinamide)

General

Early: Fatigue, muscular weakness, anorexia, indigestion, skin eruptions, depression, headaches, irritability, limb pains
Severe = pellagra: Glossitis, tremors, diarrhea, dementia, dermatitis with dark pigmentation (3 D's), confusion, memory impairment

Vitamin B$_6$ (Pyridoxine)

General

Early: Irritability, nervousness, depression, peripheral neuropathy, sideroblastic anemia, acne, fatigue
Severe: Peripheral neuritis, convulsions, nausea, vomiting, dermatitis, mucous membrane lesions, alopecia, sideroblastic anemia, arthritis, cheilosis, conjunctivitis, numbness, paresthiasis, seizures

TABLE 2 (continued)   B Vitamin Deficiency Symptoms Pertinent to Connective Tissue Healing

Specific

↓ Lysyl oxidase activity
↓ Collagen and elastin cross-links
↑ Collagen solubility (immature, weak collagen, and elastin formation)
↑ Homocysteine levels
↓ Delayed wound healing
Granulation tissues much less dense, more vascular, more cellular
Osteoporosis

Vitamin B_{12} (Cobalamins)

General

Mental depression, pernicious anemia (macrocytic anemia), fatigue, shortness of breath, weakness, peripheral neuropathy followed by irreversible neurological damage, constipation, gastrointestinal disturbances, glossitis, headaches, irritability, numbness, palpitations, spinal cord degeneration

Specific

↓ Skeletal alkaline phosphatase activity
↓ Serum osteocalcin levels
↓ Osteoblast activity
↑ Homocysteine levels

Folic Acid

General

Macrocytic anemia (fatigue, weakness, shortness of breath), gastrointestinal symptoms, glossitis, depressed ankle jerks, anorexia, apathy, constipation, growth impairment, headaches, insomnia, memory impairment, restless legs, loss of vibratory sensation in legs

Specific

↑ Homocysteine
↓ Protein and collagen synthesis (by 50%)
Collagen hydroxylation slightly decreased
Osteoporosis

Pantothenic Acid

General

Anorexia, burning feet, impaired coordination, depression, eczema, fatigue, hypotension, infections, insomnia, irritability, muscle spasms, nausea, nervousness

Specific

↓ Wound strength (by 46%)
↓ Wound fibroblasts
Osteoarthritis symptoms (cartilage calcification, osteophytes, osteoporosis)

Biotin

General

Fatigue, muscle weakness and pain, dermatitis (especially nose and mouth), depression, hair loss, anemia, anorexia, nausea, hypercholesterolemia, hyperglycemia, insomnia, gray skin, pale smooth tongue symptoms of B vitamins that affect connective tissue healing.[93,94,164,167,170,485,571-598] Of major interest are the findings of decreased wound strength in animals (by 46%) in pantothenate deficiency, osteoporosis in B_6-deficient animals, decreased wound strength in thiamin-deficient animals (by 55%), and defective collagen production, maturation, and deposition by deficiencies of thiamin, riboflavin, pyridoxine, folate, and pantothenate. These findings all indicate that healing of all connective tissues is affected adversely by deficiencies of one or more B vitamins.

IV. ASSESSMENT

Table 3 lists some of the more common measurements of B vitamin status.[170,439,571-576,599,600] Functional tests are preferred over measuring quantitative levels because of their greater sensitivity for detection of deficient status. Nevertheless, no single test is 100% accurate at finding deficient status of a particular B vitamin. Serum levels of B vitamins are notorious for not being accurate indicators of cellular or tissue status for each vitamin. Of interest is the new method of functional nutrient assessment using lymphocyte growth responses in chemically defined, serum-free media.[600,601] In general, it is far less expensive and less time-consuming to administer a clinical trial of supplementation with one or more B vitamins and note clinical responses than to exhaustively test for B vitamin status. However, a prime candidate for testing of B vitamin status would be the patient who exhibits delayed or abnormal healing.

V. INTAKES

Estimation of dietary intake of B vitamins has been characteristically unreliable.[191] However, a review on nutrition surveys of different categories of athletes found that most ingest sufficient B vitamins according to the RDA.[191] Groups at risk for deficient B vitamin intakes (usually folate, vitamin B_6, or vitamin B_{12}) were gymnasts, dancers, female runners, and wrestlers, although consistent patterns were not seen.[191] Frequent ingestion of multivitamin supplement products by athletes would almost always place intakes of B vitamins at or above the RDA.

VI. DIETARY SOURCES AND INFLUENCES

B vitamins are essential to life and are found in almost all whole foodstuffs. As foods are more refined or processed, their B vitamin content suffers. Vitamin B_{12} is unique among B vitamins since it is only present in animal foodstuffs. Folate is richest in vegetables (especially green leafy vegetables). Richest dietary sources of B vitamins and population groups at greatest risk for deficiencies are listed in Table 4.

VII. ANIMAL STUDIES

Animal studies have been quite helpful in determining that deficiencies of one or more B vitamins have deleterious effects on healing.[577-598] This section will focus on effects of B vitamin supplements on healing. Biochemical measurements of wound healing to normal rats supplemented with 1.5 mg oral thiamin per day found increased wound tensile strength (115 to 117%), but no change in collagen cross-linking.[588-590] In wound (granulation) tissue, it was found that local requirements for vitamin B_1 increased relative to increased glucose metabolism. Normal levels of vitamin B_1 in the animal's diet and tissues were insufficient to provide enough flux of energy pathways to generate sufficient ATP for increased rates of collagen synthesis. The net result was that large oral doses of thiamin accelerated wound healing by 1 to 2 d/week.

TABLE 3 Methods of Assessment for B Vitamin Status

Vitamin B$_1$ (Thiamin)

Functional Assays	Quantitative Tests
Erythrocyte transketolase activity coefficient (ETKAC)	Serum levels of thiamin (colorimetric, HPLC)
Lymphocyte growth responses	Urinary excretion
	Microbial assays of body fluids

Vitamin B$_2$ (Riboflavin)

Functional Tests	Quantitative Tests
Erythrocyte glutathione reductase enzyme activation coefficient (EGRAC)	Serum, urine, body fluid levels (fluorometric, HPLC)
Lymphocyte growth response	Urinary excretion
	Microbial assays of body fluids

Vitamin B$_3$ (Niacin, Niacinamide)

Functional Assays	Quantitative Tests
Lymphocyte growth responses	Urinary excretion of N^1-methylnicotinamide and 2-pyr
	Erythrocyte NAD levels
	Erythrocyte NAD/NADP ratio
	Microbial assays of body fluids

Vitamin B$_6$ (Pyridoxine, Pyridoxal, Pyridoxamine)

Functional Assays	Quantitative Tests
Erythrocyte enzyme activation coefficients for ALT, AST enzymes	Serum or erythrocyte pyridoxal-5-phosphate (PLP) levels
Lymphocyte growth responses	Serum vitamin B$_6$ vitamer levels
Urinary xanthurenic and kynurenic acid levels after tryptophan load	Serum or urinary 4-pyridoxic acid levels
Plasma or urinary homocysteine levels after methionine load	Microbial assays of body fluids
Plasma or urine amino acid levels and ratios	

Vitamin B$_{12}$ (Cobalamins)

Functional Assays	Quantitative Assays
Serum or urinary levels of homocysteine ± oral methionine load	Serum or erythrocyte levels of cobalamins (RIA)
Serum or urinary levels of methyl malonic acid	Microbial assays of body fluids
Lymphocyte growth responses	
Schilling test or dual-isotope variation (for vitamin B$_{12}$ absorption)	

Folate

Functional Assays	Quantitative Tests
Urinary formiminoglutamate (FIGLU) levels ± oral histidine load	Serum and erythrocyte levels of folates (RIA)
Lymphocyte growth response	Microbial assays of body fluids
Neutrophil hypersegmentation	

Pantothenate

Functional Assays	Quantitative Tests
Lymphocyte growth response	Whole blood and urine levels (colorimetric, HPLC)
	Microbial assays of body fluids

Biotin

Functional Assays	Quantitative Tests
Lymphocyte growth response	Whole blood and urine levels (colorimetric, HPLC)
	Microbial assays of body fluids

Note: HPLC = high-pressure (performance) liquid chromatography; RIA = radioimmunoassay.

TABLE 4   Dietary Sources, Influences and Persons at Greatest Risk for Deficiency of B Vitamins

Vitamin B$_1$ (Thiamin)

Dietary sources rich in thiamin (per serving) include: nutritional supplements; nutritional yeasts; Spirulina algae; rice bran; rice polish; wheat germ; pork; enriched grains and grain products (cereals); legumes (beans, peas, soybeans, lentils); other meats, milk and milk products, fruits, and vegetables have lower amounts of thiamin but can be a significant source if consumed in large quantities

Excessive ingestion of certain raw freshwater fish and shellfish, tea, coffee, blueberries, and red cabbage should be avoided, as these foods may contain antithiamin factors; the 1989 RDA for thiamin is between 1.0–1.5 mg for adults

Those at risk for thiamin deficiency include: malnutrition or starvation; malabsorption syndromes; alcoholism; elderly; restricted diets; increased metabolic rate (pregnancy, lactation, fever, infection, trauma); prolonged hemodialysis; gastric partitioning surgery; and inherited thiamin-responsive metabolic disorders

Vitamin B$_2$ (Riboflavin)

Dietary sources rich in riboflavin (per serving) include: nutritional supplements; nutritional yeasts; meats and dairy products; green leafy vegetables and enriched grains and grain products; the 1989 RDA for riboflavin is 1.2–1.8 mg for adults

Those at risk for riboflavin deficiency include: malnourished; malabsorption syndromes; elderly; hypothyroidism; and increased metabolic rate (trauma, fever, infection, pregnancy, lactation)

Vitamin B$_3$ (Niacin, Niacinamide)

Dietary sources of niacinamide are expressed as niacin equivalents, taking into account tryptophan's contribution; richest sources (per serving) include: nutritional supplements; nutritional yeasts; meats; legumes including peanuts; enriched cereals; potatoes; the 1989 RDA for niacin is between 13–20 mg for adults

Those at risk for niacinamide deficiency include: alcoholics; malnourished; malabsorption; elderly; low food intake; high consumption of corn with little protein; high consumption of sorghum or millet and increased metabolic rate (trauma, fever, infection, pregnancy, lactation)

Vitamin B$_6$ (Pyridoxal-5-phosphate, Pyridoxine)

Dietary sources richest in vitamin B$_6$ (per serving) include: nutritional supplements; nutritional yeasts; potatoes; meats; wheat germ; bananas; legumes; fortified cereal products; the 1989 RDA for vitamin B$_6$ is between 1.4–2.0 mg for adults

Those at risk for vitamin B$_6$ deficiency include pregnancy; lactation; oral contraceptive users; alcoholism; inherited metabolic disorders; malabsorption; malnourished; isoniazid therapy for tuberculosis; penicillamine therapy

Vitamin B$_{12}$ (Cobalamins)

Dietary sources for cobalamins are strictly from animal foodstuffs; vitamin B$_{12}$ is not found in plant foodstuffs; dietary supplements can also contain vitamin B$_{12}$; the 1989 RDA for vitamin B$_{12}$ is 2.0 μg for adults

Those at risk for cobalamin deficiency are malabsorption disorders; loss of gastric acidity; loss of ileum surface; long-term, strict vegetarians

Folate

Dietary sources richest in folate (per serving) include: nutritional supplements; legumes; vitamin-fortified cereals; green leafy vegetables; wheat germ; seeds; nuts; liver; the 1989 RDA for folate is 180–200 μg

Those at risk for folate deficiency include: vitamin B$_{12}$ deficiency; malnourished; malabsorption; pregnant and lactating women; increased rate of cellular division (burns, trauma, malignancies, hemolytic anemias); alcoholics; anticonvulsant therapy (phenytoin, barbiturates, primidone); folate antagonist therapy (methotrexate, 5-fluorouracil, pyrimethamine); tuberculosis therapy (isoniazid plus cycloserine); oral contraceptive users; sulfasalazine therapy; elderly; infants; inherited folate disorders

Pantothenate

Dietary sources richest in pantothenate (per serving) include: nutritional supplements; nutritional yeast; meats; legumes; whole grain products; wheat germ; vegetables; nuts; seeds; the estimated safe and adequate daily dietary intake for pantothenate is 4–7 mg for adults

Those at risk for deficiency include: malnourished; malabsorption; greatly increased metabolic rate (trauma)

**TABLE 4 (continued)   Dietary Sources, Influences and Persons at Greatest Risk
for Deficiency of B Vitamins**

Biotin

Dietary sources richest in biotin are nutritional supplements; liver; egg yolk; nutritional yeast; royal jelly; legumes; rice bran; whole grains; fish; the 1989 estimated safe and adequate daily dietary intake for biotin is 30–100 µg for adults

Those at risk for biotin deficiency include: persons consuming excessive amounts of raw egg whites; inherited disorders of biotin metabolism; extended total parenteral nutrition (biotin-free); loss of enteric gut microflora from antibiotic therapy or altered gut motility; pregnant and lactating women; antiepileptic drug therapy; alcoholics; trauma (burns and surgery); elderly; malabsorption (especially achlorhydria)

Supplemental oral pantothenate to rabbits that increased urinary excretion to 10 times normal (equivalent to 1000 to 2000 mg for humans) was studied for effects on wound healing.[593-596] A "remarkable increase" in wound strength (150 to 200%) was found, with significantly more fibroblasts in wound tissue. It was noted that, in humans, it takes at least 7 d to significantly increase serum levels at pantothenate intakes of 100 mg/d. Additional pantothenate to cultures of human fibroblasts exhibited significantly increased growth rate (up to 170%), increased collagen synthesis (150 to 220%), increased protein synthesis (150%), and increased cellular protein (up to 160%).[602,603]

VIII. HUMAN STUDIES

A. B COMPLEX MIXTURES

Work from the 1940s and later found that after severe injury, surgery, trauma, or burns, serum and urine levels of vitamins B_1, B_2, and niacin were greatly decreased for several days to several weeks postinjury, depending on severity.[604-606] With the advent of nutritional support by enteral or parenteral means, and inclusion of dietary supplements in many cases, the decreased status of B vitamins after injury has been largely reduced in hospitalized patients with major injuries. However, administration of supplemental vitamins B_1, B_6, and B_{12} (Neurobion®) to patients after gastric cancer surgery showed better improvement of depressed lymphocyte function tests, even when cells were dysfunctional before surgery.[607]

Miehlke and others, from the Rheumaklinik II in Wiesbaden, Germany, described the hypothetical basis for supplementation of neuromuscular symptoms in rheumatoid arthritis patients with oral supplementation with Neurobion Forte® (50 mg vitamin B_1, 50 mg vitamin B_6, and 250 µg vitamin B_{12} per tablet).[608] Symposiums on Neurobion detailed functional improvements in fine motor control in pentathletes (shooting accuracy),[609] reduction of NSAID (Diclofenac®) requirement in acute lumbago,[610] greater reduction in pain when combined with Diclofenac for acute lumbago,[611] and enhancement of Diclofenac effect in pain reduction for spinal degenerative rheumatic diseases,[612] in double-blind, placebo-controlled studies in hundreds of patients. Treatment periods lasted from 2 to 8 weeks, and no side effects were attributed to Neurobion. These results were supported by animal studies showing dose-dependent decreases in pain (antinociceptive effects)[612-614] and enhancement of nerve regeneration after cold lesion.[615] Thus, one oral product containing three B vitamins has documentation as an adjunct for pain relief in degenerative musculoskeletal disorders for short-term (2 to 3 month) periods. Usual daily doses were 300 mg thiamin, 300 mg pyridoxine, and 1.5 mg cyanocobalamin.

B. VITAMIN B_1 (THIAMIN)

Intravenous administration of 10 to 30 g thiamin has exhibited analgesic effects, but after a few adverse reactions to impurities in early thiamin preparations, use of intravenous thiamin ceased.[616-619] It is not known if large oral doses of thiamin have any analgesic effects. Quirin administered 1 to 2 g

TABLE 5 Niacinamide Dosage Schedules for Therapy of Joint Dysfunction

Joint Dysfunction Status	Daily Oral Dosage Schedule	Total Dose (mg)
Slight (86–95%)	150–250 mg every 3 h for 6 doses	900–1500
Moderate (71–85%)	250 mg every 3 h for 6 doses or 250 mg every 2 h for 8 doses	1500–2000
Severe (56–70%)	250 mg every 2 h for 8 doses or 250 mg every 1.5 h for 10 doses	2000–2500
Extremely severe (<56%)	250 mg every 1.5 h for 10 doses or 250 mg every 1 h for 16 doses	2500–4000

Note: Joint dysfunction was measured by the Joint Range Index, which was the range of motion in degrees determined by goniometer readings of 20 joints: neck, shoulder, hip, knee, wrist, and metacarpophalangeal joints.

1 to 2 times daily in an open field study to 133 patients with headache, arthralgia, spinal syndromes, or neuralgia that had been unsuccessfully treated with physical therapy and analgesics.[620] Overall, 73% of patients showed satisfactory or very good results in reduction of pain. Eight patients who were addicted to analgesics stopped their analgesic use after thiamin supplementation. A study by Herzog, from 1953 (when food fortification was still young, and thiamin deficiency may have been more prevalent), reported that 202/225 cases of tooth extractions had good effects for pain control and rapidity of healing after intramuscular injection of 100 mg thiamin hydrochloride 30 min before operation.[621] Similarly, 145/156 patients for periodontal surgery exhibited good results. However, this study did not use control groups and reported no objective data. Nevertheless, the clinical observations support data from other, better-controlled studies on the ability of large doses of thiamin to control pain in connective tissues.

C. VITAMIN B$_3$ (NIACIN, NIACINAMIDE)

Pioneering work by Kaufman from the 1940s and later found clinical benefits for arthritis patients with joint dysfunction after administration of oral niacinamide.[622-625] After specializing in identification and treatment of pellagra before food fortification, Dr. Kaufman noticed that after fortification, signs of niacin deficiency that remained were impaired balance, lack of joint mobility, and muscular weakness. This finding, coupled with improved flexibility of joints after niacinamide therapy for niacin deficiency observed in many patients, led to concerted studies on niacinamide and joint mobility. Initial double-blind studies found that niacinamide, and not placebo, improved joint mobility (as measured by objective parameters) by 4 weeks, with continued improvements. However, since placebo-controlled, double-blind studies were difficult to maintain in private practice, a large number of patients (842, with 663 taking niacinamide) were observed over periods of up to 20 years or more. Based on work found to be successful for treating pellagra, niacinamide was given to patients at doses of 150 to 250 mg every 1 to 3 h for 6 to 16 doses per day, depending on severity of joint dysfunction (see Table 5). The reason for frequent dosing of no more than 250 mg per dose was based on previous research showing that the ability to absorb niacinamide from single doses did not increase when over 250 mg of niacinamide was administered orally. The frequency was determined by the pharmacokinetics of niacinamide, which has a half-life in plasma of 4 to 6 h. Thus, oral dosing every 3 h or less would offer ideal pharmacokinetics of niacinamide delivery to the bloodstream and tissues.

Niacinamide therapy was successful in 70% of patients with varying degrees of either osteoarthritis or rheumatoid arthritis or both (many patients exhibit features of each condition). Thirty percent of total arthritic patients did not respond to niacinamide therapy. Ages ranged from 4 to 80 years. Rapid initial improvements in joint mobility were seen by 4 weeks, followed by slow and steady progression of increased mobility to a limit after 2 to 3 years. Usually, joint mobility improved for each individual to significantly better than age-matched controls. Joint mobility improvements were maintained as long as niacinamide therapy was continued, for over 20 years in some individuals. The kinetics of joint mobility improvement closely matched known turnover rates of cartilage in joints.[29-42] Although niacinamide does not possess analgesic or antiinflammatory effects, joint pain was slowly reduced and disappeared in the majority of patients. In over several thousand patient years of high dose niacinamide therapy, no adverse effects were reported or observed.

After conducting numerous n = 1 case studies, Dr. Kaufman determined that niacinamide dosage had to be maintained for very long time periods (even up to 20 years) to maintain improved joint mobility. When niacinamide was slowly tapered downwards and discontinued, or simply discontinued, then joint mobility worsened back to its original preniacinamide status after several weeks. Importantly, taking the same total dose of niacinamide in fewer doses (for example, 3 doses of 500 mg each per day) did not lead to similar clinical results. Thus, simply taking a single large bolus of niacinamide did not lead to improvement in joint function. Addition of other vitamins singly or in combination with niacinamide did not affect outcome of niacinamide therapy (thiamin, riboflavin, pyridoxine, pantothenate, i.m. injections of vitamin B_{12}, vitamin A, vitamin C, vitamin D). In addition, adequate calories and protein in the diet must be present, and repeated traumas or insults to joints must be avoided. Return to full mobility will be limited by prior joint damage and bone remodeling.

Thus, over 50 years of experience in frequent niacinamide doses for arthritis found long-lasting, objective improvements in joint mobility, with complete safety. The use of niacinamide has not been studied, much less confirmed, by other investigators to date, except for one report by Hoffer, which found reductions and remissions of arthritic symptoms in six patients taking 1 to 3 g/d of niacin (n = 5) or niacinamide (n = 2).[626] The time course of symptom reduction for Hoffer's patients was identical to Kaufman's data. Frequent dosing with niacinamide appeared to fit the hypothesis that metabolic activation of chondrocytes was accomplished, rather than pharmacological effects, although a mechanism of action was not sought. Nevertheless, the large number of subjects, the reproducibility of results, the congruence with known pharmacokinetics of niacinamide and cartilage physiology, the use of objective measurements of joint function, and sequential testing of individuals constituting their own controls lend considerable strength to the reported clinical observations. The use of frequent dosing with 250 mg niacinamide daily for long time periods merits further application for therapy of arthritis, degenerative joint conditions, and joint dysfunction.

D. VITAMIN B_6 (PYRIDOXINE, PYRIDOXAL-5-PHOSPHATE, PYRIDOXAMINE, 3-HYDROXY-2-METHYLPYRIDINE DERIVATIVES)

1. Carpal Tunnel Syndrome

Carpal tunnel syndrome is an increasingly common musculoskeletal/neurological disorder that is believed to be a result of tenosynovitis of flexor tendons in the carpal tunnel region of the wrist. Secondary edema, ischemia, and compression of the median nerve produces clinical symptoms of hand pain, wrist pain, tingling, numbness, night pain with sleep disturbances, positive Tinel's sign, positive Phalin's test, sensory loss, motor loss of median nerve function distal to the wrist, and muscle weakness with atrophy.[627]

During the 1970s, pioneering work on treatment of carpal tunnel syndrome with pyridoxine was initiated by Ellis and Folkers (a codiscoverer of vitamin B_6), and reported in a series of studies.[628-644] Evidence of vitamin B_6 deficiencies in many carpal tunnel syndrome patients was found, and symptoms were reduced or relieved after 4 to 12 weeks of supplementation with daily divided doses of 100 to 300 mg total pyridoxine in a majority of patients. A flurry of other studies followed, some with positive results[645-650] and some with negative results.[636,637] As an example, a very recent study will be considered. Bernstein and Dinesen of the Department of Neurology at the Kaiser Permanente Medical Center in Hayward, CA attempted to predict which patients with carpal tunnel syndrome (entrapment neuropathy) would benefit from vitamin B_6 therapy before supplementation was initiated.[650] In an open trial, 16 adult subjects with documented carpal tunnel syndrome completed a 3-month study of oral vitamin B_6 supplementation (200 mg/d of pyridoxine HCL). Standard clinical and electrophysiological measurements used in diagnosis and assessment of carpal tunnel syndrome were not predictive of clinical response. These measurements included EEG studies, motor nerve latency, sensory nerve latency, ulnar sensory conduction velocities, and pain assessments (McGill Pain Questionnaire and visual analog scale). In this study, all subjects exhibited normal EEGs before, during, and after treatment, with no differences between time intervals. Motor nerve latency across the wrist was abnormal before vitamin B_6 supplementation and did not change after treatment. However, median nerve sensory latency was significantly decreased (improved), and pain scores were decreased (improved) in all patients (55 to 30, visual analog scale, $p < 0.0001$). No toxicity (peripheral neuropathy) was noticed, as evidenced by no changes in ulnar sensory conduction velocities. Thus, vitamin B_6 at an oral dose of 200 mg/d was shown to be effective and safe for the short-term treatment of carpal tunnel syndrome. However, because motor nerve latencies were unchanged, perhaps carpal tunnel syndrome was not associated with a deficiency of vitamin B_6, but was affected by potential analgesic properties of vitamin B_6. Discrepancies between study findings can be explained by a subset of persons with carpal tunnel symptoms exhibiting a biochemical vitamin B_6 deficiency, and, therefore, respond both biochemically and clinically to pyridoxine supplementation. Other persons with carpal tunnel syndrome without vitamin B_6 deficiency may have experienced symptomatic improvement (or not) by other mechanisms of action of vitamin B_6. Very recent studies have found clinical relief of carpal tunnel syndrome from riboflavin and riboflavin plus pyridoxine supplements.[639,643] The co-administration of riboflavin and pyridoxine achieved better clinical responses than either vitamin alone. Therefore, riboflavin supplementation (50 mg/d) may be added to pyridoxine therapy for carpal tunnel syndrome.

Regardless, a consensus of research has indicated that testing of patients exhibiting carpal tunnel syndrome for biochemical vitamin B_6 status can identify those who have a high probability of response to pyridoxine supplementation. Other patients may still have beneficial responses, but probability of clinical success is unknown. When surgery was required, pyridoxine therapy was described as a useful adjunct.[647] Thus, a 3-month trial of pyridoxine supplementation at 100 mg/d ± riboflavin at 50 mg/d is warranted for patients with carpal tunnel syndrome before other treatment options are considered.

2. Other Uses for Vitamin B_6

Vitamin B_6 (100 to 150 mg/d started 4 weeks before withdrawal) has shown usefulness during withdrawal from analgesic medications (because of side effects) to prevent rebound pain.[653] Vitamin B_6 with cyproheptadine has also been used to ease symptoms of analgesic withdrawal.[653] Clinical usefulness in headache clinics and for chronic pain associated with temporomandibular joint function has also been reported.[653]

Patients with rheumatoid arthritis (n = 55) were shown to have reduced plasma levels of PLP (7.5 ± 3.9 vs. 12.4 ± 6.1 ng/ml).[654] Supplementation with 50 to 150 mg/d of pyridoxine hydrochloride for 3 months to 14 rheumatoid arthritis patients resulted in increased plasma levels of PLP (3 times baseline), but no clinical effects on sedimentation rate, rheumatoid factor, swollen joints, morning stiffness, hand grip strength, range of motion, or joint circumferences were found when compared to 7 control patients.

E. VITAMIN B_{12} (COBALAMINS)

Intramuscular injection of Adenocort® (adenosine-5-monophosphate, niacin, cyanocobalamin, and prednisolone acetate) to 75 patients with shoulder bursitis was associated with "excellent" results in 90% of subjects, especially for reduction of calcium deposits.[655] However, no control groups were studied, and the effects of a combination of components could not be ascribed to a single ingredient.

Anemia associated with rheumatoid arthritis is common. A recent study by Vreugdenhil and others of 36 rheumatoid arthritis patients found vitamin B_{12} deficiency in 7/24 (29%) and folate deficiency in 5/24 (21%) anemic patients.[656] Iron deficiency anemia was masked by concomitant vitamin B_{12} and/or folate deficiencies. Deficient status was assessed by radioassays of serum levels of vitamin B_{12} and folic acid, which are known to be less sensitive than other methods of assessment. These results suggest that careful attention to vitamin B_{12} and folate status must be given and, also, that supplementation with vitamin B_{12} and folate may be necessary in a large subset of rheumatoid arthritis patients.

F. FOLATE

Despite an abundant literature on folate, there is very little with regards to effects on human wound or connective tissue healing. A series of studies by Vogel studied the influences of folate supplementation on periodontal disease.[179] The oral mucosa is an adequate indicator of folate status due to its high rate of cell division and turnover, which is sensitive to folate status.[179,571-576] In four double-blind studies it was found that oral folate supplementation (2 mg) or topical folate administration (5 min swishing with 5 ml of 1 mg folate/ml) to normal, healthy subjects or subjects with gingivitis led to the following results: (1) increase in gingival tissue folate levels (5 to 10 times), (2) reduction in gingival fluid flow (a measure of inflammation), (3) reduction in bleeding index (another measure of tissue inflammation), and (4) no change in plaque amounts.[179] These results were found although fasting serum folate levels were in the normal range. Therefore, it was proposed that gingival tissue would benefit from increased administration of folate by enhanced ability of gingival tissue to synthesize protein (matrix) and respond to inflammation by hypertrophy and hyperplasia.[179] These studies were supported by similar findings in gingival tissues for groups known to be at risk for deficient folate status: pregnancy, oral contraceptives, and phenytoin therapy.[179] Thus, there is evidence in normal, healthy humans that local connective tissue levels of folate are insufficient to maintain an ideal healing response. It would be of great interest to extend these studies to other connective tissues, especially skin wound healing, tendons, ligaments, and joints.

G. PANTOTHENATE

One early study reported on the postoperative administration of dextro pantothenyl alcohol (with pantothenate activity) in a double-blind manner to 48 patients after serious abdominal surgery.[657] Intramuscular injections of placebo (n = 25) or *d*-pantothenol (n = 23, 200 mg each?) were given immediately after surgery, 2 h after surgery, and every 6 h until flatus was passed. The number of hours until first flatus and first feces was significantly shorter in the pantothenol group (69 vs. 77 h), and time of appearance for the first postoperative feces was also significantly shorter (106 vs. 116 h). In addition, 57% of pantothenol-treated patients rated an excellent postoperative course, while 32% of placebo patients rated excellent. Importantly, hospital stay was reduced an average of 2 days in the pantothenol group (*p* <0.0002). Thus, large doses of postoperative pantothenol were associated with improvements in surgical recovery.

A study by Aprahamian and others found that oral supplementation with 400 mg/d of pantothenate to 5 subjects for 3 weeks led to large increases in scar tissue levels of iron and copper, but not zinc, compared to 5 unsupplemented controls.[593] Iron and copper are cofactors for hydroxylase enzymes that help mature collagen.

Barton-Wright and Elliott, from St. Alfege's Hospital in London, found significantly decreased whole blood levels of pantothenate in 66 rheumatoid arthritis patients, compared to 20 mixed-diet or 9 vegetarian controls (69 vs. 107 vs. 262 μg/dl).[658] An inverse relationship was found between whole blood pantothenate levels and disease severity. Small-scale clinical trials (n = 20) of daily intramuscular injections of 50 mg calcium-*d*-pantothenate for 28 d normalized whole blood levels of pantothenate and gave temporary improvement of symptoms by 7 d. Daily injections of 50 mg royal jelly with 50 mg of pantothenate to 20 patients with rheumatoid arthritis found normalization of pantothenate levels with improvements in symptoms and a fall in the sedimentation rate. Symptoms regressed after injections were ceased. However, 10 vegetarian rheumatoid arthritis patients exhibited normalization of pantothenate levels along with disappearance of symptoms in 14 d. Only one patient had a slight recurrence 15 months later. Thus, daily administration of pantothenate (50 mg/d) with royal jelly (the food with the highest known pantothenate content) led to long-lasting relief of symptoms for a subset of vegetarian rheumatoid arthritis patients.

Annand reported on small clinical improvements for osteoarthritic patients after 12.5 mg/d of oral pantothenate supplementation.[659,660] Much later, a double-blind trial comparing placebo or 2 g of oral pantothenate for 2 months was conducted in 94 arthritic patients (47 per group).[661] Both osteoarthritis (59%) and rheumatoid arthritis (27%) patients were included. Paracetamol was the only drug allowed during the study period. For the entire group, there were no significant differences between placebo and pantothenate for morning stiffness, disability score, pain, analgesic requirements, sedimentation rate, physician assessment, and patient assessment. However, when the rheumatoid arthritis subjects were regarded separately, significant improvements in morning stiffness (8.5 to 2.8 h), disability, and pain were seen for the pantothenate group (n = 8), but not the placebo group (n = 10). Significant differences between the pantothenate and placebo groups were determined for degree of disability and pain reduction. Analgesic requirements in the pantothenate group were unchanged, but increased in the placebo group. The significant results seen with low numbers of subjects make the results remarkable. The General Practitioner Research Group concluded that pantothenate supplementation merited further trials, but none have appeared to date. This is surprising considering the safety, availability, and inexpensiveness of pantothenate supplements. Thus, it is strongly recommended that a trial of pantothenate supplementation (2 g/d in 4 divided doses), along with standard analgesics, be tried in rheumatoid arthritis patients for at least 2 months before treatments with known side effects be initiated.

IX. SAFETY

A. B COMPLEX VITAMINS

The safety of vitamins B_1 (thiamin), B_2 (riboflavin), B_3 (niacinamide, but not niacin), B_{12} (cobalamins), folate, pantothenate, and biotin has been well established after oral intakes.[571-576] Even very large daily intakes of several grams of the above-mentioned B vitamins have been well tolerated for long time periods. Thus, the practical toxicity of most B vitamins is nil. This indicates that the safety of multiple B vitamin complex products is also high, but attention must be paid to the amounts and forms of vitamins B_3 and B_6, which are discussed below.

B. SAFETY OF VITAMIN B$_6$ (PYRIDOXINE)

An increasing number of reports since 1983 have appeared concerning the potential toxicity of oral pyridoxine supplements.[662-670] An overview of findings indicated that toxicity is apparent in a time- and dose-dependent manner after ingestion of 500 mg/d or more of pyridoxine hydrochloride supplements. Doses over 100 mg, when taken for 3 years, also exhibited toxicity.[669] Most subjects were women taking pyridoxine for premenstrual syndrome symptoms. When symptoms were not alleviated, many would increase dosage until either relief or toxicity resulted. Toxicity symptoms were most often peripheral sensory neuropathy with paresthesia, hyperaesthesia, bone pains, muscle weakness, numbness, and fasciculations, usually of extremities. Interestingly, these symptoms are almost identical to vitamin B_6 deficiency symptoms.

Three hypotheses may account for observed pyridoxine toxicity with long-term, very high doses.[670] There may be a direct toxic effect of pyridoxine on peripheral nervous structures, since most peripheral sensory neuron cell bodies reside in dorsal root ganglia outside of the blood-brain barrier, and peripheral motor neurons reside in the spinal cord. Neurons in the central nervous system are protected from high plasma pyridoxine concentrations by the blood-brain barrier. Pyridines in general exhibit similar toxicity to pyridoxine, which is actually a substituted pyridine molecule. Second, the coenzymatic active form of vitamin B_6 is pyridoxal-5-phosphate (PLP). High pyridoxine concentrations may competitively inhibit activation or binding of PLP to active sites on B_6-dependent enzymes, thus resulting in functional deficiencies of vitamin B_6. Third, small amounts of toxic impurities (oxidized pyridoxine compounds?) present in pyridoxine preparations may manifest toxicity by the first or second hypothesis when high doses allow a threshold of effect to be reached. The first hypothesis has direct evidence from administration of purified pyridoxine, pyridoxal, and pyridoxamine causing inhibition of neurite growth in cell culture.[670] The second hypothesis has no direct supportive evidence in humans, and, in fact, high doses of pyridoxine routinely increase serum and tissue levels of PLP. The third hypothesis has some supportive clinical evidence, as observations on patients consuming high doses of commercially available pyridoxal-5-phosphate did not exhibit toxicity when pyridoxine did (Jaffe, R., personal communication). Since the commercial preparation of PLP involves further purification steps from pyridoxine, pyridoxal, or pyridoxamine supplement sources, it is believed that impurities found in pyridoxine preparations were removed during manufacture of PLP. Toxicity symptoms were completely reversible when daily pyridoxine doses were 500 mg or less when pyridoxine was discontinued. Higher doses were not associated with complete recovery of symptoms.

Regardless of cause, vitamin B$_6$ supplementation must be conducted carefully. Do not administer daily doses greater than 500 mg for any time period greater than 1 week. Do not administer daily doses of pyridoxine between 100 to 500 mg for more than 1 to 2 months. Daily doses of 100 mg for long time periods (up to 1 year) appear to be safe for most persons. However, after 1 year, a subset of patients may exhibit pyridoxine toxicity. It is not well known if tapering of pyridoxine doses from 100 mg daily to lower doses would maintain prevention of deficiency. It is known that doses of 10 mg or less usually do not normalize deficient vitamin B$_6$ functions. Addition of other nutrients with pyridoxine (other B vitamins singly or in combination, magnesium, zinc) did not affect toxicity findings. It is highly recommended to employ functional testing for vitamin B$_6$ status before initiation of oral doses in excess of 100 mg daily. If status is not functionally deficient, it is wise to prevent pyridoxine intakes over 50 mg daily.

C. SAFETY OF NIACIN

Niacin has a completely different safety profile than niacinamide. The large-scale, long-term use of very high oral doses of niacin as an antihyperlipidemic agent is a first-line drug therapy.[671] Doses of oral niacin greater than 20 to 50 mg cause intense flushing, tingling, and redness ("niacin flush") for short time periods after each dose. While this symptom may be pleasant or unpleasant, depending upon each individual, it is harmless. However, reports of nonspecific liver damage after time-release niacin doses and other potential toxicities after oral high-dose niacin therapy[671,672] mean that for practical purposes of healing (as described for arthritis), niacinamide should be used, and niacin should not be used. No reports of niacinamide toxicity after long-term, high-dose (up to 4 g daily in divided doses) oral supplementation have been found. Niacinamide will not cause flushing and does not normally lower blood lipid levels.

X. SUMMARY

Although B vitamins have been known to be essential nutrients since the 1920s to 1950s, specific trials with doses sufficient to affect functional status in humans during healing processes are relatively scarce compared to other lines of research for B vitamins. The large-scale use of multivitamin supplements by the U.S. population may decrease incentive for further study. Nevertheless, an increasing number of studies illustrates that high but safe doses of single B vitamins or combinations have clinical efficacy for musculoskeletal healing of certain conditions. It is also disappointing to notice clinical trials that find significant benefits and request further trials, but none appear. This is particularly true for niacinamide and pantothenate, which have shown promising effects postsurgery and in arthritis patients that have not been repeated or confirmed. Almost no studies on effects of biotin or folate on connective tissue healing can be found, unless the connection between folate and homocystinemia is considered. In short, there is an unusual paucity of information on safe, high-dose B vitamin administration for connective tissue healing. Except where noted, toxicities of B vitamins are almost nonexistent; therefore, sufficient impetus for clinical trials is apparent.

The B vitamins thiamin and pantothenate in particular may eventually be shown to have enhancing properties for healing. The question of local functional deficiencies of these two B vitamins in wounds, joints, or cartilage during periods of healing, when intense demands for energy and protein synthesis are required, has not been adequately studied. Because of their importance for production of cellular energy, and suggestive animal and human studies, thiamin and pantothenate appear to be promising enhancers of healing. Interestingly, these two B vitamins also have some evidence of ergogenic effects in athletes, definitely an energy-intensive process.[248,249]

The consistency of vitamin B_6 effects on carpal tunnel syndrome has not been expanded to other potential uses, such as osteoarthritis, osteoporosis, or fracture repair. Effects on chronic pain via serotoninergic mechanisms is another field of study with possible merits. Coadministration of B vitamins with other nutrients (such as amino acids or minerals) may prove to be even more effective.

Further work is needed on effects of short-term and long-term effects of oral B vitamin supplementation on pain and interactions with analgesics. Suggestive evidence indicated that vitamin B_6 or vitamin B_{12} may enhance effects of current NSAIDs. This opens another realm of study for B vitamins and healing — as adjuncts, rather than alternatives, to accepted drug therapies.

XI. GUIDELINES FOR USE

Table 6 lists some guidelines for use of B vitamins in injury rehabilitation and healing. When possible, a mixture of B vitamins has been listed instead of one or more single B vitamins. This is to insure adequacy of all B vitamins, and also because there are many combinations of B vitamins that are commercially available. The most striking uses of B vitamins appear to be niacinamide for osteoarthritis and pyridoxine (with riboflavin) for carpal tunnel syndrome and, thus, other fascia and joint inflammations.

TABLE 6 Guidelines for Use of B Vitamins for Injury Rehabilitation and Sports Medicine

		Condition			
B Vitamin (Daily Dose in mg)	General Trauma, Surgery, Fractures	Degenerative Joint Conditions (OA, TMJ, Invertebral Disc Conditions, etc.)	Connective Tissue Inflammations (Carpal Tunnel Syndrome, Bursitis, Tendinitis, etc.)	Autoimmune Joint Conditions (RA, etc.)	Chronic Musculoskeletal Pain
Thiamin hydrochloride	100–2000	100–2000	1000	100	1000–4000
Riboflavin	50	50	50	50	50
Niacinamide	20-100	250 mg every 3-4 h (see Table 5)	20-100	20-100	20-100
Pyridoxine hydrochloride	50	50	100	50	100-150
Cyanocobalamin	0.1	0.1	0.1	0.1	0.1–1.0
Folate	0.4–0.8	0.4–0.8	2-5	2-5	0.4
Pantothenate	1000	1000	1000	2000	1000
Biotin	0.1–1.0	0.1–1.0	0.1–1.0	0.1–1.0	0.1–1.0

Chapter 7

VITAMIN C (ASCORBIC ACID)

I. INTRODUCTION

Few single nutrients have attracted as much popular attention as vitamin C (ascorbic acid). Vitamin C is the generic term for L-ascorbic acid and its close molecular relatives. Ascorbate is a reducing, 6-carbon sugar (hexose derivative) with many specific and nonspecific functions. Biological activity is exhibited by L-ascorbate and dehydroascorbate, since dehydroascorbate can be reduced back to ascorbate.[673] L-Ascorbate can be oxidized to the monodehydroascorbate free radical, which quickly dismutes or is converted to dehydroascorbate. However, upon exposure to oxygen or heavy metals, especially under alkaline conditions, dehydroascorbate is converted to diketogulonic acid (dioxogulonate). Diketogulonate has no biological vitamin C activity and its formation represents an irreversible loss of ascorbate; hence, the reason the essentiality of vitamin C. Erythorbate (D-iso-ascorbate) exhibits about 5% of ascorbate biological activity, but is an equally effective antioxidant as ascorbate *in vitro*.[673] Erythorbate, which does not occur naturally, is in large-scale use as a food preservative, meaning many persons have a significant intake.

Since vitamin C is an essential dietary component only for humans, primates, guinea pigs, fruit bats, some birds, most fish, insects, and invertebrates, most lab animals are inadequate for comparative studies of ascorbate. Thus, most animal experiments with ascorbate have utilized guinea pigs.

II. ROLES AND FUNCTIONS

Table 1 lists some of the more pertinent roles and functions of ascorbate for connective tissue healing.[93,94,163,164,170,179,439,485,673-679] The major role of ascorbate in connective tissues is in activation of α-ketoglutarate linked, iron-containing hydroxylases (prolyl hydroxylases and lysyl hydroxylases). These enzymes are critical for proper posttranscriptional modification of collagen chains by formation of hydroxyproline and hydroxylysine residues. These modified amino acids confer shape and biological function for collagens throughout the body, which are the major component of connective tissues, and essential for repair and healing processes to occur. Ascorbate is also a direct antioxidant and can "recharge" other antioxidants, especially tocopherol. Thus, ascorbate may play protective roles during expression of free radicals in pain and inflammation. Ascorbate is a potent reducing agent or oxidizing agent, depending upon conditions, and can participate in a nonspecific manner in many enzymatic reactions. Ascorbate appears to have noncofactor effects on regulation of collagen gene transcription. This means that ascorbate is more than a simple redox compound. Most of the functions of ascorbate are directly applicable to the health of connective tissues and their responses to injury.

III. DEFICIENCY SYMPTOMS

The classical deficiency disease of ascorbate lack is scurvy.[93,94,163,164,170,179,439,485,673-679] Scurvy exhibits severe disruption of connective tissues because newly formed collagen and tissues are not structurally sound. Table 2 lists known symptoms of ascorbate deficiency. Scurvy exhibits the most extreme ascorbate deficiency symptoms, but some symptoms may manifest before outright scurvy

TABLE 1   Ascorbate Functions Pertinent to Connective Tissue Healing

1. Specific cofactor for α-ketoglutarate-linked, iron-containing hydroxylases
   - Cofactor for prolyl hydroxylase (modifies collagen, elastin, and osteocalcin proteins)
   - Cofactor for lysyl hydroxylase (modifies collagen)
   - Carnitine synthesis
   - Complement C1q modification
   - Protein C modification (involved in blood clotting)
2. Nonspecific reducing agent
   - Stimulates activity of many enzymes
   - Preserves enzyme-iron or enzyme-manganese complexes in reduced, active state
   - Maintains iron in reduced state on transport and storage proteins
   - Increases iron and manganese mobilization from food and intestinal tract
3. Electron donor for some reactions
   - Steroid hormone synthesis
4. Direct antioxidant
   - Quenching of superoxide, singlet oxygen, hydroxy radical, free radicals
   - Protection of retinoids, carotenoids, tocopherols, B complex vitamins, lipids
5. Direct stimulation of collagen synthesis by gene regulation
   - Regulates formation and maintenance of collagen and intercellular matrix
6. Specific cofactor for copper-containing hydroxylases (catecholamine synthesis, pituitary peptide hormone amidation)
7. Immune system effects (immunostimulatory)
8. Reduces prostaglandin F_2 (antiinflammatory effects)
9. Involved in nonenzymatic histamine degradation (with oxygen and copper)
10. Detoxification of toxic heavy metals and xenobiotics
11. Stimulates fibroblast growth and matrix production *in vitro*
12. Stimulates chondrocyte anabolism *in vitro*
13. Stimulates proteoglycan and collagen production of chondrocytes *in vitro*

TABLE 2   Ascorbate Deficiency Symptoms on Human Connective Tissues

- Skin, gum, bone lesions
- Impaired wound healing (by 50%, decreased wound strength, collagen formation, lack of scar formation)
- Polysomes in fibroblasts not formed
- Petechiae and hemorrhages, capillary fragility
- Joint pain and effusions
- Edema
- Anemia (usually iron-deficient, but folate-deficient may overlap)
- Bone pain and osteopenia
- Bilateral femoral neuropathy
- Muscle weakness
- Fatigue and lassitude
- Depressed fibroblast functions
- Decreased hydroxylation of lysine and proline
- Decreased resistance to infection
- Impaired wound neovascularization
- Elevated plasma histamine (proinflammatory, vasodilatory)
- Increased membrane lipid peroxidation
- "Biochemical" scurvy temporarily induced by severe injury

(especially fatigue). Interestingly, minimal body stores of ascorbate were sufficient to heal small, simple, uncomplicated wounds at a slower than normal rate in humans.[678]

Biochemical scurvy is a term that refers to observations of reduced serum and urinary levels of ascorbate after trauma, injury, surgery, burns, or other major stressors.[604,605,673] The clinical significance of biochemical scurvy is not clear, but appears to have some short-term detriments for healing processes.

IV. ASSESSMENT

The most common method of assessment of ascorbate status is serum, whole blood, urine, or leukocyte ascorbate levels.[673-676] Plasma or serum ascorbate levels below 0.2 to 0.3 mg/dl (<17 mM) are indicative of deficient status. Leukocyte ascorbate levels <8.2 pmol/10^6 cells (<0.5 µg/10^6 cells) also signify deficient tissue stores. Knowing the differential count of leukocytes is essential, since different white blood cell types exhibit different ascorbate levels. Urinary hydroxyproline levels have been advocated as a functional measure of ascorbate status, since hydroxyproline formation is dependent upon ascorbate status. However, many diseases and conditions can influence urinary hydroxyproline levels independent of ascorbate status. Determination of the total body pool of ascorbate and fractional rate of loss is a research methodology that is not practical for routine use. Finally, a very simple and practical assay, lingual decolorization time of 2,6-dichlorodiphenol is subject to many interferences, and results must be interpreted with caution. An overview of assessments for ascorbate status reveals that serum or leukocyte ascorbate is useful for finding severe deficiencies. However, a test for status of ascorbate function has not been adequately developed. Thus, the testing for ascorbate status is less than ideal at this time. Again, a clinical trial of ascorbate supplementation is less expensive and may have potential clinical benefits compared to testing for ascorbate status.

Ascorbate intake can interfere with other diagnostic tests. High intakes (over 100 mg/d) can inhibit glucose oxidase methodology on urine dipsticks, preventing detection of urinary glucose.[673-677] Conversely, ascorbate intake can cause artificial positive values for urine-reducing sugars by the alkaline copper method (which is used only infrequently). Tests for fecal occult blood as a screen for colorectal cancer are blocked by ascorbate when blood is present.

V. INTAKES

The dietary requirement for ascorbate in humans ranges from 30 to 80 mg daily, depending upon what endpoints are being considered.[673-677] The lower dose of 30 mg daily is to prevent scurvy and prevent impairment of wound healing, with a reasonable (3 to 4 month) buffer if ascorbate intake drops to zero. The higher figure of 80 mg is to account for lifestyle variables such as smoking or drug intakes that are known to adversely affect status of ascorbate. Only a small percentage of ascorbate intakes in the U.S. is below 70% of the RDA of 60 mg/d.[439,673-677] Thus, frank deficiencies of ascorbate are uncommon in the U.S. in general, although certain population groups may be at increased risk for deficient intake or status (biochemical scurvy?). Average intakes are insufficient to saturate tissues with ascorbate, which may play a role in possible enhancement of healing. Table 3 lists groups at increased risk for ascorbate deficiency via intake or other causes.

VI. DIETARY SOURCES AND INFLUENCES

The richest dietary sources of ascorbate are fresh fruits and vegetables.[763-767] Since vitamin C is labile to heat, storage, cooking, and processing, plant foods must be eaten fresh to ensure adequate intake of ascorbate from foods. Citrus fruits, acerola cherries, and rose hips in particular are rich dietary sources of ascorbate. Another problem with ascorbate intake is the large variability of ascorbate content between separate pieces of fruit or vegetables. Therefore, even eating two to three servings of fresh citrus fruits daily is not a guarantee of obtaining adequate dietary intake of ascorbate.

Ingestion of high doses of aspirin, corticosteroids, tetracyclines, or oral contraceptives was associated with reduced serum and/or leukocyte levels of ascorbate.[679] Supplementation with 1 g or more of ascorbate daily was required to bring depressed tissue levels of ascorbate into reference ranges for each group.[679]

TABLE 3   **Factors Contributing to Risk
for Ascorbate Deficiency**

Inadequate food intake (anorexics, elderly, dieters, invalids)
Malabsorption syndromes
Moderate to severe physical injury or emotional stress
Pregnancy and lactation
Smoking tobacco products
Obesity and indolence
Alcoholics
Rheumatoid arthritis
Kidney dialysis (hemodialysis and peritoneal dialysis)
Diabetes
Oral contraceptives
Salicylates
Corticosteroids
Tetracycline

VII. HUMAN STUDIES

A. SURGERY AND WOUND HEALING

The use of ascorbate for human healing conditions dates back to the 1940s. During World War II, the population of Great Britain was subjected to rationing of fresh foods and to bombing which produced a large number of surgical cases in persons with marginal or deficient ascorbate intake.[680] At St. Bartholomew's Hospital in London, routine use of 1000 mg/d ascorbic acid for 3 d before surgery was made, followed by 100 mg/d of ascorbic acid.[680] Wound disruption was decreased 76% after ascorbate was supplemented to surgical patients. Experimental and clinical ascorbate depletion in human subjects found a 50 to 60% decrease in wound strength.[678-687] When leukocyte ascorbate levels decreased by 50% or more, there was an eight times higher incidence of wound dehiscence.[685] Similar findings when serum ascorbate dropped below 0.2 mg/dl were reported by Bartlett.[683] Also, surgery itself decreased both serum and leukocyte ascorbate levels by 50%.[675] Thus, there is biochemical rationale for repletion of vitamin C to postsurgical patients.

Repletion of volunteers made scorbutic by lack of dietary ascorbate intake with 4, 8, 16, or 32 mg/d of ascorbate did not find any differences between doses for effects on wound healing.[686] Supplementation with 100, 300, 700, or 1100 mg/d of ascorbate to humans with adequate vitamin C intake and status found that experimental wounds were equally strong at all doses.[683] However, when surgical patients were repleted with 1000 mg ascorbate/d, a 3- to 6-fold increase in wound strength was found, compared to no increases after 100 mg/d.[683] Similarly, a decrease in serum ascorbate between days 6 to 9 postsurgery was found in patients supplemented with 500 mg ascorbate daily.[688] In patients that were not supplemented with ascorbate, serum levels decreased sooner, greater, and longer than supplemented patients. All 82 patients with complicated cholecystectomy in Russia exhibited low serum levels of ascorbate in one study.[689] In 50 patients given intravenous ascorbate (200 to 250 mg/d), the serum levels were normalized by day 6 postsurgery, and patients were discharged 1 to 2 d earlier than nonsupplemented patients (whose serum ascorbate never returned to normal).

A classic study by Ringsdorf and Cheraskin studied the effects of ascorbate supplementation in wound healing of normal, healthy males.[690] Two healthy dental students consuming a diet adequate in vitamin C were given a standardized gingival surgical lesion, and the time to complete closure (healing) was measured. The subjects then received 1 or 2 g daily of vitamin C after similar surgical lesions. Both doses of ascorbate led to significantly reduced healing times (10 or 9 vs. 18 d). Thus, supplementation with large doses of ascorbate (1 to 2 g/d) was associated with enhancement of small wound healing by 40 to 50%.

Many other studies on the effects of ascorbate supplementation on periodontal disease (gingival inflammation) can be found. A thesis by Mallek reported that supplementation with 1 g/d of ascorbate to 11 healthy subjects with slight to little periodontal disease increased gingival ascorbate concentration 3-fold.[691] Decreased tissue permeability and increased collagen synthesis of gingival cultures was found after ascorbate supplementation. Serum and leukocyte levels of ascorbate did not correlate with gingival levels and did not correlate with intake of ascorbate. Another study administered 1 g ascorbate daily to 10 healthy subjects for 7 weeks.[692] No difference in periodontal status was found. A review of 11 studies on ascorbate administration and periodontal conditions also found that plaque formation was not altered by ascorbate, and 5/6 studies found decreased gingival inflammation and reduced gingival permeability at doses of 1 g/d of ascorbate.[179] Another study measured the effect of experimental vitamin C deficiency (5 mg ascorbate per d), followed by vitamin C adequacy (65 mg/d), followed by high doses of vitamin C (605 mg/d).[693,694] Upon probing, the deficient ascorbate intake resulted in bleeding gums and inflammation. Adequate doses of ascorbate reduced bleeding and inflammation, but not completely. High doses of ascorbate almost completely eliminated bleeding and inflammation. Thus, ascorbate induced healthier gingival tissue in a dose-dependent manner. As with other studies, doses needed to be >600 mg/d to find clinical benefits. Another report found that gingival hydroxyproline and proline synthesis was increased after 100 mg ascorbate was given daily to subjects with marginal vitamin C status.[695]

In the only study that reached bowel tolerance doses of ascorbate, Lytle found clinical benefits in reduction of chronic pain in 21 subjects with sensitive gums.[696] Bowel tolerance was reached by ingesting 1 tsp of sodium ascorbate (2.4 g) every 15 min until watery diarrhea was reached (do not stop at mere rumbling, auscultations, or flatus). This amount for each patient was recorded, and 1 tsp less than that amount was ingested on day 2 in divided doses. Ascorbate dose was reduced by 1 tsp each day. Ascorbate administration was for 4 d. The median intake of ascorbate for bowel tolerance was 19 g (9 to 47 g or 4 to 20 tsp). After retesting, 10/21 patients were completely free from sensitivity, 9/21 were improved, and only 2/21 patients were unchanged.

This study is important because it is the only one to reach true bowel tolerance of ascorbate, which is the maximum tolerated dose, as opposed to tissue saturation by about 100 mg ascorbate daily. It is not well known that at intakes over 100 mg ascorbate per day, tissue levels do not rise further. Rather, intercellular fluids (plasma, connective tissue fluids, vitreous humor) exhibit further increases in ascorbate concentration.[673] Serum concentration is limited by removal of ascorbate by the kidney. Therefore, other fluids (intercellular) are able to reach higher levels of ascorbate after large oral doses. Bowel tolerance doses are thought to saturate both tissues and extracellular fluids. Thus, results in only 4 d (relief of pain) may be quite possible when maximum doses of ascorbate are reached. These doses have not been systematically studied on other models of human healing, and such studies would be difficult to perform in a double-blind manner. Nevertheless, preliminary research indicates that maximum doses of ascorbate deserve further scrutiny.

Experiments on wound healing and surgery in humans points to several consistent conclusions. First, either surgery itself, or preceding health conditions leading to surgical intervention, decreases ascorbate status in the short term (biochemical scurvy). Second, deficiency of ascorbate can adversely affect wound healing and strength. Third, supplementation of surgical patients or healthy subjects with 1 g ascorbate or more per day results in enhancement of healing for minor wounds, improved ascorbate status, reduced inflammation, and improved recovery. Fourth, either a dose-response or threshold of effect may be apparent for ascorbate. Thus, it seems prudent to administer at least 1 g daily to surgical patients (regardless of prior ascorbate status) before, during, and after surgery.

B. SKIN ULCERS

Four studies have found enhanced healing in various types of skin ulcers. Hunter and Rajan found that administration of 1 g/d of ascorbate for 5 to 6 d to paraplegics with pressure sores resulted in a significant increase in ulcer collagen synthesis.[697] In a series of 99 paraplegics, Burr and Rajan found that 23% exhibited low leukocyte ascorbate levels.[698] Compared to unsupplemented controls, addition of 1 g/d of ascorbate for 3 d resulted in significant collagen synthesis in ulcers. Afifi and others conducted a double-blind, placebo-controlled crossover study in 8 patients with thalassemia leg ulcers of 2 to 4 year duration.[699] Administration of 3 g daily (in 3 doses) for 8 weeks resulted in complete healing in 7/14 ulcers and partial healing in 5/14. In the placebo group, only 4/12 ulcers showed partial healing. After crossover, 4 patients switched from ascorbate to placebo saw complete healing, while 9/12 former placebo subjects were totally healed. Thus, ascorbate was associated with healing responses not previously seen by other methods in leg ulcers in thalassemia patients. Taylor and colleagues studied the effects of ascorbate on pressure sores in 20 subjects.[700] While ten subjects received placebo, another 10 received 1 g/d of ascorbate for 4 weeks. An 85% reduction in ulcer size (healing rate 2.47 cm^2/week) was seen in ascorbate-supplemented subjects, while placebo subjects showed a 43% reduction in ulcer size (healing rate 1.45 cm^2/week). The placebo group exhibited the following reductions (%) in ulcer area: 4, 14, 22, 39, 45, 50, 54, 60, 60, and 80; the ascorbate group exhibited reductions (%) of 21, 72, 81, 87, 87, 90, 100, 100, 100, and 100, a highly significant difference. Thus, doses of ascorbate at 1 g or more daily were associated with enhanced healing of skin ulcers from various causes.

C. DEGENERATIVE JOINT DISEASES

While the study of ascorbate on wound healing and surgery has enjoyed research interest for over five decades, the study of ascorbate effects on degenerative joint diseases is virtually nil. Even though a substantial amount of *in vitro* work has found that ascorbate stimulates collagen and proteoglycan synthesis of chondrocyte cultures in a dose-dependent manner, and stimulates transcription of collagen genes,[93,94,673-679] there are no controlled studies of ascorbate supplementation in human degenerative joint disease. Anecdotal case reports by Greenwood on himself and his patients suggested that daily oral doses of 1 to 4 g ascorbate for long time periods were safe, and reduced symptoms in a majority of patients.[701] Unfortunately, no objective data was presented. Likewise, a review of therapeutic effects of vitamin C suggested a "possible therapeutic potential of vitamin C in the management of back pain as it relates to degenerative disc disease." [702] Another case study by Biskind and Martin described the influence of ascorbate and bioflavonoid supplementation on a severe case of subpatellar bursitis.[703] A 38-year-old male presented with severe pain, tenderness, swelling, heat, and limited mobility from severe subpatellar bursitis. After initiating therapy with vitamin C and bioflavonoids every 4 h, swelling and pain were significantly reduced by 24 h and almost completely normal by 72 h.

Animal research in beagles[704] and guinea pigs[522] showed that additional dietary ascorbate in excess of adequate amounts (150 mg/d instead of 2 to 4 mg/d required for prevention of scurvy in guinea pigs) led to greatly reduced symptoms and anatomical findings of osteoarthritis in supplemented animals.

It is known that ascorbate levels in serum and leukocytes are significantly reduced in rheumatoid arthritis patients by a combination of inflammatory and pharmacological effects.[439] A single report used the controversial lingual test for ascorbate status and found that 76% of patients with neuromusculoskeletal disorders exhibited ascorbate deficiencies.[705] Thus, there is some evidence to suggest that ascorbate status is not adequate in humans with degenerative joint diseases.

It is difficult to understand the lack of studies on ascorbate effects on osteoarthritis and other degenerative joint diseases in humans. Ascorbate is inexpensive, well tolerated, has biochemical rationale, *in vitro* supportive evidence, and animal supportive evidence. Based on animal and *in vitro* findings, ascorbate can be considered as a chondroprotective agent, similar to vitamin E and other substances to be discussed later in this book. Studies on the effects of large oral doses of ascorbate (at least 1 g/d and preferably over 4 g/d) for effects on degenerative joint diseases are a gaping hole in both musculoskeletal and nutritional research knowledge.

VIII. SAFETY

The results of recent studies have clarified the safety of ascorbate supplementation in humans.[673-675] An acceptable daily intake (ADI) with no risk of harm for long-term ingestion is 1050 mg/70 kg/d, as determined by the Joint Expert Committee on Food Additives of the FAO/WHO.[675] Consensus of recent reviews has found excellent safety from 1 to 5 g/d administered in divided doses. Even doses of 10 g ascorbate daily are not considered to be a serious health risk for humans. Previously, high doses of ascorbate were hypothesized to increase formation of oxalate stones in urine, destroy vitamin B_{12} in the gut, increase urine urate levels, increase toxicity of iron, increase mutagenicity, and induce rebound scurvy. There has been no human clinical evidence supporting these hypotheses, as determined by recent studies which have specifically addressed these concerns.[673-675] The only practical safety concerns for ascorbate are gastrointestinal distress and diarrhea (osmotic) from very large single doses (ranges from 2 to 20 g among individuals) or very large daily doses (over 10 g daily). A possible concern is the coadministration of large doses of ascorbate with aluminum-containing products (antacids) in renal failure, since ascorbate may enhance intestinal uptake of aluminum, which is nephrotoxic.[674] Otherwise, daily doses of 1 to 5 g of ascorbate should be considered for future clinical trials.

IX. SUMMARY

Long-term administration of ascorbate is associated with safety and possibly with protective effects on cancer and cardiovascular diseases which have not been considered here.[8,673-677] With regards to musculoskeletal healing, the use of ascorbate has not kept up with its scientific and public popularity. Potential benefits for reducing length of stay in hospitalized surgical patients should be studied more closely at this time of intense focus on health care costs and outcomes. From the available data, supplementation with at least 1 g daily of ascorbate appears to be helpful for skin wounds or ulcers. The application of ascorbate to degenerative joint disease is supported by all lines of research except controlled human studies. Given the benefits shown in other types of healing, and the known safety, availability and inexpensiveness of ascorbate argues strongly in favor of inclusion for nutritional support of joint conditions.

One factor not considered in great detail is that various forms of ascorbate are available commercially. Vitamin C is available as ascorbic acid, sodium ascorbate, calcium ascorbate, mixtures of other minerals with ascorbates (zinc, magnesium, manganese, copper, iron), esterified ascorbate (polymers of calcium ascorbate), and any conceivable combination of the above forms. Thus, it is possible to coadminister essential minerals along with ascorbate. Mineral ascorbates are thought to provide a buffering capacity to reduce acidity of ascorbate and, thus, reduce potential gastrointestinal distress from large doses of ascorbate. The forms of tablets, capsules, powders, and effervescent products added to foods mean that ascorbate supplementation is quite flexible.

Ascorbate is safe, plentiful, readily available, inexpensive, and documented to exhibit some moderate benefits for connective tissue protection or healing. The lack of human trials of ascorbate for degenerative joint diseases is deplorable. The use of large doses of ascorbate in clinical practice for possible enhancement of connective tissue healing is justified, based on current research.

X. GUIDELINES FOR USE

Table 4 lists some clinical applications for ascorbate supplementation during injury rehabilitation and musculoskeletal damage. Daily doses of 1 g can be initiated in almost every person and maintained for long time periods. If desired, increases in dosage to 4 to 5 g daily (in divided doses) can be administered during periods of additional stress. The use of bowel tolerance ascorbate doses is not recommended for routine practice since considerable expertise and practice is necessary to monitor patient compliance. The long-term effects of bowel tolerance doses are not well known. In short, although relatively few specific studies of ascorbate supplementation for specific musculoskeletal conditions are available, the known mechanisms, pharmacokinetics, and results from clinical trials suggest that the use of ascorbate can be expanded into many healing conditions.

TABLE 4   Guidelines for Use of Ascorbate in Musculoskeletal Healing

Daily Doses

500–1000 mg 2–4 times daily as ascorbic acid, sodium ascorbate, calcium ascorbate, or
  mixed ascorbates

Conditions

Documented Need or Benefits
  Surgery
  Skin damage (ulcers, burns, lacerations, abrasions)
  Periodontal inflammation or disease
Speculative Need or Benefits
  Degenerative joint conditions (osteoarthritis, invertebral disc degeneration,
    temporomandibular joint syndrome, bursitis, tendinitis, tenosynovitis)
  Joint inflammation (rheumatoid arthritis, spondylitis, joint surgery)
  Chronic musculoskeletal pain (low back pain, joint pain, stress fractures)
  Sports injuries (sprains, strains, bruises, hematomas, contusions, ligament tears)

Chapter 8

CALCIUM AND MAGNESIUM

I. CALCIUM

A. ROLES AND FUNCTIONS

The average adult human contains 20 to 25 g of calcium per kilogram of body weight, or 1 to 1.5 kg calcium. Calcium is the most abundant cation in the body, and the fifth most common inorganic element in humans. Over 99% of body calcium resides in the skeleton (bone) as an insoluble, hydroxyapatite-like crystalline structure deposited on an organic osteoid matrix. The remaining 1% of body calcium is solubilized in plasma, body fluids, and cells. Soluble calcium is an essential control and signaling mechanism for many biological activities, listed in Table 1. The regulatory roles of calcium are so vital to health and life that plasma calcium levels are carefully maintained at near 2.5 mM (10 mg/dl), even at the expense of the skeleton. Calcium in plasma and bone is in rapid equilibrium in order to ensure a steady level of soluble calcium. Plasma calcium is either bound to protein (40%), mostly on albumin, or is free, ionic calcium (35%), which possesses biological activity. The other plasma calcium is bound as organic complexes to simple molecules such as citrate. The intracellular environment is almost calcium-free, with concentrations 1,000 to 10,000 times lower than plasma. This concentration gradient is used to advantage by cells to maintain regulatory roles of calcium.

Many excellent reviews have been written describing the roles and functions of calcium in general.[170,705,706] There are so many vital functions of calcium that it is easier to find physiological processes that are not affected by calcium. This chapter is intended to give an overview of calcium effects on musculoskeletal healing pertinent to injury rehabilitation and sports medicine. Thus, the focus will not be on postmenopausal osteoporosis, for which a huge literature has accumulated. Rather, the focus will be on effects of calcium supplementation on bone loss in athletic amenorrhea. For reviews on bone mass, osteoporosis, and health, the reader is referred to a few of the many excellent reviews.[705-711]

B. DEFICIENCY SYMPTOMS

Deficiency symptoms of calcium can be divided into two basic categories: acute and chronic. Acute calcium deficiencies may arise from excessive sweating during heavy exercise.[712] Muscle cramps result from altered neuromuscular functions from lack of calcium homeostasis. Intake of calcium-containing electrolyte beverages can quickly correct sweat-induced muscle cramps when calcium loss is the culprit. Usually, sodium, potassium, and magnesium are more important for causing muscle cramps by depletion.

Chronic deficiency of calcium leads primarily to bone loss (osteoporosis).[705-711] While many factors affect bone mass, calcium deficiency is definitely associated with progressive bone loss that is responsive to calcium supplementation. The long-term effects of osteoporosis are usually not seen until later in adult life (over 60 years of age). However, athletic amenorrhea is usually associated with osteoporosis at young ages and will be discussed later in this section.

C. ASSESSMENT

Routine outpatient assessment of calcium status is difficult. Calcium levels are maintained at the expense of skeletal reserves of calcium, so serum, plasma, and, usually, urinary calcium levels are not helpful indicators of calcium status. Rather, calcium status is most often determined by other factors that

TABLE 1   Roles for Soluble Calcium

Muscle contraction
Nerve impulse conduction
Synaptic transmission
Hormone actions
Gastric and digestive secretion
Blood coagulation
Cellular adhesiveness
Cell membrane maintenance and function
Enzyme activities
Buffer for acidosis

regulate calcium absorption, metabolism, and excretion. Current tests available on an outpatient basis include whole blood calcium level, blood cell calcium levels, serum vitamin D measurements (1,25OHD), urine γ-carboxyglutamic acid levels, parathyroid hormone (including C- and N-terminal portions), serum ionized calcium levels, urine calcium levels, hair calcium levels, bone mineral density, X-ray spectral analysis of buccal cells, and lymphocyte growth responses.[600,705,713] No single determination is a valid indicator in all circumstances. Rather, a combination of several tests can give a picture of calcium status. As with other nutrients, it may be more clinically efficient and practical to initiate a trial of calcium supplementation and note clinical responses.

D. INTAKES

This section will focus on calcium intakes of athletes. In general, calcium intakes of male athletes are usually adequate (according to the RDA) unless total food intake is lowered during periods of weight loss.[191] However, calcium intakes of females athletes in general frequently showed deficient intakes.[191,714-719] Furthermore, calcium intakes of female amenorrheic athletes, or in groups of female athletes with high prevalence of amenorrhea (dancers, gymnasts, long-distance runners), have shown frequent deficiencies.[191,715,720-730] Calcium intake is a definite concern of most females athletes, especially thinner athletes (ballet dancers, dancers, majorettes, gymnasts, long-distance runners, some bodybuilders).

It is acknowledged that intake of calcium in younger persons (adolescents and adults less than 30 years old) has become a major health issue, since it is now clear that peak bone mass is attained before age 25 to 30. Peak bone mass is important because of the almost obligatory bone loss which occurs later in life, especially significant in women. Thus, attention to calcium intake in adolescent and young adult years is of particular importance.

E. DIETARY SOURCES AND INFLUENCES

Food sources richest in calcium are calcium supplements; bone meal; egg shells; multiple vitamin/mineral products with calcium; milk and milk products; dairy products (yogurt, cheese, ice cream); canned salmon, sardines, or anchovies with bones; tofu; green leafy vegetables, and fortified foods. Perhaps of equal or more importance than dietary intake of calcium are the factors that influence calcium uptake and absorption. Table 2 lists some dietary factors that either enhance or diminish calcium absorption, as well as other nondietary factors that alter calcium excretion or metabolism to produce a deficient state or increased dietary requirement.[402,705]

F. HUMAN STUDIES
1. Bone Loss and Athletic Amenorrhea

Perhaps the most prevalent aspect of calcium and healing in sports medicine is bone loss associated with amenorrhea. Athletic amenorrhea is the absence of menstrual cycles or periods (no more than one period in the last 6 months).[731] Incidence of athletic amenorrhea ranges from 7 to 71%, depending upon the group studied.[731,732] Athletic amenorrhea is classified as secondary amenorrhea, meaning menstrual

TABLE 2 Dietary and Other Factors Influencing Calcium Uptake and Status

Dietary Factors

Enhance Uptake	Inhibit Uptake
Lysine	High fatty acid (fat) content
Arginine	High oxalate foods (cocoa, soybeans, kale, spinach, rhubarb)
Vitamin D	High phosphate foods (unpolished rice, wheat meal, bran)
Lactose	High phytate foods (whole grains)
Glucose polymers	High fiber intakes
	Alkali ingestion (antacids)
	Vitamin D deficiency
	Magnesium deficiency
	Chronic ingestion of aluminum hydroxide phosphate-binding gels
	Protein-rich diets (enhance excretion)
	High sodium diets (increase excretion)
	Magnesium-rich diets (enhance excretion)

Nondietary Factors

Enhance Status	Inhibit Status
Ultraviolet light exposure	Increased gut transit time
Younger age	Stress
Males	Cortisol and corticosteroids
Androgens	Cushing's Disease
Some antibiotics (penicillin, neomycin)	Immobilization
	Anticonvulsants
	Thyroid hormones and hyperthyroidism
	Older ages
	Long-term thiazide diuretics
	Growth hormone excess and acromegaly
	Estrogen loss
	Metabolic acidosis
	Achlorhydria, hypochlorhydria
	Hyperparathyroidism
	Sarcoidosis, metastatic bone disease
	Familial hypercalciuria

cycles were existent, but a secondary situation (exercise?) precipitated loss of cycles. Primary amenorrhea means no menstrual periods have occurred.

Low body fat percentage, training, age of menarche, and hormonal responses were not predictive factors for athletic amenorrhea.[731] However, athletic amenorrhea has been linked to major affective disorders manifested as eating disorders and compulsive behavior about foods, training, and thinness.[731,733-735] Compulsive behavior leads to decreased food intake (fewer total calories and less energy),[731,733,736-739] lower fat intakes,[727,737] and a higher rate of strict vegetarianism.[731,739] A low-calorie vegan diet has been associated with higher incidence of amenorrhea and reduced levels of reproductive hormones in sedentary and athletic females.[731]

Athletic amenorrhea is associated with bone loss, especially lumber spine bone loss.[731,735,737,740] Female amenorrheic athletes with chronological ages in the 20s frequently exhibited lumbar bone age of women in their 50s.[735] Irregular menses during adolescence has been associated with lower peak bone mass formation in female athletes.[741] Amenorrhea can lead to osteoporosis in young female athletes.[740-742] Athletic amenorrhea has also been associated with increased incidence of stress fractures and scoliosis.[735,736,743,744]

Calcium intakes of female athletes in general and groups prone to amenorrhea in particular are apt to be low (see previous section on calcium intakes). Intake of other nutrients was often deficient. In combination with findings that deficient calcium intakes are a contributing factor to osteoporosis,[705-711] it appears that calcium intake in amenorrheic athletes needs special attention to prevent deficient intakes.

Since calcium supplementation alone has not been entirely successful for repletion of lost bone mass, other dietary factors must be necessary for proper calcium utilization.[745] Bone repletion (synthesis) can be thought of as a chain of events. Many links in the chain are nutrients. In addition to calcium, other nutrients are essential for proper osteoid formation and mineralization.[711,745] Therefore, if a chain is strengthened by calcium supplementation, a weak link in the form of inadequate magnesium, zinc, copper, manganese, boron, ascorbate, B vitamins, or energy can negate the beneficial effects of additional calcium. The dietary practices of amenorrheic athletes strongly indicate multiple deficiencies. Thus, calcium supplementation to prevent or reverse bone loss is but one important dietary factor in athletic osteoporosis.

At this time, there are no specific studies showing effects of calcium supplementation on osteoporosis of amenorrheic athletes. However, athletic amenorrhea is reversible, and bone mass may be returned towards or to normal in approximately 2 years after return of regular menses.[735]

G. SAFETY

In general, daily doses of 1000 to 2500 mg of calcium are safe for long-term administration. Exceptions are persons with renal disease, sarcoidosis, or persons prone to kidney stone formation. Milk-alkali syndrome is possible after consumption of two or more quarts of milk daily along with large amounts of calcium carbonate antacids. Calcium deposition in soft tissues and formation of kidney stones are symptoms of milk-alkali syndrome. Intakes of calcium greater than 2 to 4 g daily have the potential to depress uptake of magnesium, iron, zinc, manganese, and other minerals.

H. SUMMARY

Calcium is an essential nutrient that is strictly controlled and regulated by the body for its nonskeletal functions. Thus, frank calcium deficiencies (acute) are rare. During injury (even fractures), calcium can be mobilized from bone stores to maintain supply to injured tissues. Therefore, calcium supplementation to enhance healing of fractures has not met with success, nor have benefits for wound healing in surgical settings been found for calcium. The most common form of calcium deficiency is bone loss (osteoporosis), which may take years to develop and progress, even in young female athletes. Osteoporosis secondary to athletic amenorrhea appears to be the chief concern of calcium in sports medicine and should always be a concern to females regardless of age.

One confusing aspect of calcium supplementation is the ever-increasing number of chemical forms of calcium from which to choose. Calcium carbonate is the least expensive supplement, and appears to have equivalent absorption to other forms in normal, healthy young persons. Since calcium carbonate is 40% calcium by weight, the smallest tablets or smallest number of tablets can be given in the carbonate form. Taking calcium carbonate supplements with meals or orange juice enhances absorption. Calcium citrate and calcium citrate-malate are two other forms of calcium with improved absorption in several studies.[746-751] Calcium hydroxyapatite products have also become available recently. These products are equivalent to purified bone meal and represent another bioavailable form of calcium along with phosphate and other minerals found in bone. Bone meal (Ossopan®) will be discussed separately from calcium later in this section. Other acceptable forms of calcium supplements are calcium lactate and calcium gluconate. Calcium salts of tricarboxylic acid cycle intermediates have recently become available as a mixture. Calcium phosphates and calcium chloride are unacceptable forms of calcium supplementation. A more important aspect of calcium supplementation is the dissolution times of calcium supplement tablets. Personal experience has indicated that most calcium supplements exhibit very long dissolution times (unpublished data). If calcium products do not release their contents before transit past the duodenum and proximal ileum, then calcium absorption will not be complete. Anyone can test whether their calcium supplement dissolves adequately by placing the tablet in a glass of water with 1 tsp of vinegar, and gently stirring the tablet every 5 min. If the tablet has not started breaking up by 10 min, then it will not release its calcium at the sites of maximum absorption. Of course, this quandary can be avoided by chewing calcium tablets, which is not favorable for most persons. Also, effervescent tablets, chewable wafers or tablets, capsules, or powders will bypass potential problems with calcium supplement tablets.

I. GUIDELINES FOR USE OF CALCIUM

Calcium intake should be increased by dietary means first. The section on dietary sources lists foods richest in calcium — their consumption should be increased. However, dairy products (the richest source of dietary calcium) contain large amounts of phosphorus, which may defeat the effects of calcium over long time periods. Since milk and dairy products are less concentrated in other minerals (particularly magnesium) than calcium, a first attempt should be made to increase dietary calcium by nondairy means. If desired, calcium supplements can be added, and taken with each meal. Usually, doses of 500 mg of elemental calcium daily with a meal are sufficient to bolster calcium intake into the recommended intakes of 800 to 1200 mg/d. Calcium intake should be increased for cases of athletic amenorrhea and for adolescents with insufficient dietary intake of calcium (usually dancers, gymnasts, ice skaters, majorettes, or long-distance runners). Other persons exhibiting deficient dietary intake of calcium or bone loss regardless of cause should increase calcium intake.

II. BONE MEAL (OSSOPAN, MICROCRYSTALLINE HYDROXYAPATITE, MCHC)

A. INTRODUCTION

Common sense dictates that the chief source of calcium in primitive man's diet was probably bones from fish and other animals. Since bones have been a human dietary option for millennia, and a staple of carnivorous animals, it is not surprising to find that modern medicine has studied the effect of a diet enriched in bone on the health of damaged or diseased skeletal systems. Bones are a common byproduct of slaughterhouses, and it is relatively easy to collect and process bones into bone meal. One such product, named Ossopan®, from Robapharm, Switzerland, is derived from crushing of defatted, raw veal bones under cold temperatures to yield a form of bone meal sufficiently standardized to merit medical study. Ossopan has been administered as both powder and tablets. Presently, many similar products are available in the U.S. as dietary supplements.

Bone is a logical choice for a dietary form of calcium intake. Ossopan contains approximately 120 mg/g of calcium, 82 mg/g phosphorus, 215 mg/g collagen, 75 mg/g noncollagen proteins, fluoride (4 µg/g),[751] and other trace minerals normally found in bone.[752] Drivdahl and others, of the V. A. Medical Center and University of Washington, examined the effects of aqueous extracts of embryonic chick femorae and tibiae on *in vitro* bone cell growth.[753] Calvarial cells isolated from 17-d-old chick frontal and parietal bones were cultured in the presence of chick bone extracts and showed significant increases in bone dry weight, hydroxyproline incorporation (collagen synthesis), and thymidine incorporation (DNA synthesis). Effects were specific for calvarial cells and were not seen for cultures of liver, skin, or kidney cells. Effects were attributed to intact bone, and not marrow. Thus, embryonic bone contained a specific, mitogenic protein for stimulation of osteoblast activity.

Another effort to isolate bone-specific growth factors from Ossopan examined the effect of guanidine-Tris-EDTA extractable proteins from Ossopan on cultures of human bone cells (osteoblasts) isolated from the trabecular bone of femoral head samples taken from hip replacement surgery.[754] This study, from Stepan and others at Loma Linda University, found 36 mg of acid-soluble protein extractable from 1 g of Ossopan. The protein extract itself caused a large increase in human osteoblast DNA synthesis (up to 581%) and alkaline phosphatase activity (up to 178%), both markers for bone formation. In addition, measurable levels of IGF-I, IGF-II, TGF-β, and osteocalcin were found. These proteins are known bone growth factors. Table 3 illustrates the relative levels of these proteins in Ossopan and human bone.

**TABLE 3   Comparative Levels of Bone Growth
Factors in Bone Meal (Ossopan) and
Human Bone**

Growth Factor	Level (µg/g) Bone Meal (Ossopan)	Human Bone
IGF-I	0.20 ± 0.02	0.085
IGF-II	0.10 ± 0.01	1.26
TGF-β	0.025 ± 0.002	0.46
Osteocalcin	7.0 ± 0.7	

Adapted from Štěpán, J., Mohan, S., Jennings, J., Wergedal, J.,
Taylor, A., and Baylink, D., *Life Sci.,* 49, 79, 1991.

Note: IGF-I = insulin-like growth factor; IGF-II = insulin-like growth
factor II; TGF-β = transforming growth factor beta.

Thus, bone itself contains specific growth factors that are preserved in a commercial product (Ossopan). Is presence of these proteinaceous growth factors of practical significance when bone meal is given orally? Interestingly, TGF-β is activated by acid or proteolysis and stimulates differentiation of intestinal epithelial cells.[754] IGF-I has specific receptors on colonic epithelial cell membranes.[754] Thus, proteinaceous bone growth factors present in bone meal may exert a practical effect by indirectly improving intestinal absorption of calcium (from concomitant bone meal presence or other dietary sources). This concept is further supported by several studies, all showing increased absorption of calcium from Ossopan compared to synthetic, microcrystalline hydroxyapatite,[755,756] compared to calcium gluconate in elderly osteoporotic patients,[757] and compared to calcium gluconate in healthy males.[755,758] Furthermore, clinical results from oral administration of Ossopan or ashed Ossopan (organic matrix removed) showed that intact Ossopan produced significantly better clinical results (*vide infra*). Thus, many researchers feel that intact bone meal (Ossopan) offers more than minerals for nutriture of skeletal systems.

B. ANIMAL STUDIES

Early studies from Europe demonstrated that experimentally induced fractures in rats, rabbits, or dogs healed sooner after administration of Ossopan than after administration of bone ash or no treatment.[759-763] An example of animal results is the report of Annefeld and others, from the Department of Research and Development of Robapharm in Basel, Switzerland, and the Institute of Medical Statistics and Documentation, University of Mainz, Mainz, Germany.[764] Divided into 4 groups of 15 rabbits each, 60 rabbits were given a standardized bony defect in the distal femoral epiphysis. One group served as controls, one group received 830 mg/d of Ossopan (178 mg calcium/d), one group received 510 mg/d of bone mineral ash (179 mg calcium/d), and the last group received 650 mg/d of calcium carbonate (Os-Cal®) supplying 189 mg/d of calcium. Fluorescent bone markers were given to all animals during four different time periods, and animals were sacrificed on the 35th, 56th, and 84th postoperative days. Overall scores of bone healing were significantly increased in all calcium supplement groups compared to the control group; however, the Ossopan group was significantly increased compared to either bone mineral ash or calcium carbonate.[764] These results further suggest that Ossopan possesses more than just mineral content.

C. HUMAN STUDIES

1. Fracture Healing

Mills and others, of St. Boniface Hospital in Winnipeg, Manitoba, Canada, and British hospitals, reported on the administration of Ossopan (9 g/d) or placebo on time to union of tibial shaft fractures in 97 patients for 6 weeks.[751] In patients under 55 years, mean union time for Ossopan (11.5 weeks) did not differ from mean union time for placebo (12.5 weeks). In patients over 55 years, mean union time for Ossopan (11 weeks) was significantly less than the placebo group (14.2 weeks). Number of nonunion cases were Ossopan 3, placebo 9. Ossopan was also given to 28 patients with very delayed union after more complicated fractures of various long bones. After 12 weeks, 25/28 patients showed reunion of bones. Thus, Ossopan was shown to be helpful in cases of fracture in the elderly and in stubborn cases of nonunion. However, except in the more severe fractures, younger patients did not show a significant improvement following Ossopan supplementation.

2. Postmenopausal Osteoporosis

Durance and others, of King's College Hospital in London, England, divided 14 patients (58 to 88 years) with documented osteoporosis (severe pain, recent fractures, analgesic use, elevated urinary hydroxyproline excretion, increased plasma alkaline phosphatase activity) into 2 groups of 7 each.[765] One group was given 1500 mg of calcium per day from Ossopan, while the other group was given 1500 mg of calcium per day from ashed Ossopan (organic matrix removed) for 9 months. Percentage increase in plasma calcium (107.6 vs. 100.6%) and calcium-phosphorus product (115.6 vs. 104.7%) was significantly higher in the Ossopan group. The Ossopan group showed a steady decline in urinary hydroxyproline excretion, whereas the ashed Ossopan group did not. Patients taking Ossopan reported less bone pain, and eventually ceased analgesic use in 6/7 subjects. The ashed Ossopan group ceased analgesic use in 3/7 subjects. However, measures of bone mass (radiological metacarpal index and bone biopsy) were not different between the two groups, although 4/6 patients on Ossopan showed increases in metacarpal index, compared to 3/7 for ashed Ossopan. Thus, Ossopan was associated with improvements in calcium metabolism and bone mass in severely osteoporotic patients.

Galasko and co-workers from the Department of Orthopedic Surgery of the University of Manchester in England carried out a randomized, controlled study on 107 patients between 60 to 89 years of age with Colles' fracture of the distal radius.[766] Half of the patients were given 10 g of Ossopan daily for 24 months. The mean cortical area and width were measured radiographically in the uninjured hand, and although the difference between the groups was not statistically significant, for patients aged 60 to 69 years, the Ossopan group exhibited no net bone loss (+0.0274 mm/year change) while the untreated group lost bone (–0.054 mm/year). Since bone loss in these patients was slower than that induced by corticosteroids or liver disease, a longer time period of observation may be needed before statistical significance between the two groups is reached.

Dambacher and Rüegsegger of the Research Laboratory for Calcium Metabolism at the University of Zurich in Switzerland studied the effects of Ossopan supplementation (7.47 g/d) for 2 years to 11 osteoporotic patients compared to 14 untreated controls.[767] Trabecular and total bone density of the distal tibia and radius were measured by computerized tomography. Ossopan treatment did not change total or trabecular bone density (both were +0.2 ± 0.2%), but controls lost both trabecular (-5.8 ± 1.9%) and total (-3.3 ± 1.4%) bone. Thus, Ossopan exhibited the ability to halt progression of bone loss in osteoporotic patients.

Stepan and colleagues at the Charles University Faculty of Medicine in Prague, Czechoslovakia administered nothing (n = 20) or 10 g/d of Ossopan (n = 28) for 3 years to women (mean of 46 years) made postmenopausal by surgical removal of the ovaries during hysterectomy operations at least 1 year prior to study entry.[752] After 2 years, 14 patients treated with Ossopan did not show any differences to the control group, and these patients were given estrogen replacement therapy and continued Ossopan supplementation. Table 4 lists the results of Ossopan supplementation. Cortical bone loss was much less during Ossopan supplementation, and biochemical indices of bone resorption (abnormal at the start of the study) returned close to normal values. Estrogen replacement therapy to Ossopan nonresponders returned biochemical indices to normal by 6 months in 6 subjects. Thus, Ossopan decreased bone loss and decreased bone resorption in half of the women with early postmenopausal osteoporosis. In women receiving both Ossopan and estrogen therapy, all showed favorable biochemical indices indicating net bone resorption was greatly decreased. This illustrates that Ossopan and estrogen therapy are compatible. Thus, although Ossopan supplementation by itself seems to be less effective than estrogen therapy, half of women with osteoporosis showed benefits that are surmised (over time) to prevent the morbidity associated with osteoporosis (fractures).

TABLE 4   Changes in Biochemical Bone Parameters in Surgically Induced Postmenopausal Women

Measurement	Control Group		Ossopan® Group	
	Pre	Post	Pre	Post
Urinary hydroxyproline/ creatinine ratio (mmol/mol)	28.2	26.1	31.6	22.0[a]
Plasma tartrate-resistant acid phosphatase (U/l)	6.51	6.65	6.88	5.58[a]
Serum bone alkaline phosphatase (U/l)	19.6	17.5	19.9	13.9[a]
Serum calcium (mmol/l)	1.29	1.28	1.27	1.27
Urinary calcium/ creatinine ratio (mol/mol)	0.43	0.33	0.50	0.26
Cortical area (mm²)	47.0	43.7	48.0	47.0
Cortical area (% change from baseline)	0	-6.94	0	-2.04[a]

Note: Adapted from Reference 752. Women made postmenopausal by surgical removal of ovaries for benign uterine disease were given either nothing (control group n = 20) or 9 g/d of Ossopan (n = 28) for 3 years.

[a]   Significantly different from control group ($p < 0.01$).

TABLE 5   Changes in Bone Parameters in Corticosteroid-Treated Rheumatoid Arthritis Patients

Measurement	Control Group	Ossopan® Group
Mean loss of stem height (cm ± SD)	1.16 ± 0.71	0.87 ± 0.58[a]
Mean loss of radial bone density (Bone mineral content ÷ bone width ± SD)	0.06 ± 0.03	0.04 ± 0.03[a]
Back symptoms		
Better	6	8
Same	15	20
Worse	11	4

Note: Adapted from Reference 768. Seventy-two corticosteroid-treated rheumatoid arthritis patients were divided into two groups: controls and Ossopan-treated. Ossopan was given at a dose of 6 g/d for 12 months. Stem height refers to the crown to seat distance while sitting in a standard chair. Bone density and width was measured by photon absorption densitometry.

[a]   Significant difference from control group ($p < 0.05$).

3. Corticosteroid-Induced Osteoporosis

Nilsen and others, from the University of Bristol and Royal National Hospital for Rheumatic Diseases in Bath, England, studied 72 patients with rheumatoid arthritis who had been treated with corticosteroids. They were divided into two equal groups of controls (no supplement) and Ossopan (6 g/d) for 12 months.[768] Table 5 lists the results for each group. Ossopan showed "a significant prophylactic effect in preventing the development of osteoporosis in corticosteroid-treated rheumatoid patients."[768] Particularly important is the slowing of the loss of spinal column height by Ossopan.

Pines and co-workers from Hertford County and East Herts Hospitals in Hertford, England studied the effects of administration of 6 to 8 g/d of Ossopan to 29 patients (average 55 years old) on long-term (average 6.3 years) prednisolone treatment (5 to 20 mg/d) of respiratory disorders for 12 months, compared to an untreated control group (n = 8).[769] Back pain was initially present in 19 treated and 4 untreated patients. After 12 months, 17/19 Ossopan-treated patients had no back pain (severity scores changed from 1.66 to 0.08), while 0/4 untreated patients had no back pain, which was increased in 3/4 (severity scores changed from 1.38 to 1.88). The difference between groups was highly significant. Mean cortical thickness of metacarpals did not change in the Ossopan group (3.94 to 3.93 mm), but decreased greatly in the untreated group (4.13 to 3.86 mm). Although half of the Ossopan group expressed organoleptic dissatisfaction with the taste of Ossopan powder, an equivalent amount of tablets was well tolerated. No fractures occurred in either group during the study period. Thus, prophylactic treatment with Ossopan appeared to slow or stop the progression of osteoporosis caused by long-term corticosteroid therapy. The almost total ablation of back pain was described as "dramatic."

Stellon and others from St. Thomas' Hospital and King's College Hospital in London, England studied the effect of Ossopan treatment (8 g/d) on 18 patients treated with corticosteroids for chronic active hepatitis compared to 18 patients serving as controls.[770] Prednisolone treatment (9 mg/d average) was given for at least 1 year before entry into the study. In the two patients treated with Ossopan exhibiting lower back pain upon study initiation, one had no pain after 6 months. In one untreated patient, back pain persisted throughout the 2-year study period, and two additional controls exhibited back pain during the study period. No Ossopan-treated patients exhibited fractures during the study period, but three untreated controls developed vertebral fractures. Bone mineral content decreased significantly in the controls (0.91 to 0.88 g/cm), but there was no change in the Ossopan-treated group (0.93 to 0.93 g/cm). Trabecular bone volume increased in the Ossopan-treated group (18.6 ± 5.1 to 20.3 ± 3.1%), but decreased in the untreated controls (19.7 ± 4.2 to 18.9 ± 4.6%). Cortical plate thickness (assessed by bone biopsy) decreased significantly in both groups, but significantly less in the Ossopan-treated group. Thus, Ossopan treatment prevented bone loss associated with long-term corticosteroid treatment.

4. Metabolic Bone Diseases

Dent and Davies, of the University College Hospital in London, England, administered 8 g/d of Ossopan to 3 young patients with different types of Osteogenesis Imperfecta, all with previous or current fractures.[771] After 16 d of Ossopan supplementation, 0.1 to 0.25 mg/d of vitamin D_2 (dihydrotachysterol) was started. Patients were followed for up to 2 years. Calcium balance immediately became positive and was made more so after vitamin D_2 administration. The positive calcium balance lasted throughout the observation period. No new fractures occurred, and the Ossopan was well tolerated. No hypercalcemia was noted. Thus, in children, large doses of Ossopan were well tolerated and produced large positive changes in calcium balance. These events suggest that Ossopan may have possible utility for other bone loss disorders, such as osteoporosis.

Epstein and co-workers, of the Royal Free Hospital in London, England, studied the prophylactic effect of Ossopan or calcium gluconate on cortical bone thinning in 64 postmenopausal women with primary biliary cirrhosis.[772] Patients with primary biliary cirrhosis exhibit premature cortical bone loss partly because of inactivity, renal tubular acidosis, steatorrhea, and the malabsorption of calcium, phosphorus, and vitamin D. The 64 patients were divided into 3 groups: controls (n = 21), Ossopan-treated (n = 15), and calcium gluconate-treated (n = 17). All patients received monthly injections of vitamin D_2 (100,000 IU). Either 8 g/d of Ossopan (supplying 35 mmol of calcium) or 4 tablets of calcium gluconate (supplying 40 mmol of calcium) were given daily, and patients were followed for up to 18 months. Changes in cortical bone mass were followed by quantification of radiologic images of metacarpal thicknesses. After 14 months, controls showed a significant decrease in cortical bone (–0.08 ± 0.03 mm), the calcium gluconate-treated group showed no change (–0.02 ± 0.05 mm) and the Ossopan-treated group showed a significant increase (+0.08 ± 0.07 mm). No changes in serum calcium or phosphorus were measured. These results indicate that Ossopan was better absorbed than a soluble calcium salt (calcium gluconate), with practical benefits. Since Ossopan contains phosphate, and phosphate is malabsorbed during primary biliary cirrhosis, it appears evident that the presence of phosphate with calcium and vitamin D confers a therapeutic advantage over calcium alone. Since the bone loss associated with primary biliary cirrhosis resembles that of postmenopausal osteoporosis,[772] only accelerated, these findings are of significance to other bone loss disorders.

D. SUMMARY AND GUIDELINES

Ossopan, the commercial form of bone meal, has been studied with some success for disorders of bone loss. Ossopan appeared most effective in reversing bone loss from disorders where bone loss is rapid (corticosteroid therapy, primary biliary cirrhosis). Postmenopausal osteoporosis showed a slowing or even a halt in the progression of bone loss, but given the length of time for symptoms to develop in postmenopausal osteoporosis (5 to 20 years) compared to the length of studies utilizing Ossopan (up to 3 years), a final conclusion on whether the beneficial changes in bone mass seen from Ossopan supplementation would result in fewer fractures and less loss of stature is not available. However, Ossopan supplementation did produce the necessary biochemical changes which are associated with maintenance of bone mass above the critical threshold level for fractures. It is likely that Ossopan supplementation, if continued for a long enough time period, would prevent to a large extent the later complications of osteoporosis. The implication of considerable savings of human suffering and medical costs is significant if widespread use of Ossopan was practiced. Ossopan may also play a role in enhancing healing of long bone fractures when expected healing is delayed, meaning that Ossopan may have usefulness in cases where the opportunity for prevention of bone loss is already lost.

Also, evidence to support Ossopan as being a superior form of calcium supplementation for prevention of bone loss includes greater absorption than other sources of calcium, presence of proteinaceous factors that enhance intestinal calcium absorption, and presence of phosphate and other trace minerals. Thus, Ossopan is more than just a calcium supplement.

For conditions where bone loss is expected, successful doses of Ossopan ranged from 8 to 10 g/d. Ossopan powder was frequently mixed in carbonated drinks or hot cereals to make it more palatable. Ossopan tablets at equivalent daily doses were well tolerated, but 8 to 10 tablets daily are necessary to reach required dosage. Ossopan was administered either all at once in the evening or in two separate doses, one in the morning and one in the evening.

Ossopan represents a simple means to replenish nutrients needed for maintenance of bone mass and fracture healing. Apart from a large amount of material to consume, no side effects have been noted in extensive human studies. Use of Ossopan in bone loss disorders should be strongly considered, given its safety and numerous successful studies.

III. MAGNESIUM

A. ROLES AND FUNCTIONS

Like calcium, magnesium is involved in hundreds of reactions of essential importance to life. Whereas calcium is primarily an extracellular cation, magnesium is primarily an intracellular cation. Magnesium and calcium share many reciprocal roles. As described by an ever-increasing number of excellent reviews,[170,773-778] the myriad of functions for magnesium are so important as to be taken for granted. In many respects, magnesium is the forgotten mineral. Magnesium's ubiquity is not matched by research commensurate with its importance, especially when compared to other minerals, such as calcium, iron, and zinc. Magnesium is now being shown to have a major impact on all aspects of health, and magnesium nutriture will one day become more important than calcium.

Table 6 lists some of the hundreds of functions of magnesium pertaining to healing.[170,773-778] Magnesium is the fourth most abundant cation in the body, and second to potassium as the major intracellular cation. An average human (70 kg) contains 20 to 28 g of magnesium, with 60 to 65% in bone mineral, 27% in muscle, and 6 to 7% in other cells. Only 1% of total body magnesium is in

**TABLE 6   Magnesium Functions Pertinent
to Connective Tissue Healing**

Cofactor or essential for activity for over 300 enzymatic reactions
Alkaline phosphatase activity
Complexation with high-energy phosphate compounds
Regulator of cellular energy metabolism
Complexation with phospholipids in membranes
Complexation with nuclei acids
Roles in protein synthesis
Roles in amino acid metabolism
Interactions with calcium and calciferol metabolism
Second messenger for hormonal responses
Activation of hormone receptors
Inhibition of parathyroid hormone release
Enhanced solubility of octacalcium phosphate in plasma
  (role in driving calcium into bone synthesis)

extracellular fluids (including plasma), with 55% free, 32% bound to proteins, and the remainder associated with low molecular weight ligands such as phosphate and citrate.

Magnesium fulfills so many essential functions that it is almost impossible to single out any one function as being critical for healing. Therefore, the status of magnesium function becomes important for its effect on overall magnesium function (and thus, overall cellular function).

B. DEFICIENCY SYMPTOMS

Table 7 lists some deficiency symptoms of magnesium relevant to connective tissues.[170,773-778] Keep in mind that many other health problems are associated with magnesium deficiency, especially cardiovascular diseases. The most visible deficiency symptoms concern the skeletal system and interactions with calcium metabolism. However, the extent to which soft tissues are affected is not fully known and may be more disadvantageous than previously thought. The main concerns for a sports medicine patient base are excessive sweating with loss of magnesium, and chronic magnesium intakes for proper maintenance of neuromuscular functions and prevention of bone loss.

Certain population groups are at increased risk for magnesium deficiency.[170,439,773-778] Trauma, sepsis, burns, starvation, major surgery, renal disease, malabsorption syndromes, alcoholism, diabetes, malnutrition, and cardiovascular diseases have all been associated with varying degrees of deficient magnesium status.

C. ASSESSMENT

The assessment of magnesium status in humans is still controversial. At this time, no consensus has been reached for a practical laboratory assessment of magnesium status. Several markers are in use and can give information of value if results are abnormal. However, a characteristic of magnesium assessment is that many times magnesium markers appear normal, but responses are still found to magnesium repletion.[439] Table 8 lists some of the more common methods of magnesium assessment. In general, measurement of levels in serum, erythrocytes, leukocytes, or hair will find deficient status if deficiency is prolonged or severe. The correlation between magnesium indicators has a long history of unreliability. As with other nutrients, perhaps the best measure of assessment is a clinical trial of magnesium supplementation, followed by careful examination for changes in magnesium deficiency symptoms, including mood and neuromuscular findings.

D. INTAKES

The intakes of magnesium are equally controversial as assessment methods.[439,773-778] For the general population, intakes for magnesium appear to be low for females at all age groups.[439,774,779] The large variability of magnesium intakes for a given population means that a subset (20 to 70%) of any group

TABLE 7   Deficiency Symptoms of Magnesium Relevant to Connective Tissues

Acute Deficiency Symptoms	Chronic Deficiency Symptoms
Fatigue	Fatigue
Abnormal neuromuscular functions (tics, muscle tremors, bruxism, irritability, muscle spasms, Trousseau signs, Chvostek signs, muscle fasciculations, progressing to myoclonic jerks, tetany, convulsions, and coma)	Reduced plasma and cellular levels of magnesium
	Decreased excretion of magnesium in feces and urine
	Hypokalemia and hypocalcemia
	Abnormal neuromuscular functions (tics, muscle tremors, bruxism, irritability, muscle spasms, muscle tension)
Personality changes (usually depression, anxiety, nervousness, confusion, disorientation)	Personality changes (usually depression, anxiety, nervousness, confusion, disorientation)
Nausea and vomiting	Anorexia
Muscle weakness, pains	Bone loss (osteoporosis)
	Impaired wound healing
	Depressed immune function
	Edema
	Insomnia
	Decreased plasma alkaline phosphatase activity
	Vitamin D resistance, skeletal inactivity

TABLE 8   Methods of Assessment for Magnesium Status

Plasma or serum magnesium levels
Erythrocyte magnesium levels
Leukocyte (peripheral blood mononuclear cell) magnesium levels
Skeletal or muscle levels (biopsy)
24-h urinary magnesium levels
Magnesium challenge test (% retention of an IV magnesium dose followed by urine levels)
Lymphocyte growth responses

will have deficient intakes. In athlete groups, since most athletes eat more than average persons, and magnesium is present in most foods, a high incidence of deficient magnesium intake was not found.[191] However, magnesium intakes of female gymnasts, female runners, female triathletes, and wrestlers were sometimes found to be deficient.[191] Any population with reduced food intake is subject to risk for magnesium deficiency.

The magnesium status of athletes is also controversial, with conflicting findings.[780-787] Since almost all determinations of magnesium status were made from serum or erythrocyte levels, there may be considerable discrepancy with tissue levels and functions. Thus, a clear consensus is not available on the magnesium status of athletes, but there is cause for concern that status may not be ideal in a large subset of athletes.

E. DIETARY SOURCES AND INFLUENCES

Magnesium is widely distributed among foodstuffs.[788] Since magnesium is the primary mineral associated with chlorophyll, vegetables have relatively high contents of magnesium. Food sources richest in magnesium are nutritional supplements, seeds (especially pumpkin seeds), nuts, soybeans, legumes, whole grains, and fresh vegetables. Refining and processing of foods tends to remove large amounts of magnesium.

Of perhaps greater impact than dietary sources of magnesium are other factors that compromise magnesium status. Persons at risk for deficient magnesium status are listed in Table 9.[170,439,773-779]

Unlike other minerals, there is not a clear-cut distinction between magnesium uptake from inorganic and organic salts. Magnesium salts of oxide, sulfate, chloride, and carbonate are associated with adequate absorption in most individuals. Organic chelates of magnesium (ascorbate, aspartate, citrate, gluconate, lactate, malate, orotate) also offer adequate absorption and tolerance.

TABLE 9   Groups at Risk for Magnesium Deficiency

Inadequate dietary intakes
  (all women, elderly, anorexics, dieters)
Malabsorption disorders
Severe injury
Alcoholics
Diabetics
Renal disease and dialysis
Hyperthyroidism
Hyperparathyroidism
Hyperaldosteronism
Protein-calorie malnutrition
Diuretic use
Excessive lactation
Metabolic acidosis
Potassium depletion
Nephrotoxic drugs
Cardiovascular diseases
Paget's disease
Pregnancy
Long-term antibiotic therapy
Chemotherapeutic and immunosuppressive medications
Cirrhosis
Osteoporosis
Digitalis therapy
Athletes (strenuous exercise)?

F. HUMAN STUDIES

The study of magnesium in athletics has lagged behind other areas (such as cardiovascular disease). However, at this time documentation for two areas of interest to healing can be found. The first is excessive sweating and acute magnesium deficiency. One case report described a female tennis player with severe carpopedal spasms and decreased serum magnesium levels.[789] Muscle cramps were alleviated after administration of 500 mg/d of magnesium gluconate.

The other aspect of magnesium and injury rehabilitation is bone health. Although specific studies in athletes are not available, sufficient research has been performed to document a pivotal role for magnesium nutriture in bone loss. Of primary importance are findings of repletion of bone mass after magnesium supplementation, which was not documented after calcium and/or estrogen administration. First, magnesium deficiencies in serum or bone of groups with bone loss (osteoporosis) have been determined by various investigators.[773,774,790-799] Second, supplementation with magnesium has been associated with increases in bone mass compared to control groups.[793,794,800-802] In a landmark study, Abraham and Grewal, in practice at Women's Life Care in Anaheim Hills, CA, studied the effect of a multiple vitamin/mineral supplement emphasizing magnesium instead of calcium on bone mass in postmenopausal women on hormonal replacement therapy.[801] A multiple vitamin/mineral supplement containing 500 mg of calcium as citrate and 200 mg of magnesium as oxide, in addition to zinc, iron, copper, manganese, and other trace elements at RDA levels was given to 19 women. An additional 400 mg of magnesium (as oxide) was added daily. Thus, women received 50% of the RDA for calcium and 200% of the RDA for magnesium via supplementation. Seven women served as controls. Measurements of calcaneous bone density by single photon absorptiometry before supplementation and 1 year later found that control women exhibited a nonsignificant 0.7% increase in bone density, while supplemented women exhibited an increase in bone density of 11% ($p <0.01$). This magnitude of bone density accretion has not been found after calcium, estrogen, and vitamin D administration. Thus, this study reiterated the importance of many other nutrients in addition to calcium for reversal of bone mass. Magnesium was the primary ingredient, and based on evidence from deficient status in bone loss syndromes, and preliminary clinical success, it appears that magnesium supplementation, along with adequate mineral status, may be a primary therapy for bone loss syndromes. Unfortunately, the extrapolation of these results to osteoporosis seen in athletic amenorrhea is not clear. However, the encouraging results argue for close attention to be paid to magnesium status in all athletes.

G. SAFETY

Oral administration of magnesium salts appears to be safe at daily intakes of 400 to 1000 mg/d.[773-778] Magnesium salts have been in use for many years as cathartics and antacids; so, one effect of overdosing is nausea, diarrhea, and vomiting. However, doses greater than 1000 mg of elemental magnesium at once may prove cathartic. Acute toxicity can be obtained after very large doses of magnesium salts, and consists of hypotension, nausea, vomiting, flushing, and mental status changes. These symptoms are not seen until serum levels are increased by three times (which is difficult). Care in patients with renal diseases must be taken with any additional magnesium. Thus, supplemental magnesium is generally safe in divided doses of 200 to 1000 mg daily.

H. SUMMARY AND GUIDELINES

At this time, it is difficult to reliably ascertain magnesium intake or status in athletes. Although magnesium intakes do not appear to be a problem, magnesium status of athletes remains suspect, especially for thin female athletes, although male athletes are not immune to deficits in magnesium status. It is logical to administer magnesium when calcium supplements are given, since excess calcium and vitamin D intakes may increase tendency to soft tissue calcification. More health care advocates are urging a dietary goal of 1:1 ratios of calcium to magnesium, instead of the 2:1 ratio commonly accepted at present. After review of the prodigious (and largely forgotten) research on magnesium, it is prudent to include magnesium-rich foods, or include a magnesium supplement of 200 to 400 mg daily during strenuous exercise. For athletes with bone loss or unexplained symptoms listed in Table 7, magnesium supplementation at doses of 400 to 1000 mg daily should be considered.

Chapter 9

TRACE MINERALS

I. IRON

A. ROLES AND FUNCTIONS IN HEALING

Iron is a required cofactor in lysyl and prolyl hydroxylases, necessary for proper posttranscriptional modification and cross-linking of collagen and elastin molecules.[93,95-97,100,163,164,485] As such, iron deficiency may impair wound healing by an effect on hydroxylases. This has not been conclusively determined to this date. Also, severe anemia may impair oxygen transport to wound sites and impair healing. Except in cases of extreme anemia requiring transfusions, there has been no clear-cut effect of anemia on wound healing.[163,164,485] In fact, noniron aspects of anemia (increased blood viscosity, hypovolemia), rather than oxygen transport, are believed to account for effects of severe iron-deficiency anemia on wound healing. Defects in immune function during iron deficiency have not been correlated with increased risk of infection and impaired wound healing.[163,164,458] Therefore, iron deficiencies do not appear to be a factor to consider for healing of connective tissues.

Iron deficiency and resulting anemia is of practical concern to runners and other athletes.[731,732] As this aspect of iron does not directly involve healing, it will not be discussed further. The reader is referred to other excellent reviews on iron deficiency and anemia in sports.[191,731,732,785,803,804]

B. ROLES AND FUNCTIONS IN INFLAMMATION

Iron may actually be more important to the healing process by its presence or excess via effects on inflammatory processes. Recent research, which has been performed mostly since 1981, has determined that iron may exacerbate inflammation by catalysis of free radical formation.[549,805] Iron is known to catalyze the formation of hydroxyl, ferryl, and perferryl free radicals in the presence of superoxide and hydrogen peroxide by the Fenton reaction (see Table 1). Numerous studies have shown that the hydroxyl radical is capable of damaging any biological macromolecule, including hyaluronan, proteoglycans, collagens, proteins, lipids, DNA, and RNA.[305-307,549,805] Hydroxyl radical, along with hydrogen peroxide and superoxide, has been shown to exert damaging effects on macromolecular components of synovial fluid and cartilage.[305-307,549,805] Proinflammatory effects of free radicals are also well known.[305-307,549,805] It turns out that iron is removed from ferritin in an unbound form. The unbound iron can then react with hydrogen peroxide and superoxide in a catalytic fashion to generate hydroxyl radicals.[805] At high levels of ascorbate (>100 μmol) *in vitro*, iron salts can generate superoxide and initiate further free radical formation, although this concentration is rarely reached *in vivo*.[806] Thus, ascorbate can be exonerated from being a prooxidant *in vivo*,[806] but iron cannot.[805,806] Since ferritin is ubiquitous in tissues, and concentrates in inflamed joint synovium,[805] the mere presence of normal amounts of ferritin are sufficient to initiate and promulgate free radical reactions destructive to tissues. The superoxide and hydrogen peroxide are ably supplied by activated neutrophils and macrophages (also by macrophage-like synoviovytes).[805] Generation of free radicals by ferritin-unbound iron is enhanced when the usual iron binding proteins (whose function is to keep iron bound, and thus safe from forming free radical reactions) become saturated with iron. A greater degree of ferritin saturation during rheumatoid arthritis has been found.[805] Thus, an excess of iron or conditions of inflammation (which are produced by exercise[512]) may produce free radicals that damage connective tissues. In inflammatory diseases, even if levels of antioxidant protectors and chelators are normal, those levels are insufficient to prevent free radical formation and tissue damage.[805] This is the free radical hypothesis of tissue damage.

TABLE 1   Fenton Reaction (Iron Catalysis of Free Radicals)

$$H_2O_2 + O_2^- \xrightarrow{Fe} \cdot OH + O_2 + OH^-$$

Hydrogen peroxide (H_2O_2) and superoxide (O_2^-) in presence of free iron react to form
hydroxyl radical ($\cdot OH$), molecular oxygen (O_2), and hydroxide ion (OH^-).

C. SUMMARY AND GUIDELINES

Because of the recent illumination of the inescapable role of iron in free radical formation during inflammation, it is wise to prevent needless iron intake or supplementation. Especially during the healing process, when inflammation is likely, iron intake is not required and may prolong recovery. Therefore, no additional iron intake aside from usual dietary sources is recommended. Almost every multiple vitamin/mineral product contains 15 to 18 mg of iron, usually as inorganic salts (ferrous sulfate). Thus, if supplementation is desired during healing, the absence of iron is desirable, and other sources of multiple supplementation without iron need to be found. At present, it is difficult, but not impossible, to locate multiple vitamin/mineral products containing no iron. Usually, these products can be found in health food stores or mail-order companies that cater to health care providers.

II. ZINC

A. INTRODUCTION

Zinc is a transition metal with a molecular weight of 65.2. Zinc compounds appear to be the oldest form of therapy for connective tissue disorders, dating back to the topical use of calamine (an impure form of zinc oxide) for skin wounds in the Ebers Papyrus from 1550 B.C.[807] To this day, calamine is still in use as an agent for healing of topical skin wounds, and use of pharmaceutical grades of zinc oxide in topical preparations evolved from calamine applications. The modern study of zinc as an essential agent for wound healing began in 1953 with the serendipitous observation by Strain that burned rats accidentally fed a diet high in zinc healed faster than burned rats fed a diet with normal zinc content.[807] This observation led to further studies, which came at a time when zinc was considered more of a passive contaminant in bodies than an essential nutrient. Realization of the importance of zinc nutriture after conclusive studies of zinc-deficient young men in Iran during the 1960s underscored the roles found for zinc in animals.[808] Realization of the essentiality of zinc in humans fostered an explosion of research on zinc roles, functions, and effects, which has continued into the 1990s unabated. This section will examine the use of zinc compounds on the healing of connective tissues, with emphasis on human studies.

An average human body contains 2 to 3 g of zinc, with the majority located in muscles, bones, skin, and liver.[808] Prostate and ocular tissues contain the highest concentrations of zinc (600 to 800 μg/g), with bone (200 μg/g) and muscle (50 μg/g) having higher zinc concentrations than most other tissues (30 μg/g). Thus, most body zinc (70 to 80%) resides in musculoskeletal tissues.

B. ROLES AND FUNCTIONS

As a well-studied, essential nutrient, many roles and functions have been discovered for zinc. Table 2 lists the roles for zinc that have particular interest for musculoskeletal healing.[93,140,163,164,167,808,809] The main functions of zinc are to activate a large number of zinc metalloenzymes (over 120 known), stabilize structural conformation of polysomes, stabilize membranes, regulate cytoskeleton structures, and provide activity for thymic hormones necessary for proper immune function.[93,140,163,164,167,808,809] Since zinc is a component of the key enzymes involved in basic cellular events, such as DNA synthesis, RNA synthesis, protein synthesis, and numerous regulatory and degradative functions, zinc is essential for overall cell function, even more so when cell growth is required. Wound healing invariably involves cell growth (fibroblasts, endothelial cells, epithelial cells, immune cells, osteoblasts, etc.), making zinc paramount for proper healing responses of all tissues.

**TABLE 2 Zinc Roles with Particular Interest
for Connective Tissue Healing**

Activation of zinc metalloenzymes necessary for healing responses
  DNA polymerases (cell growth)
  RNA polymerases (cell growth, protein synthesis)
  Nucleotide transferases (cell growth, protein synthesis)
  Alkaline phosphatase (bone mineralization)
  Thymidine kinase (cell growth)
  Carbonic anhydrase (pH control)
  Copper-zinc superoxide dismutase (antioxidant protection)
  Lactic dehydrogenase (LDH) (cell energy, lactate removal)
Polysome conformation
  Protein synthesis
  Cell growth
  Collagen synthesis
Stabilization of cell membranes and cytoskeletons
  Nutrient and waste transport

In addition to cell growth and replication, zinc has more specific roles in sexual maturation (gonadal hormone synthesis), fertility, reproduction, night vision, immune functions, taste, and appetite. Zinc-dependent enzymes of particular importance for connective tissue healing include alcohol dehydrogenase, alkaline phosphatase, carbonic anhydrase, copper-zinc superoxide dismutase (CuZnSOD), DNA polymerase, deoxynucleotidyl transferases, lactic dehydrogenase, and thymidine kinase.[808,809] Metallothionen exhibits specific zinc (and copper) binding affinity, providing cells a flexible way to regulate intracellular zinc levels and functions, which is finally beginning to be understood.[810] Zinc effects on retinol-binding proteins may have more practical influence on vitamin A status than vitamin A itself in trauma situations.

C. DEFICIENCY SYMPTOMS

The list of zinc deficiency symptoms is exceptionally long, so attention will be paid to those that relate to musculoskeletal healing in humans. Primary signs of zinc deficiency include impaired wound healing, skin lesions (eczema, ulcers, acne, seborrhea, pustules, rashes), hypogeusia (decreased taste), anorexia, immune deficiencies (less resistance to infections), alopecia, and growth retardation.[808,809,811] All of these clinical symptoms are reversed by zinc supplementation. A zinc deficiency may promote deficiencies of other nutrients by virtue of its effects on behavior, taste, and appetite, with possible adverse ramifications for healing.

Laboratory findings in zinc deficient states are listed in Table 3. Of particular interest are decreased collagen synthesis, impaired glucose metabolism, reduced albumin synthesis, and reduced insulin response. These findings are of primary importance for energy utilization, nutrient transport, and nutrient utilization on a broad regulatory scale. Thus, zinc deficiency will show relatively nonspecific delays or hindrances of healing that may be difficult to notice or attribute to zinc.

The primary finding of zinc deficiency with interest to this book is impaired wound healing. Numerous studies in animals have definitely found delays in skin wound healing during zinc deficiency.[807,808] The effect of zinc deficiency is mostly on epithelialization, which occurs during the second phase of wound healing. For example, tensile strength of surgical wounds was not significantly different between control and zinc-deficient rats 6 d after surgery, but were quite different 12 d after surgery.[812,813] In addition, there were fewer fibroblasts and less collagen deposition at 12 d in the zinc-deficient rats. The timing of maximum zinc effects on wound healing in animals was 12 to 15 d after injury, during epithelialization and granulation tissue formation. This finding indicates that zinc is involved during the portion of wound healing when synthesis of extracellular matrix (i.e., collagen and proteoglycans) is greatest. This is entirely logical and consistent with the known roles and functions of zinc in DNA, RNA, and protein synthesis.

TABLE 3   Laboratory Findings in Zinc Deficiency

Decreased Values	Increased Values
Serum zinc	Serum ammonia
Serum alkaline phosphatase	Serum RNAse
Collagen synthesis	HMG CoA-reductase
Albumin synthesis	
Glucose metabolism	
Insulin response	
Lymphocyte proliferation	
Lymphocyte nucleoside phosphorylase	
T lymphocyte functions	
Leukocyte chemotaxis	
Serum thymic factors	
Serum testosterone	
Platelet aggregation	

D. ASSESSMENT

The assessment of zinc status has never been fully satisfactory. Serum and plasma levels of zinc have been measured repeatedly for many years, but since zinc exists mainly as an intracellular component of enzymes and other proteins, the serum level of zinc does not necessarily correlate with zinc tissue status.[814,815] For instance, 98% of total body zinc (2 to 3 g) is intracellular. Of the 0.1% of total body zinc present in plasma, about 55 to 90% is loosely bound to albumin, 5 to 40% is firmly bound to α_2-macroglobulin, 5 to 10% is loosely bound to various low molecular weight ligands (peptides, amino acids), and 3% is present in leukocytes.[809,814]

Many factors influence serum levels of zinc (see Table 4).[808,814-816] These factors make the estimation of tissue zinc function difficult to determine from a single specimen. Serum zinc levels average around 100 µg/dl (15 µM) in apparently healthy individuals. Combination of serum zinc levels with levels from a nucleated tissue (leukocyte, liver, bone, muscle) may yield a better idea of zinc status. Zinc levels in serum are reduced by most types of inflammation and stress that releases corticosteroids. Serum zinc appears to be sequestered into the liver by binding to induced metallothionen as a normal sequelae to inflammation. Liver sequestration of zinc is thought to be a defense response against bacterial growth and to assist in synthesis of acute phase proteins.[808,810] Usually, assessment of zinc:copper ratios may give information on the presence or extent of inflammation (see also Section III. Copper). During stress and inflammation, zinc excretion is increased, which may also lead to further losses of body zinc. Thus, serum or plasma zinc is unreliable as an indicator of zinc status.

Other practical methods of assessment of zinc status include measurement of zinc levels in urine, hair, nails, saliva, erythrocytes, and leukocytes (neutrophils).[814,815] Simultaneous measurement of zinc levels in these body fluids and cells provides information on both short-term and long-term zinc status. Ideally, tissue biopsies of liver, bone, muscle, and kidney would more accurately reflect intracellular levels of zinc in the tissues that contain most body zinc; however, these tissues are not practical for routine examinations.[814] Likewise, the determination of zinc status by measuring metabolic balance, turnover rate, and exchangeable pools of zinc after administration of radioactive zinc-65 is also not practical.[814] Measurement of zinc-dependent enzyme activities (alkaline phosphatase, carbonic anhydrase, δ-aminolevulinic acid dehydratase) has not been shown to correlate with tissue zinc status.[814]

A zinc tolerance test (rise in serum zinc levels after a zinc dose of 5 to 50 mg) has been proposed as a means of zinc status assessment, as well as absorption.[815] Taste disorders of zinc deficiency may be utilized as a measure of zinc status. The taste (or lack thereof) of a zinc sulfate solution may identify zinc-deficient individuals.[817] Recently, the functional status of cellular zinc has been determined by lymphocyte growth response to a graded dose-response curve of zinc in a chemically defined medium.[600]

TABLE 4   Factors Influencing Serum Levels of Zinc

Factors Decreasing Zinc Levels

Dietary Factors
  Degree of fasting
  Decreased food intake
  Insufficient intake (malnutrition)
  Fiber, phytate intake
  Geophagia
  Excess calcium, magnesium, copper
  Alcohol
  Extended total parenteral nutrition without zinc
Drugs and Chemicals
  Corticosteroids
  Cytostatics
  Oral contraceptives
  D-penicillamine
  Tetracyclines
  Anticonvulsants
Diseases and Health Conditions
  Inflammation (including rheumatoid arthritis)
  Burns
  Surgery
  Acute infections
  Malignant diseases
  Liver disease
  Diabetes
  Chronic diarrhea
  Malabsorption disorders (ulcers, Crohn's, sprue,
    inflammatory bowel syndrome, pancreatitis, etc.)
  Renal diseases
  Hypoalbuminemia
  Anemias (especially sickle-cell)
  Osteoporosis
  Acrodermatitis enteropathica
  Ehlers-Danlos Syndrome
  Epilepsy
  (Rare) congenital disorders of zinc metabolism
Physiological Factors
  Aging
  Pregnancy
  Stress (adrenal corticosteroid release)
  Growth hormone therapy
  Circadian and diurnal rhythms

Factors Increasing Zinc Levels

Dietary Factors
  Zinc supplements
  Intake of zinc-rich foods
  Chelation to or coadministration of picolinate, citrate,
    histidinate, aspartate, cysteine, pancreas powder
Drugs and Chemicals
  Diuretics
Diseases and Health Conditions
  Diabetes
Physiological Factors
  Circadian and diurnal rhythms
  (Rare) congenital disorders of zinc
  Metabolism

Other promising tests with practical attributes include *in vitro* erythrocyte uptake of zinc-65, and response to zinc supplementation. Cunnane[815] has stated:

> "The method of assessing zinc nutriture that is considered most reliable is that of clinical evaluation of the individual's response to zinc supplementation. Regardless of plasma zinc concentration, enzyme activities, apparent zinc absorption, or zinc balance, if the clinical symptoms suggestive of zinc depletion are alleviated by zinc supplementation, then zinc depletion should be considered to have existed."

Thus, measurement of zinc levels in serum or plasma offers the most facile means to determine whether a zinc deficiency exists, but there are so many factors influencing plasma zinc levels that caution must be exercised during the interpretation of results. Usually, another measure of zinc status should be performed, especially if conditions in Table 4 are encountered. The empirical observations of change in clinical symptoms resulting from a trial of zinc supplementation still offer the least expensive and, perhaps, most reliable indicator of zinc status. The symptoms in Table 5 (and findings in Table 3) may be used to gauge zinc status.

**TABLE 5   Clinical Signs of Zinc
Deficiency in Humans**

Impaired wound healing
Immune deficiencies
Behavioral disturbances
Skin lesions (eczema, rashes, seborrhea, acne)
Alopecia
Hypogeusia (less taste)
Delayed sexual maturation
Hypogonadism, hypospermia
Growth retardation
Anorexia

Note: These deficiency symptoms have been
shown to be responsive to zinc
supplementation in humans.

E. INTAKES

Surveys of zinc intakes in the U.S. have found that many people may not be ingesting sufficient zinc to meet 1989 RDA levels (12 to 15 mg/d for adults).[809] Zinc intakes have averaged from 47 to 67% of the RDA in some recent studies.[779,809,818,819] Women in particular seem to have lower zinc intakes than males.[779] Wide variations in zinc intake for every population were seen in each study, which confounds generalizations about zinc intakes of individuals. Although more discrete data on the estimated percentage of persons ingesting deficient or marginally deficient zinc levels is still unavailable, there is a consensus that marginal zinc intake and, thus, marginal zinc status is common in an apparently well-nourished U.S. population. Dietary analysis over 3 or 7 d may provide an indication of an individual's zinc intake.

Several studies on zinc intakes of athletes have found results from adequate to deficient.[804] A common trend, regardless of average intakes, was that from 20 to 40% of each population studied exhibited deficient intakes. Likewise, studies measuring serum or plasma zinc levels in athletic groups found that a large subset of subjects (8 to 35%) exhibited deficient levels.[780,783,784,804,820] Exercise itself has an unclear effect on zinc status, but, again, a consistent trend is that if weight (muscle mass) declined, so did zinc status.[804] Otherwise, zinc appeared to be redistributed from plasma to erythrocytes and liver metallothionen. The implications for zinc status of this apparent adaptation to stress are not completely known at this time. Exercise may influence zinc in a manner similar to inflammation — sequestration with less availability to connective tissues. Thus, athletes recovering from trauma or surgery may be at increased risk for deficient zinc status and, therefore, suboptimal healing.

F. DIETARY SOURCES AND INFLUENCES

In addition to total zinc intake, the bioavailability of zinc from food or supplemental sources can vary considerably. Estimates of percentage of zinc absorbed from foods ranged from 12 to 59%.[809] Factors that affect zinc bioavailability are listed in Table 6.[808,809] From the large number of influencing factors, it can be seen that simple knowledge of dietary zinc intake levels may not be sufficient to determine dietary adequacy of zinc status.

Foods richest in zinc concentration per serving include: oysters, red meats, grain germs, seeds, nuts, soybean products, legumes, and potatoes.[808,809] Zinc-fortified cereal products are also a rich dietary source of zinc. Although cow milk is an important quantitative source of dietary zinc, the difficulty in digestion of casein leaves much zinc unavailable for absorption.[809]

Of particular interest are the effects of zinc chelates such as zinc monomethionine, zinc histidinate, zinc citrate, zinc aspartate, and zinc picolinate. These compounds appear to be zinc ligands *in vivo*[808,809] and also improve bioavailability over zinc sulfate.[822] It is believed that organic zinc salts would have less potential toxicity and less interference from and with other minerals. For example, zinc monomethionine uptake is independent of fiber intake, unlike zinc sulfate, which exhibits depressed

TABLE 6   Factors Influencing the Bioavailability of Zinc

Factors That Increase Zinc Uptake	Factors That Decrease Zinc Uptake
Muscle meats (heme content?)	Phytates (whole grains)
Picolinate	Excess dietary calcium, iron, copper
Citrate	Very high levels of EDTA
Amino acids	Oxalates (rhubarb, spinach)
Methionine	Intestinal metallothionen (induced by zinc or copper excess)
Cysteine (and glutathione)	Prostaglandin $F_{2\alpha}$
Histidine	
Lysine	
Glycine	
EDTA	
Prostaglandin E_2	
Lymphokines	
Corticosteroids	

uptake with fiber intake. An animal study compared zinc sulfate to zinc cysteamine-*N*-acetate during bone healing and found better results and less toxicity from the organic chelate.[823] Thus, preliminary evidence indicates that organic zinc salts behave quite differently from zinc sulfate. Therapeutic trials with organic zinc chelates may offer a significant difference in results from zinc sulfate trials and are therefore worthy of further attention.

G. ANIMAL STUDIES

Numerous studies have been performed on several species of animals in the study of zinc and wound healing.[824] Zinc was found to be essential for normal healing of skin, bones, gingiva, and gastric mucosa. In animals with adequate zinc status, supplemental zinc did not accelerate wound healing. Acceleration of wound healing was only seen in zinc-deficient animals. The early animal studies that found enhancement of wound healing from supplemental zinc were performed before dietary requirements of zinc were known and established. In retrospect, these studies measured zinc supplementation during zinc-deficient diets. These studies spurred research into human wound healing and zinc.

H. HUMAN STUDIES
1. Zinc and Wound Healing

Zinc has earned an association with wound healing, starting with the reports of Pories from 1966.[825] After determining that zinc was essential for proper wound healing in animal models, and unable to perform the same invasive measurements on humans, Pories chose the wounds made by excising pilonidal sinuses as a model of human wound healing. Pilonidal sinuses occur mostly in young, healthy males believed to consume an adequate diet and, therefore, not to have a deficient zinc intake. Healing of pilonidal sinus surgery is by second intention, with granulation tissue formation, offering a close comparison to animal models of wound healing. Eight subjects were studied, aged 16 to 27. After excision and cleaning of the wound, a cast of the wound was made with dental materials, and the wound volume measured by displacement of water volume. Wounds were completely healed in 36 to 63 d. A correlation between the healing rate and hair zinc levels was found, suggesting that zinc status played a role in human wound healing.

Pories and co-workers, from Wright-Patterson Air Force Hospital and the University of Rochester, published a landmark study in 1967 of the effect of zinc supplements on human wound healing.[826,827] There were 20 young airmen (18 to 40 years) with pilonidal sinuses randomly allocated into two groups of 10 subjects each — controls and zinc-treated. Endpoints were rate of wound healing determined by measurements of wound volume and time to complete healing (complete coverage with epithelium). Zinc treatment was 220 mg t.i.d. of zinc sulfate heptahydrate ($ZnSO_4 \cdot 7H_2O$), supplying 150 mg of elemental zinc per day. The time for complete healing was significantly sooner in the zinc-treated group (45.8 ± 2.6 vs. 80.1 ± 13.7 d, $p < 0.02$), an acceleration of 43%. Healing rates were also significantly faster (threefold) in the zinc-treated group (1.25 vs. 0.44 ml/d, p <0.01). Visual observation of healing wounds noted "cleaner, pinker and healthier granulations with considerably less purulent exudate."[827] The results are more remarkable considering that the average size of zinc-treated wounds was 54.5 ml compared to 32.3 ml for control wounds. Similar to animal studies, the acceleration of healing by zinc was seen only after 15 d. No toxicity from zinc sulfate was seen for the study period (43 to 61 d), and zinc sulfate was given after meals or with milk. One subject noted mild transient gastric discomfort when he ingested zinc before meals. Zinc status was not assessed in these subjects, so it was not known if the results were due to repletion of hidden zinc deficiencies or a pharmacological effect.

An extension of the previous study by Pories to 17 hospitalized patients with indolent wound healing was reported in 1969.[828] Patient wounds were as follows: 8/17 skin ulcers; 6/17 amputation sites; and 3/17 surgical wounds. Six patients were diabetics. All patients were given 150 mg elemental zinc daily as 220 mg $ZnSO_4 \cdot 7H_2O$ t.i.d. for 1 month or more. Serum zinc levels were determined before and after therapy. Patients who responded to zinc (11/17 by complete healing of wounds) all had serum zinc levels <100 µg/ml, and the 6/17 patients who did not exhibit complete wound healing all had serum zinc levels over 100 µg/ml. All patients except one ended with serum zinc levels over 100 µg/ml after zinc therapy. Positive changes in wound healing in responders usually occurred within 1 week, even if serum values took 4 to 6 weeks to enter normal ranges.

Henzel and others studied zinc levels in serum, erythrocytes, urine, skin, and wounds in normal controls and surgical patients.[829] Surgical patients were then given 220 mg $ZnSO_4 \cdot 7H_2O$ t.i.d., along with 500 mg ascorbic acid and a multiple vitamin supplement. In the first 2 weeks following major surgery, 11 subjects showed an average increase in urinary zinc excretion of 128%. In 16 patients with wound healing problems, skin zinc levels were 7.5 µg/g, while surgical patients with normal wound healing and controls averaged 16.8 and 16.6 µg/g, respectively. Granulation tissue from healing wounds in controls averaged 11.7 µg/g, while granulation tissue from surgical patients with normal wound healing showed 11.2 µg/g of zinc. Patients with wound healing problems showed zinc levels in granulation tissue of 6.6 µg/g. After zinc supplementation, controls and patients with normal wound healing showed an accumulation of zinc in granulation tissue, but patients with poor wound healing showed a smaller accumulation of zinc in granulation tissue. It was found that zinc supplementation was concentrated in healing wounds before repleting serum and skin levels of zinc in patients with poor wound healing. Furthermore, patients with poor wound healing showed a lag in increased urinary zinc excretion after supplementation, whereas control subjects immediately showed hyperzincuria after supplementation, indicating that deficient body zinc stores were being repleted. In the 16 patients with delayed wound healing, zinc supplementation improved healing to normal limits, concomitant with increased zinc levels in skin and wound sites. Again, these data indicate that zinc-deficient subjects exhibit impaired wound healing, which can be normalized after zinc supplementation. Subjects with adequate zinc status did not exhibit stimulation of wound healing, but did accumulate additional zinc at the wound site.

Barcia, from the Department of General Surgery at Martin Army Hospital in Fort Benning, Georgia, attempted a repeat study similar to that of Pories.[830] As in the previous study, 20 subjects with pilonidal sinus disease were divided into two groups: controls and zinc-treated. Zinc therapy was 220 mg $ZnSO_4 \cdot 7H_2O$ t.i.d., until wound healing was complete. The endpoint of complete epithelialization was used, and showed that there was no difference between control and zinc-treated groups for time to heal (59.6 vs. 63.7 d, respectively). In addition, three subjects reported nausea and epigastric distress from zinc sulfate therapy.

Buerk and others, from Tufts University School of Medicine, fed a zinc-deficient diet (1.0 mg/d) to four volunteers and measured wound healing from an experimental wound on the forearm as soon as serum zinc reached 0.8 µg/ml.[831] After the initial wound was healed, 150 mg of zinc per day was given, and another identical wound was studied for healing time. Although plasma zinc levels decreased from 1.15 to 0.62 µg/ml, and erythrocyte zinc also decreased (15.0 to 11.8 µg/ml), only one patient exhibited a prolonged healing time during zinc deficiency (48 vs. 36 d). This patient exhibited a cumulative, negative zinc balance of 58 mg, whereas the other three subjects did not show a significantly negative zinc balance. Thus, results indicate that a true zinc deficiency is associated with delayed wound healing in humans, and supplemental zinc to persons of adequate zinc status does not accelerate wound healing.

In otolaryngology, the formation of contact granulomas after laryngeal trauma or surgery has been difficult to resolve.[832,833] Pullen and others reported that 7/8 patients with respiratory tract granulations responded rapidly with elimination of granulomas and no residual granuloma formation.[832] Pullen also reported on a number of case reports (12) that found 7/10 patients responsive to zinc sulfate therapy (150 mg elemental zinc daily) within 5 months, but usually sooner.[833]

In six patients with bilateral adrenalectomy followed by corticosteroid therapy, wound healing 6 months to 2 years after the initial surgery was poor.[834] These patients exhibited low serum levels of zinc (probably due to corticosteroid therapy). Zinc supplementation was given to three patients, with complete healing noticed by 8 weeks. The three control patients showed little or no healing by 16 weeks. Rate of healing was positively correlated with serum zinc levels. Again, subjects with a zinc deficiency exhibited "enhanced" healing rates after zinc repletion. These results are consistent with zinc repletion normalizing wound healing.

Several reviews of zinc effects on wound healing in humans all reached the same conclusions: (1) studies had relatively few subjects, were poorly controlled, and most did not assess zinc status; (2) patients deficient in zinc were benefitted from zinc supplementation; (3) patients replete in zinc did not show enhanced healing; (4) assessment of zinc status was difficult and unreliable; and (5) zinc deficiencies were not uncommon in surgical patients.[807,824,835-837] Due to the uncertain incidence of marginal zinc deficiencies in the general population, even in apparently healthy subjects, it seems prudent to initiate zinc supplementation immediately after surgery. Since effects of zinc would be apparent only after 15 d, this allows sufficient time to replete most zinc-deficient subjects. Consult the section on zinc guidelines for an explanation of dosage and forms of zinc supplements.

2. Zinc and Skin Ulcer Healing

Closely allied with studies of zinc on wound healing are even more studies on the effects of zinc supplements for healing of skin ulcers from various causes (diabetes, venous insufficiency, arterio-venous insufficiency, decubitus [pressure sores], sickle-cell disease). Two British studies reported in 1968 found that zinc sulfate was effective for healing of decubitus ulcers, but no control groups were studied.[838,839] In 1969, Husain, from the Department of Dermatology, Southern General Hospital in Glasgow, reported on the effects of oral zinc supplementation in a double-blind manner to 104 patients with chronic lower limb ulcers.[840] All patients received bed rest and topical therapy consisting of sodium sulfate, calamine lotion, or eusol dressings. Ulcer healing was measured by volume determinations and planimetry of ulcer area until complete healing (no scab formation). Determinations of serum zinc before, during, and after the study quickly unblinded the investigator. Serum zinc levels rose from 102 to 189 µg/dl after zinc supplementation, which indicates that many subjects were initially zinc deficient, and compliance was good. Patients treated with zinc healed in 32.3 d (12 to 71 d), and placebo patients healed in 77.2 d (35 to 232 d), a significant difference ($p < 0.001$). The healing rate for zinc-treated ulcers was 90 mm^2 and 422 mm^2 for placebo patients. The only side effects noticed were three subjects with diarrhea after zinc therapy. This study found significant benefits from zinc supplementation in a population of chronic ulcer patients that did not respond to topical therapy.

Another study, by Greaves and Skillen, from the University Departments of Dermatology and Clinical Biochemistry at Newcastle upon Tyne, followed 18 patients with chronic venous leg ulcers of over 2 years duration.[841] All patients did not respond to conventional treatments and were ambulatory. All patients were given 220 mg of $ZnSO_4 \cdot 7H_2O$ t.i.d. for at least 4 months. After 4 months, 13/18 patients exhibited complete ulcer healing, and serum zinc rose by 25% or more in 10/15 subjects. Side effects noted were transient mild nausea in three subjects. Ulcer patients exhibited significantly lower serum zinc levels than normal controls (15 vs. 18 µM), indicating zinc deficiency was common in the ulcer group. Thus, this study offered further evidence that repletion of zinc-deficient patients with leg ulcers resulted in improved healing, but no control group was examined.

Serjeant and others, from the University of the West Indies in Kingston, Jamaica, studied the effects of zinc supplementation in 29 patients with sickle-cell disease leg ulcers.[842] Once again, 17 subjects received 220 mg/d of $ZnSO_4 \cdot 7H_2O$ t.i.d. for 12 weeks. All patients received topical eusol dressings. Initial serum zinc levels were 85 µg/dl for each group, significantly less than the 101 µg/dl serum zinc levels seen in non-sickle-cell relatives. Zinc supplementation raised levels to 143 µg/dl throughout the study period. Results showed that 6/15 zinc-treated subjects had complete healing, compared to 3/14 in the placebo group. Likewise, improvement in healing was noted for 13/15 zinc-treated subjects and 8/14 placebo subjects. The healing rate was faster in the zinc group (8.1 mm² vs. 2.8 mm²). Although all patients exhibited low serum zinc levels, this finding is endemic to sickle-cell anemia. Although the healing rate in sickle-cell patients with zinc was slower than previous studies of venous leg ulcers, it was significantly faster than the placebo. This study offers further evidence that leg ulcer healing is enhanced when a zinc-deficient state is encountered.

Myers and Cherry, from Louisiana State University School of Medicine in New Orleans, studied 40 ambulatory patients with chronic stasis ulcers of 3 months to 25 years duration (4.7 years mean).[843] All patients received compressive dressings and bed rest, and 16 received the usual dose of zinc sulfate (220 mg/d of $ZnSO_4 \cdot 7H_2O$ t.i.d.) for an average of 13 weeks. Zinc-treated subjects were compared with the untreated group, and themselves, before zinc therapy. The healing rate was determined by planimetry of wound area with time. Serum zinc levels were in the normal range before therapy. Results did not show any significant benefits from zinc therapy, nor was there an association between serum zinc and subsequent healing. Statistical reanalysis of the raw data from Myers and Cherry by more appropriate nonparametric testing did find a significant improvement in healing in the zinc group.[807] In addition, the significantly larger ulcer size in the placebo group biased results in favor of the placebo group.[835] Even so, an enhancing effect of zinc on ulcer healing was still found.

Norris and Reynolds reported on an ambitious double-blind, crossover study of zinc therapy for chronic decubitus ulcers in 14 geriatric patients, with 12-week placebo and zinc periods.[844] Unfortunately, half of the patients died before completion of the study, and only three subjects finished the entire 24-week study. Even so, Norris used incorrect statistical analysis to conclude there was no effect from zinc therapy when, in retrospect,[835] there was no proper way to analyze the data, since so many paired observations were lost.

Clayton reported on the results of a double-blind study of 10 patients with leg ulcers observed for 4 weeks.[845] In this study, the healing rate was faster in the placebo group, and not the zinc group, which was attributed to the significantly larger ulcer sizes in the placebo group (66 cm²) compared to the zinc group (45 cm²), a difference of 47%.[835] Since larger ulcers will heal relatively faster due to their larger size, this study was biased towards an effect for the placebo group. In addition, other studies all reproducibly showed that 4 weeks was an insufficient time interval to fully evaluate zinc effects, which routinely occurred after 30 d of zinc supplementation. Also, the group of ten patients was quite small to subdivide. Thus, the study of Clayton was biased towards the placebo group and cannot be compared to other studies.

Greaves and Ive conducted a double-blind study on 38 patients with chronic venous leg ulcers.[846] Zinc therapy was given for 4 months, or until ulcers were healed. Although the zinc group had a greater healing rate, the difference was not statistically different from the placebo. However, this study has been criticized for using a measurement of ulcer size which was less accurate than other methods.[835]

Hallböök and Lanner, from the Department of Surgery, University of Lund, in Lund, Sweden, conducted a double-blind trial in 27 patients with chronic venous leg ulcers.[847] All patients received the same topical dressings and were ambulatory; 13 subjects received 600 mg/d of effervescent zinc sulfate for 18 weeks. Ulcer size was measured by planimetry, and serum zinc levels were determined. Patients were divided into two groups based on their initial serum zinc levels, with a cutoff of 110 µg/dl. Each group was further subdivided into placebo and zinc-treated sets. In zinc-deficient patients (95 µg/dl serum zinc), zinc sulfate produced a highly significant improvement in healing, compared to placebo subjects. In the zinc-sufficient group, there was no difference between zinc and placebo sets. Zinc-treated subjects from each group were not different in their healing rates. A zinc effect was not seen until after 4 weeks of therapy, and zinc therapy evaluation was recommended no sooner than 7 to 8 weeks. This study reconfirmed the previous findings that zinc supplementation could normalize healing in deficient subjects, but not enhance healing in subjects with normal zinc status.

Haeger and co-workers studied the effects of zinc sulfate therapy on chronic venous leg ulcers from 53 subjects.[848] All subjects received topical silver spray with compressive bandages and were ambulatory.

Subjects were given either placebo, zinc sulfate capsules, or effervescent zinc sulfate (200 mg/d t.i.d.) until healing was complete. Completely healed ulcers ranged from 17/17 in the effervescent zinc group to 11/12 in the zinc capsule-treated group to 11/19 in the placebo group, a significant difference in favor of zinc groups. After 30 d, the healing rate was significantly faster in the zinc groups. Three patients on zinc sulfate capsules discontinued treatment after some mild side effects were noted, and the same percentage of dropouts was found in the placebo group. Healing of chronic leg ulcers from venous insufficiency was significantly enhanced by zinc sulfate therapy, after 30 d of therapy.

Husain studied 90 additional chronic lower limb ulcer patients (duration of 3 to 5 years) that were refractory to conventional topical therapy.[849] All subjects showed a low serum zinc level (93 µg/dl), and all were given topical treatment with compressive dressings. The usual dose of zinc sulfate (220 mg/d of $ZnSO_4 \cdot 7H_2O$ t.i.d.) was given for 112 d. At the end of the study period, 62/80 subjects were completely healed. Uptake of radioactive zinc-65 into ulcer areas was not different than non-ulcer areas. In one patient with no improvement in healing, corticosteroid-induced malabsorption of zinc was proven.

Pories and Strain referred to two studies by Brewer from 1966 and 1967 on patients with decubitus ulcers.[807] An initial study found 7/16 patients treated with zinc sulfate were completely healed in 8 weeks, with no changes in 4/16 patients. A second double-blind study with 14 patients found no differences between placebo and zinc-treated groups in healing of decubitus ulcers.

Merchant and co-workers studied the effects of zinc supplementation on 32 patients with idiopathic oral ulcerations (recurrent aphthous ulcers).[850] Zinc therapy (50 mg/d of elemental zinc from sulfate) was given to 17/32 patients. Supplementation was increased to 150 mg/d of zinc after 3 weeks if no changes were observed. Nine zinc-treated patients had serum zinc levels < 110 µg/dl. Overall, all nine subjects with low serum zinc levels were improved (less frequency, more remissions, less pain). Control patients (15/32) showed no decrease in the frequency of ulcer incidence. Again, this study showed that lower zinc status was associated with improvements upon zinc repletion which were not seen to the same extent in subjects with higher serum zinc levels.

Watkinson and others from the Medical Research Council Dunn Nutrition Unit in Cambridge, England, and Keneba, Gambia carried out a double-blind trial of zinc therapy in 28 children with acute tropical leg ulcers.[851] Although serum zinc levels were increased by zinc supplementation, initial values were not deficient, and no difference between the placebo and zinc groups was found for healing rates of ulcers.

Subsequent studies attempted to determine the prevalence of zinc deficiency in patients with leg ulcers from various causes. Ågren found that Swedish patients with arterial and venous leg ulcers showed lower serum zinc levels than a control group.[852] Bruske did not find significantly altered serum levels of zinc in venous leg ulcer patients in Germany,[853] while Thomas found a suboptimal zinc status by lowered leukocyte zinc levels in long-stay, elderly inpatients, 14/21 of which had leg ulcers or pressure sores.[854] Also, patients with healing problems exhibited lowest zinc status. In Russia, institutionalized elderly were shown to have lowered serum and leukocyte zinc levels, although no statistical relationship was found for zinc levels and presence of leg ulcers or unhealed wounds.[855] A Polish study found that only 10 to 15% of 20 patients with varicose ulcers exhibited deficient levels of plasma or erythrocyte zinc.[856] An Israeli study found that levels of zinc in varicose ulcers were less than unaffected leg skin, but equal to arm skin levels, suggesting a defect in zinc distribution.[857] A comprehensive review of nutritional intake and status of patients with pressure sores reported from 1943 to 1989 found a clear demonstration of malnutrition (including zinc) in such patients.[858] Likewise, general malnutrition, including subnormal plasma zinc levels, was found in a population of tube-fed nursing home patients with decubitus ulcers.[859] Thus, zinc is but one nutrient deficiency found in the average elderly skin ulcer patient. According to these findings, zinc would be expected to enhance healing in a subset of patients, which may or may not reach statistical significance. These findings are consistent with the literature on zinc and ulcer healing. Thus, zinc is important, but not singular, for enhancing skin ulcer healing.

Overall, many subjects with various types of recalcitrant leg ulcers were shown to have less than optimal zinc status and also shown to have benefits from oral zinc supplements. In cases where adequate zinc serum levels were found, zinc supplements tended not to benefit skin ulcer healing. Effects of zinc were apparent after 30 d of treatment, which is a rather slow effect that might be missed in impatient subjects. The ability of zinc to normalize, rather than stimulate, healing was supported by the majority of studies on zinc and leg ulcers in humans.

3. Zinc and Gastric Ulcer Healing

Healing of gastric and duodenal ulcers is not directly applicable to injury rehabilitation and sports medicine. Nevertheless, the healing of gastric mucosa (an epithelial tissue) is sufficiently similar to skin and loose connective tissues commonly encountered in sports medicine to briefly mention aspects of gastric ulcer healing and zinc. This section offers further data and evidence for a zinc effect on healing tissues that support the information on wound healing and skin ulcers.

Interest in zinc as a therapeutic agent for gastric ulcer healing started after zinc-deficient humans subjects exhibited gastrointestinal disorders, including ulcers.[808] Various zinc salts were examined for antiulcer effects in animal models and then human studies. Dozens of animal studies identified several potential mechanisms for antiulcer effects of zinc salts, including prostaglandin synthesis, antioxidant activity, membrane stabilization, and prevention of release of vasoactive substances known to precipitate ulcerogenic changes.[301,860-862] Human studies routinely revealed faster healing (compared to placebo) and less relapse (compared to H_2-blockers) after zinc salt treatments.[860,863-865] Zinc sulfate, zinc acexamate, and zinc carnosine[295-301] have been successfully used in gastric-duodenal ulcer therapy. Excellent tolerability and safety have been found with zinc salt use on gastric ulcers. Effects were seen, even though evidence of zinc deficiency was not found in most subjects.[861] Overall, the results further support the function and use of zinc to improve epithelial tissue healing.

4. Zinc and Burns

Another interaction of zinc and skin has been found in thermal burn patients. Usually, serum zinc levels drop quickly and remain depressed for several weeks or months, depending on severity and depth of burns.[866] Losses of zinc from burn wounds are large and can amount to 5 to 10% of total body stores per week.[866-869] Pories and Strain measured the hair zinc levels at various times after thermal burns (3rd degree, 3 to 40% of body surface) in 6 patients.[825] A rapid and large decrease in hair zinc was seen for at least 40 d to levels 20 to 50% below the lower reference range. A slow increase to preburn levels by 100 d was seen for 7/8 patients. This observation spurred closer studies of zinc as therapy after burns in humans. Usually, a correlation of zinc status with healing rates has been found in burned patients.[869] The effects of zinc supplements appear to benefit the patients with the least adequate zinc status, and not benefit those with adequate zinc status and intake.[869] These results mirror the findings of zinc and other skin conditions.

5. Zinc and Arthritis

After early surveys of rheumatoid arthritis patients found consistent decreases in serum zinc levels,[870-874] a clinical trial of zinc supplementation to patients with rheumatoid arthritis was conducted.[875] Simkin, from the Department of Rheumatology at the University of Washington in Seattle, administered 220 mg/d of $ZnSO_4 \cdot 7H_2O$ t.i.d. or placebo to 24 patients with rheumatoid arthritis, in addition to existing therapies, for 12 weeks.[875] The double-blind period was followed by an open period in which each subject received zinc sulfate for another 12 weeks. The results of this study and others are given in Table 7. This trial found a beneficial effect on symptoms of rheumatoid arthritis and initiated a series of studies by other investigators.[876-886] In addition to the studies listed in Table 7, Heinitz reported on the excellent response of a single patient to zinc aspartate.[887] Out of five double-blind studies, three found some significant benefits from zinc sulfate therapy, compared to the placebo group. One study was a double-blind, crossover design, and two also showed improvements in placebo subjects who were given zinc sulfate after the blinded study period in an open period. In each study that measured serum zinc levels, increases were noted, and serum alkaline phosphatase activity also increased. All studies examined relatively small numbers of subjects (13 to 35), and clear evidence of zinc deficiency was not

TABLE 7   Results of Oral Zinc Therapy in Rheumatoid Arthritis

Reference	n	Dosage	Study Design	Results
875	12 placebo 12 experimental	220 mg/d t.i.d. $ZnSO_4 \cdot 7H_2O$ 12 weeks + 12 weeks	rdb and open	Significant ↓ Joint swelling; ↓ joint tenderness; ↓ morning stiffness; ↓ walking time; overall patient assessment; ↑ serum zinc, alkaline phosphatase Not significant Grip strength; erythrocyte sedimentation rate; routine lab parameters
884	13	200 mg/d t.i.d. $ZnSO_4 \cdot 7H_2O$	Open	Significant ↓ Erythrocyte sedimentation rate; 5/9 subjects responded favorably
880 (psoriatic arthritis)	24 dbco 12 open	220 mg/d t.i.d. $ZnSO_4 \cdot 7H_2O$ 12 weeks + 24 weeks	rdbco and open	Significant ↓ Morning stiffness; ↓ joint pain; ↓ joint swelling; ↑ joint motility; ↓ analgesic usage; overall patient assessment; ↑ serum zinc, albumin; ↓ serum immunoglobulins Not significant Grip strength; psoriatic skin involvement; erythrocyte sedimentation rate; routine lab parameters
882	17 placebo 18 experimental	200 mg/d t.i.d. $ZnSO_4 \cdot 7H_2O$ 16 weeks	rdb	Significant ↑ Serum zinc, alkaline phosphatase, 5'-nucleotidase Not significant Morning stiffness, night awakening, joint pain, joint size, grip strength, articular index, functional index, patient assessment, investigator evaluation, prednisone dosage, erythrocyte sedimentation rate, fibrinogen, rheumatoid factor
878	9 placebo 9 experimental	250 mg/d t.i.d. $ZnSO_4 \cdot 7H_2O$ 12 weeks	rdb	Significant ↓ Joint swelling; ↓ joint tenderness; ↓ morning stiffness; ↑ walking time; ↓ analgesic, prednisone usage; onset of fatigue; overall assessment; ↑ serum zinc, alkaline phosphatase
883	9 placebo 12 experimental	220 mg/d t.i.d. $ZnSO_4 \cdot 7H_2O$ 24 weeks	rdb	Significant ↓ Ring size; ↑ alkaline phosphatase Not significant Joint pain; morning stiffness; articular index; grip strength; patient assessment; routine lab parameters; erythrocyte sedimentation rate
885	22	220 mg/d t.i.d. $ZnSO_4 \cdot 7H_2O$ 2–24 months	Open	Significant Initial subjective assessment (deteriorated later) Not significant Investigator evaluation; number of affected joints; ARA grading; functional classification; erythrocyte sedimentation rate; routine lab parameters
881 (psoriatic arthritis)	18	200 mg/d t.i.d. $ZnSO_4 \cdot 7H_2O$ 6 months	Open	Significant ↓ Number of swollen joints; ↓ joint tenderness; ↓Ritchie articular index; ↓ analgesic usage; ↓ erythrocyte sedimentation rate; ↓ plasma copper level

Abbreviations used: rdb = randomized, double-blind; dbco = double-blind, crossover; rdbco = randomized, double-blind, crossover; $ZnSO_4 \cdot 7H_2O$ = zinc sulfate heptahydrate.

found in almost every study. Thus, the hypothesis that repletion of zinc deficiency would affect rheumatoid arthritis was not fully tested. Two other open trials of zinc sulfate and rheumatoid arthritis were equivocal — one showed benefits from zinc, the other did not.[884,885] One additional open study on zinc and psoriatic arthritis showed significant benefits after 6 months of therapy, similar to earlier findings in a double-blind study.[881]

Thus, results from equally well-designed and comparable studies found different results for zinc sulfate supplementation in rheumatoid arthritis. Since serum levels of zinc are an unreliable indicator of zinc status, no study adequately assessed zinc status. Thus, differences in observed results among studies could be related to undetected differences in zinc status. Differing medications could also account for some variability, since penicillamine and corticosteroids are known to affect zinc status and were used in some patients. Subsequent research has indicated that decreased plasma zinc levels are a nonspecific consequence of inflammation.[810,874] Thus, variable findings in serum zinc levels from subjects with rheumatoid arthritis (5/9 studies showed decreased levels)[878] are obviously influenced to a large degree by other factors not taken into account in studies to date. For example, zinc excretion was significantly increased in two studies of rheumatoid arthritis patients,[878] and erythrocyte and leukocyte zinc levels were decreased in rheumatoid arthritis patients.[874] Interactions with histidine and copper are also suspected to influence zinc roles in rheumatoid arthritis.[878] Thus, a rationale for zinc therapy in rheumatoid arthritis is unclear at this time and may relate more to inflammation in general than specific antirheumatic effects. Empirical testing of zinc sulfate in rheumatoid arthritis has yielded equivocal results. Unfortunately, zinc chelates, such as zinc histidinate, zinc monomethionine, zinc picolinate, zinc citrate, or zinc aspartate, have not been tested in rheumatoid arthritis. Since these zinc salts have different pharmacokinetics than zinc sulfate, their attributes may be different than zinc sulfate. Thus, the question of whether zinc is beneficial for inflammatory joint diseases remains unanswered.

6. Zinc and Bone Healing

The effects of zinc status on bone health stem from the essential role of zinc in bone calcification.[888] Bones are one tissue where zinc is concentrated relative to other tissues. Zinc deficiencies delay bone healing in animal models.[888] Zinc supplementation to animals with experimental bone fractures has enhanced healing rates.[823,888] Loss of zinc and bone mass has been found in humans immobilized by accidents, skeletal trauma, or bed rest.[889-892] These occurrences start immediately after injury or rest, and persist for long time periods.

Higashi and others, from the Department of Pediatrics in Kumamoto University Medical School in Kumamoto, Japan, studied the relationship between zinc status and bone demineralization in 74 disabled persons (ages 16 to 45 years).[893] Their results showed that as disability increased, bone mineralization decreased, and the distribution of body zinc in the skeleton diminished. All subjects were institutionalized at the same facility and fed diets containing 6.7 ± 1 mg/d of zinc. Bone mineral density of the lumbar spine was determined by X-ray densitometry, and subjects were placed into three groups according to their disability (Group 1 = able to walk with assistance; Group 2 = able to crawl; Group 3 = bedridden). Importantly, zinc status was measured by kinetic studies of zinc clearance and fractional excretion, a dynamic means of assessing zinc status. Results found that serum zinc, a measure of zinc status used previously in many studies, was not different between groups, offering further evidence of the futility of using serum zinc measurements to assess tissue zinc status. However, studies of zinc kinetics after intravenous administration found that peripheral tissues (presumably including the skeleton) took up more zinc than controls, indicating deficient status of zinc in tissues. The bone mineral density was negatively correlated with the distribution volume of zinc (-0.387, $p < 0.005$), and as disability progressed, so did zinc deficient status and loss of bone mineral density. Urinary calcium excretion was significantly higher in the bedridden group. The results taken together suggest that zinc deficiency exists in tissues of disabled or bedridden persons at usual dietary intakes (7 mg/d). These results argue in favor of zinc deficiency being a major factor in bone density loss after immobilization, consistent with findings from multiple studies. The implications for active persons suddenly immobilized by an injury, and wishing to minimize bone loss, are to pay close attention to zinc status and consider prophylactic zinc supplementation.

I. SAFETY

Zinc therapy is not without toxicity.[894] Like many other trace elements, zinc was initially thought to be toxic until its essentiality was proven. Therefore, use of zinc supplements must follow certain guidelines to prevent possible toxicity. Numerous studies have administered oral zinc sulfate (600 to 660 mg $ZnSO_4 \cdot H_2O$, for 150 mg of elemental zinc) daily in 3 divided doses for long time periods (up to 2 years) to patients in various health states. About 5 to 10% of subjects given this amount of zinc sulfate exhibited signs of gastric distress, such as nausea, epigastric pain or burning, and occasional vomiting. However, these effects were almost always encountered when subjects did not follow directions and ingested zinc sulfate on empty stomachs. When zinc sulfate supplements were consumed with meals or a glass of milk, very few immediate side effects were noticed. Long-term effects (3 to 6 months) on clinical laboratory parameters after zinc supplementation were almost always unchanged. However, three separate studies have found long-term side effects from high doses of zinc sulfate. All three results appear to be explained by the effects of zinc on reduction of copper status, perhaps by induction of intestinal metallothionen to counteract excess zinc, which then binds to dietary copper, rendering it unavailable. Also, symptoms of zinc excess are similar to symptoms of excess prostaglandin synthesis (gastrointestinal distress, diarrhea, nausea), which may be related to the known roles of zinc in prostaglandin synthesis.[894]

Anemia due to copper depletion by excess zinc intake (150 to 5000 mg/d) has been observed repeatedly.[894] Anemia is seen after several months of high-dose zinc supplementation and resolves after cessation of zinc, or by copper supplementation (at least 1 mg/d). The second long-term zinc side effect is suppression of immune function in human volunteers after several months of ingesting over 150 mg elemental zinc daily.[895] Third, zinc supplementation (160 mg/d and greater) has been associated with reductions in serum HDL cholesterol levels.[896] Each of these observations was after large doses of zinc sulfate, an inorganic salt. It is not known whether organic zinc chelates would exhibit similar results.

J. SUMMARY

The role of zinc in wound healing has become common knowledge; however, the clinical use of zinc has not. Despite some studies showing significant benefits for healing of surgical wounds, skin ulcers, bone fractures, burns, and gastric ulcers, clinical use of zinc has never progressed into routine use. Part of the reason is that studies have not been reproducible (some studies showed benefits, others did not). A major problem is that assessment of zinc status is still not reliable or suited for routine testing. While the most reliable test is a supplementation trial, this does not offer predictive information on zinc status and, therefore, benefit from zinc supplements. Another problem is the universal use of zinc sulfate in human studies instead of other zinc chelates that are now known to be more bioavailable with less interactions and side effects. Zinc sulfate is not an ideal choice for oral zinc therapy, but almost no studies in humans have used anything else. Increasing recognition of malnutrition and benefits of nutritional repletion in hospitalized patients means that inclusion of zinc in enteral or parenteral supplements can help prevent problems associated with zinc deficiencies.

The question of whether zinc supplementation is beneficial to healing of traumatic injuries commonly seen in sports medicine cannot be answered conclusively at this time. Strong evidence indicates that when zinc deficiency is present, zinc supplementation is extremely beneficial. However, when a definite zinc deficiency is not found or not suspected, does zinc have therapeutic value? Again, studies are equivocal. Most studies examined populations of older, diseased adults, with dubious relevance to younger, apparently more healthy athletes. One has to examine the incidence of zinc deficiency in athletic populations, where one again finds conflicting results. Nevertheless, subsets of every group studied have shown definite zinc deficiencies, even if the population as a whole averages adequate zinc status. Thus, without extensive, expensive, and time-consuming testing, one cannot predict the zinc status of an individual with any accuracy. Thus, it is prudent to insure adequate zinc supply during critical healing times for almost any injury or condition. This is, in effect, a supplementation trial, with healing as an endpoint, which may be the most useful indicator of zinc status. It is less expensive and may induce a positive placebo effect. If zinc deficiency is present, then its correction

TABLE 8   Guidelines for Zinc Supplementation

Daily dosage:	25–50 mg in 1 or 2 doses
Supplemental forms:	Zinc monomethionine, zinc histidinate, zinc citrate, zinc picolinate, zinc aspartate, zinc cysteinate, zinc carnosinate

Injuries/conditions for which zinc supplementation is indicated:
- Surgical wounds
- Bone fractures
- Immobilizing injuries or conditions
- Lacerations
- Abrasions
- Skin ulcers or damage
- Bone loss (osteoporosis)
- Corticosteroid therapy
- Thermal burns (2nd and 3rd degree)
- Gastric or duodenal ulcers
- Delayed wound healing
- Delayed healing of connective tissues

would normalize healing. If zinc status is not deficient, then side effects become a major issue. Side effects can be prevented by use of lower doses of more modern zinc chelates instead of zinc sulfate.

K. GUIDELINES FOR USE

Zinc supplementation is easily accomplished by one of two means. First is the inclusion of a multiple vitamin/mineral product that contains zinc. These products usually supply 10 to 15 mg of zinc daily, although careful attention must be paid to the label. Also, multiple vitamin/mineral products frequently use inorganic salts (such as zinc oxide or sulfate), which are known to be less bioavailable and more prone to interferences in uptake. Second, use of specific zinc supplements can be considered. Preferred zinc supplements would be in the following forms: monomethionine; picolinate; citrate; aspartate; histidinate; or cysteinate. Daily doses should range from 25 to 50 mg, in 1 or 2 doses daily. Although almost no data exist to confirm the utility of adding copper to zinc supplements (to prevent possible depressions in copper status), the use of organic zinc chelates with additional copper is sound nutritional practice. The ratio of elemental zinc to copper can range from 10 to 25:1. These ranges are well within safety limits for each mineral. Use of organic chelates is recommended to prevent possible interactions with each other and other minerals. Table 8 lists some conditions where it is more feasible to ensure adequate zinc status by supplementation than to wait for possible delays in healing.

III. COPPER

A. INTRODUCTION

Copper has had a long history of medicinal uses, including treatment of arthritic conditions.[808] Total body copper content ranges from 70 to 99 mg, and is richest in liver and brain tissues.[808] Total body percentage of copper is distributed as follows: skeletal muscle, 25 to 40%; skeleton, 19%, bone marrow, 15%; skin, 15%; liver, 8 to 15%; and brain, 8 to 10%.[808,897] As can be seen, musculoskeletal tissues contain the majority of total body copper. Copper was shown to be essential for humans in 1966, and its importance in nutrition has increased yearly. Copper ions (cupric or Cu^{2+}) are potent oxidizing agents, which contribute to activity of copper-containing enzymes and peptides.

B. ROLES AND FUNCTIONS

Copper functions primarily as a component of metalloenzymes (cuproenzymes) with essential functions and also activates other enzymes. Table 9 lists some cuproenzymes and their respective

TABLE 9   Functions of Copper Pertinent to Connective Tissues

Roles	Functions
Component of lysyl oxidase	Collagen and elastin cross-linking (structural integrity of collagen, elastin, connective tissues, arteries; formation of osteoid)
Component of copper-zinc superoxide dismutase	Antioxidant functions
Component of cytochrome *c* oxidase	Cellular energy production
Component of ceruloplasmin (ferroxidase I)	Antioxidant functions, acute phase reactant

physiological functions.[93,808,897] All copper metalloenzymes involve molecular oxygen or oxygen species in their reactions. Of particular importance to connective tissues are copper-zinc superoxide dismutase (CuZnSOD) and lysyl oxidase. CuZnSOD protects tissues from superoxide anion damage by converting superoxide into hydrogen peroxide ($2O_2^- + 2H^+ \rightarrow H_2O_2 + O_2$).[898] Lysyl oxidase catalyses cross-linking of collagen, which is necessary for proper collagen formation, osteoid formation, and integrity of all connective tissues.[93,899] Thus, copper is essential for formation and maintenance of connective tissues and skeletal mineralization.

Cytochrome c oxidase is the terminal enzyme in oxidative phosphorylation, consuming oxygen and generating ATP, thus being vital for production of cellular energy.[900] Ceruloplasmin is also an acute phase reactant that catalyzes oxidation of ferrous ions to ferric ions and, in so doing, possesses weak antioxidant properties.[901]

C. DEFICIENCY SYMPTOMS

Most deficiency symptoms of copper have been observed in infants or patients receiving TPN without copper and represent acute copper deficiency symptoms. These symptoms are listed in Table 10. However, increasing evidence suggests that chronic low intake or function of copper may be associated with connective tissue disorders in adults.[902] Acute copper deficiency in humans is associated with bone loss and fractures, in addition to anemia and neutropenia. [808,897,903-914] Specific findings in infants were marginal spur formation (Pelken's sign), metaphyseal radiolucency (Truemmerfeld zone), double epiphyses, generalized osteoporosis (ground glass appearance), calcification at ossification centers (Wimberger's rings), subperiosteal calcification, and undisplaced fractures in various stages of healing.[904] In Menke's Disease, a congenital defect in copper absorption and utilization, children exhibit osteoporotic bones.[93,904,915] Ehlers-Danlos Syndromes V and IX exhibit decreased lysyl oxidase activity, resulting in greater collagen degradation, with connective tissue abnormalities.[93] In this instance, an effective deficiency of copper in connective tissues is mimicked by decreased lysyl oxidase activity. In fact, osteopenia of copper deficiency closely resembles osteoporosis of scurvy, which probably reflects the commonality of function for ascorbate and copper to catalyze collagen cross-link formation by two different mechanisms. Thus, osteopenia of copper deficiency is clearly linked to the essential function of the cuproenzyme lysyl oxidase.

D. ASSESSMENT

At this time, there is no single marker for copper status that is accepted as sensitive and accurate. Obvious measurements of copper status include serum (plasma) copper levels, hair copper levels, and erythrocyte copper levels.[808,916,917] Static measurements of copper levels are not trustworthy for finding deficiencies, since many factors not related to copper nutriture affect copper levels (see Table 11). However, static copper levels of body fluids are acceptable for determining copper excess, as in Wilson's Disease. Usually, if serum copper or serum ceruloplasmin levels are low, then a copper deficiency is indicated, subject to constraints in Table 13. Normal ranges for human serum copper are 12 to 23 μmol/l, and for ceruloplasmin, 20 to 60 mg/dl.

Hair mineral analysis is an accurate method to determine copper deficiency when environmental copper contamination (air, soaps, shampoos, conditioners), rate of hair growth, and length of hair from scalp are controlled, provided conditions in Table 13 are not evident.[808]

TABLE 10   Deficiency Symptoms of Copper in Humans

Anemia (microcytic, hypochromic)
Neutropenia
Skeletal demineralization (osteoporosis, bone fragility, fractures)
Subperiosteal hemorrhages
Depigmentation of hair, skin
Defective elastin formation (arterial aneurysms, decreased tensile strength of skin)
Cerebral, cerebellar degeneration
Hypotonia
Hypothermia
Clinical findings include:
   ↓ Erythrocyte CuZnSOD activity
   ↓ Lysyl oxidase activity (tissue culture)
   ↓ Liver glutathione peroxidase activity
   ↓ Glucose tolerance
   ↓ Immune function
   ↓ Serum copper levels
   ↓ Serum ceruloplasmin levels
   ↓ Lecithin:cholesterol acyltransferase (LCAT) activity
   ↑ Serum cholesterol
   ↓ Serum HDL cholesterol
   ↑ Cell membrane lipid peroxidation
   ↓ Insoluble elastin
   ↓ Collagen fiber maturation
   ↑ Collagen degradation
   ↓ Tensile strength and stretch modulus of elastin
   ↓ Extractable hexosamines

Note: Most of these symptoms have been documented in infants, patients receiving
long-term total parenteral nutrition, Ehlers-Danlos Syndrome V and IX, or
Menke's disease (congenital abnormality of copper metabolism).

Functional indices of copper status include determination of enzymatic activity of cuproenzymes. Serum ceruloplasmin activity (as a ferroxidase) represents short-term copper status, since ceruloplasmin has a serum half-life of 3 to 5 days.[916] However, since ceruloplasmin contains up to 95% of total serum copper, estimation of ceruloplasmin activity has little benefits over total serum copper determinations and the same interferences (see Table 11). However, the ratio of ceruloplasmin levels determined by enzymatic and radial immunodiffusion methods may be indicative of short-term copper status.[917]

Erythrocyte CuZnSOD activity has become the method of choice for determination of copper status. Ease of collection, ease of determination, and good correlation with tissue copper levels make CuZnSOD an accurate indicator of copper deficiency, less subject to variables seen in Table 13.[916,917] CuZnSOD activity represents a long-term reflection of copper status since the lifespan of erythrocytes is approximately 3 months. The reference range for erythrocyte CuZnSOD activity will vary with methodology and laboratory.

Clinical symptoms of copper deficiency (sideroblastic anemia, bone demineralization) appear after a long-term, chronic deficit of copper has been maintained. Of course, perhaps the simplest and least expensive means of assessing copper status is to administer a copper supplement and monitor copper status, both biochemically and clinically. Unfortunately, this method is retrospective, but does combine diagnosis and treatment at one time.

E.   INTAKES

The 1989 RDAs list a range of 2 to 3 mg/d for the Estimated Safe and Adequate Daily Dietary Intake (ESADDI), although recent research suggests that copper balance in humans is met at 1.2 to 1.4 mg Cu per day.[808] If the latter figures are applicable, then the low copper intakes found for women may have less practical significance.

TABLE 11 Factors Affecting Determination of Copper Status

"False" Elevations	"False" Depressions
Inflammation	Long-term corticosteroid therapy
Infection, sepsis	Decreased ceruloplasmin synthesis (liver diseases)
Third-degree burns	Zinc deficiency ($\downarrow$ erythrocyte superoxide dismutase,
Estrogen therapy	$\downarrow$ protein synthesis)
Oral contraceptives	
Pregnancy	
Cigarette smoking	
High-dose corticosteroids	
Contamination	
Hemolysis	
Wilson's disease	
Advancing age	
Females	
Diurnal variation (morning peak)	

Note: These factors affect serum levels of total copper. "False" elevations or depressions are in relation to nutritional status and actual tissue stores of copper.

Table 12 lists estimated dietary intakes of copper for women in the U.S. It can be seen that the majority of women do not consume even the lower limit of the ESADDI of copper, with most consuming about half of the ESADDI. Males consumed amounts of copper within the ESADDI, but there is still a significant proportion of males with intakes well below the ESADDI. Overall, most studies have found suboptimal intakes of copper in the U.S.[918]

F. DIETARY SOURCES AND INFLUENCES

Dietary sources richest in copper are oysters, shellfish (lobster, shrimp, crab, clams, mussels), soybean products, legumes, nuts, seeds, brans, liver, and potatoes.[788] Copper is widely distributed in foods with variable levels. Milk, eggs, and rice are very low in copper, which may be detrimental to some infants.

Nonfood sources of copper can significantly add to copper intakes. Copper pipes carrying drinking water and cooking with copper and brass utensils can add a significant amount of copper to a daily dietary intake. Inhibitory dietary factors include (1) uncooked meat, (2) cellulose fiber, (3) ascorbic acid excess [vitamin C], (4) zinc excess, (5) iron excess, (6) phosphate excess, and (7) possibly fructose.[808,919] Sucrose, and especially fructose, when fed to male rats at high dietary intakes (60% of calories), decreased bioavailability of copper by 30%, compared to isocaloric starch intakes.[919] Applicability of these results to humans is unclear at this time, although a diet with 20% sucrose does not appear to affect short-term copper status in man.[919] Factors that enhance copper uptake are (1) breast milk, (2) histidine, and (3) other single amino acids. Knowledge on dietary influences on copper uptake and absorption is still in seminal stages.

G. ANIMAL STUDIES

Reviews by Carnes summarized earlier work on animals made deficient in copper.[920,921] Osteoporosis, cortical and trabecular thinning, lack of osteoid, spontaneous fractures, excessive joint mobility, swelling of the ends of long bones and joints, physical deformities, lameness, stiffness of gait, reduced tensile strength of skin, depigmentation of hair (achromotrichia), and growth impairment were seen. Many similarities to ascorbic acid deficiency were seen, which suggests that an as yet unidentified copper-associated protein may interact with ascorbic acid metabolism, or that a common mechanism of defective collagen cross-linking is apparent. Most defects were seen in young, growing animals (calves, lambs, swine, dogs, rats, mice) and fowl (chicks, turkey poults), rather than adult animals. Copper depletion frequently resulted in death of adult animals from aneurysms or hemorrhages before osseous abnormalities were evident.

TABLE 12   Dietary Copper Intakes in Adult Women in the U.S.

Ref.	Subjects	Copper Intake (mg/d)
976	1989 Safe and Adequate Daily Intake	2.0–3.0
955	High protein hospital diet	<0.20
953	15 high school ♀	0.34
955	General hospital diet	0.42
953	28 college ♀	0.58
779	Selected Minerals in Foods Survey	
	14–16 years ♀	0.77
	25–30 years ♀	0.93
	60–65 years ♀	0.86
819	28 adults (both genders)	1.2
918	Standard diet, Minnesota	1.3

Strause and Saltman, of the University of California at San Diego in La Jolla, fed weanling rats a diet low in manganese (2.5 ppm) and low in copper (0.5 ppm) in a series of studies, and examined long-term parameters of bone status.[922-924] A low-copper diet, rather than a completely copper-deficient diet, was chosen to prevent premature deaths from aortic aneurysms, and also to more closely mimic a chronic, marginal intake of copper that may be prevalent in human females. Decreased femur calcium (200 ± 30 vs. 333 ± 111 mg/g), increased serum calcium, increased serum phosphorus, reduced ability to calcify demineralized bone implants, and reduced ability to resorb implanted bone powder were recorded. These results all signify that a combined low intake of copper and manganese leads to detrimental changes in bone health and metabolism in rats. These findings are important given the possible low copper intakes of women throughout a lifetime.[779]

However, Massie and others, of the Masonic Medical Research Laboratory in Utica, New York, found that elderly mice with decreased bone density exhibited progressively higher bone levels of copper (by 61%) than younger animals, and that excess femur copper correlated better than other parameters (calcium, iron, boron, collagen) with decreased bone density. Further work is necessary to determine whether or not copper is accumulated as an adaptive but futile response to decreasing bone mass because of other limiting factors.

A naturally occurring tripeptide with growth factor properties isolated from human plasma was determined to be the curpic salt of glycyl-histidinyl-lysinate (GHL-Cu).[925] GHL-Cu possessed SOD and angiogenic activities. Effects of GHL-Cu on rat skin wound healing was reported by Pickart and others from the University of Washington at Seattle.[925] A 2-cm circular patch of skin was removed from the back of rats, and 50 μg GHL-Cu was injected around the wound. Wound healing was significantly enhanced, so that after 15 d, 6/10 GHL-Cu-treated wounds were fully healed, while 0/10 control wounds were healed. Results were similar in mice and pigs. GHL-Cu doubled the migration of human capillary endothelial cells in a Boyen chamber model. Thus, GHL-Cu may minimize tissue damage from oxidants while simultaneously providing a chemoattractant stimulus for neovascularization.

Numerous studies of copper compounds on animal models of gastric ulcers have found significant enhancement of healing.[926] Compounds with highest activity were copper complexes with nonsteroidal antiinflammatory agents. These and other studies suggest that endogenous copper may facilitate action of NSAIDs. Thus, copper compounds, both nature-identical and synthetic, assist and enhance wound healing in animal models.

H. HUMAN STUDIES
1. Arthritis and Inflammatory Conditions

Use of copper jewelry (usually bracelets) to alleviate arthritis symptoms has been a folk medicine practice for many years.[927] Walker and Keats, of the University of Newcastle Shortland, New South Wales, Australia, selected 166 subjects with arthritis/rheumatism that responded to a newspaper notice.[927,928] Seventy-seven subjects were given both a copper bracelet and an identical-looking aluminum bracelet to wear in consecutive 1-month periods in a random order. Subjects evaluated perceived effectiveness of each bracelet and results were compared to a control group of 41 subjects. Significantly more subjects perceived the copper bracelet to be more effective at reducing arthritic symptoms. Of the 77 subjects with bracelets, 10/77 (13%) judged the aluminum bracelets were better, 30/77 (39%) judged the bracelets were the same, and 37/77 (48%) judged the copper bracelets were better. Only 7/41 (17%) controls became "better" without bracelets during the study period. Interestingly, control subjects who were previous users of copper bracelets fared significantly worse when not wearing their bracelet (11/19, 58%). The average weight loss of bracelets was 13 mg, indicating that approximately 0.4 mg/d of copper was potentially available for dermal absorption. In addition, dietary analysis revealed that most subjects consumed "low" amounts of copper and seldom ate foods rich in copper (liver, shellfish, mushrooms, nuts). Dermal absorption of copper was shown to be previously documented. Long-term use of copper bracelets could add the total amount of body copper via dermal transfer in a year's time. Thus, it is feasible that copper bracelets may actually have therapeutic value for reduction of arthritic symptoms. The use of copper sebacate as a source of copper for nutritional supplements reflects the concept of copper bracelets solubilized by sweat.

Another folk medicine treatment for arthritis based on copper therapy was apple cider vinegar, which was traditionally made in copper-lined vessels.[929] Small amounts of copper from the vessel would be solubilized by organic acids from apple juice (malate). If consumed with quantity and regularity, then intake of organic copper chelates may be sufficient to replete physiological functions, similar to copper bracelets. However, simply consuming commercially available apple cider (not produced in copper vessels) would not have a chance to add copper to a person's diet, nor would therapeutic benefits follow.

Rheumatism in Finland is common, but Finnish copper miners rarely suffered from rheumatism.[930] Furthermore, purulent infections were uncommon. Therefore, there are substantial anecdotal observations to indicate further studies on the role of copper as therapy in rheumatic diseases be scrutinized.

Values of serum copper and ceruloplasmin are consistently elevated in inflammatory conditions and represent a part of the Acute Phase Response.[931] Ceruloplasmin contains 95% of serum copper, with most of the rest bound to albumin.[810] Serum copper and ceruloplasmin levels have been repeatedly documented to be elevated in patients with rheumatoid arthritis, ankylosing spondylitis, psoriatic arthritis, and sarcoidosis with joint involvement,[932-935] but seldom in osteoarthritis. At present, the increase in copper (ceruloplasmin) is thought to represent an attempt to increase antioxidant activity by converting ferrous ions to ferric ions, thereby short-circuiting production of hydroxyl radicals from superoxide radicals and hydrogen peroxide.[810] Ceruloplasmin can also scavenge superoxide, albeit at low efficiency compared to CuZnSOD, and can also transport copper to cells for synthesis of CuZnSOD and other essential cuproenzymes.[810] Other antiinflammatory effects of copper are listed in Table 13.[810,929,936-938]

Rheumatoid arthritis patients showed an inverse relationship between erythrocyte CuZnSOD activity and severity of disease,[934] and decreased activity of erythrocyte CuZnSOD compared to control subjects.[939] Copper supplementation (2 mg Cu/d as copper glycinate for 4 weeks) led to a significant increase in erythrocyte CuZnSOD activity (2934 ± 456 to 3448 ± 446 Units/ml erythrocytes) in 18/23 rheumatoid arthritis subjects, resulting in identical values to supplemented controls (3486 ± 443 U/ml erythrocytes).[939] This study suggests that even in spite of elevated levels of serum copper, a relative copper deficiency in tissues occurred which was sufficient to decrease cuproenzyme functions. Although clinical outcomes were not reported, these results argue for serious consideration of copper supplementation to rheumatoid arthritic patients at safe, dietary levels for repletion of tissue copper stores.

Clinical trials of copper supplementation to patients with rheumatoid arthritis have a long and overlooked history, even before the role of copper was even barely understood. Copper complexes derived from tuberculosis research around 1940 were tried as a series of intravenous injections in patients with rheumatoid arthritis.[940,941] Cupralene (sodium 3-(allylcuprothkouredo) 1-benzoate) and Dicuprene (Cuprimyl, cupric bis[8-hydroxyquinoline di(diethylammonium sulfonate)]) were the two compounds studied initially.[940] Doses of 0.25 to 0.5 g per injection and 2 to 5 g per series were routinely administered for 10 to 14 series. Total doses of copper ranged from 0.4 to 1.0 g over a period of several months (about 10 mg Cu/d).

TABLE 13 Antiinflammatory Effects of Copper

Superoxide dismutase (CuZnSOD) mimic (copper complexes with amino acids and other low molecular weight
  ligands possess significant superoxide dismutase activity and are found *in vivo*)
Catalase mimic (copper–polyamine complexes possess catalase activity)
Ceruloplasmin ferroxidase activity oxidizes free ferrous ions to less reactive ferric ions to reduce formation of
  highly reactive hydroxyl radicals from peroxide
Ceruloplasmin possesses direct superoxide dismutase activity (less efficient than CuZnSOD)
Ceruloplasmin may transfer copper to cells for synthesis of CuZnSOD
Copper–histidine or copper–cysteine complexes stabilize gamma globulins and reduce Rheumatoid Factor
  formation
Copper salts inhibit kinin generation by kallikrein inhibition
Catecholamine synthesis is dependent on the cuproenzyme β-dopamine hydroxylase
Indirect effects on eicosanoid synthesis ($\downarrow$ PGE$_2$, $\uparrow$ PGF$_2$ by affecting redox capacity
Possible counterirritant effects promote inflammation and resulting repair
Generation of peroxide with thiols to inhibit lymphocyte and fibroblast proliferation
Induce metallothionen synthesis, which sequesters zinc and copper away from microbes
Specific antimycoplasma activity from copper complexes
Stabilization of lysosomal enzymes by decreased lysosomal permeability
Enhances histamine activity by forming copper–histamine complex
Lysyl oxidase induction by copper supplements in animals to enhance collagen and elastin production

Several investigators, using the established medical research practice at the time of physician evaluation, found that intravenous Cupralene or Dicuprene resulted in clinical improvements (Very Good, Good, or Moderate) in 60 to 83% of patients with rheumatoid arthritis or other arthritides.[940-949] Symptoms were ameliorated rapidly (2 to 4 weeks) and apparent remissions occurred, lasting for at least 1 year. Results were seen regardless of whether gold salts were used previously or not. Infrequent, minor toxicities (nausea, vomiting) were encountered, and laboratory values of liver and kidney function and blood counts were not adversely affected, and often normalized. Thus, intravenous copper compounds were as successful or superior to gold salts and much less toxic for treatment of rheumatoid arthritis.

However, in 1950, Tyson published only the second English-language publication on intravenous copper compound therapy for rheumatoid arthritis and found only 2/27 "typical" rheumatoid arthritis patients improved after Cupralene treatment.[950] Toxicities were frequent and severe, which discouraged further research on intravenous copper compounds in the U.S. However, there were several flaws in the study of Tyson. First, larger doses than European contemporaries were used (0.5 g per injection). Second, a garlic taste and odor was encountered, unlike other investigators. These spurious findings indicate that the Cupralene used by Tyson had degraded, releasing allicin, the major odor and taste component of garlic, which occurs after chemical decomposition via intramolecular rearrangement and subsequent oxidation.[940]

Thus, an unusual set of circumstances conspired to discourage further research on copper compounds as therapeutic agents for rheumatoid arthritis: (1) the most accessible study in the U.S. was unknowingly fatally flawed and unsuccessful; (2) successful European studies were unfamiliar; (3) no mechanisms of action were known or suspected; (4) at the time, there was no knowledge of the essentiality, physiological need, or roles of copper; (5) there were no convenient sources for dissemination of information (easy computer access to large databases was 30 years away); (6) criticism over lack of controlled studies (although gold salts and corticosteroids earned their reputations from uncontrolled studies); and (7) simultaneous advent of corticosteroid therapy, which rapidly captured almost all rheumatological clinical research efforts because of convenient oral usage and apparent cures. Thus, testing of copper compounds for rheumatoid arthritis never progressed to more controlled clinical studies and was quickly relegated to unproven or unsuccessful status.

In 1950, the German physician Hangarter, on the Faculty of Medicine at the University of Kiel, started clinical research on Permalon (cupric chloride-salicylic acid complex, 2.5 mg per vial) for treatment of rheumatoid arthritis.[940,941] Intravenous injections of one vial were given daily for 8 to 14 days. Pain, redness, and joint swelling were quickly and markedly reduced, while joint mobility rapidly improved (2 to 4 injections).[930,940,941] No toxicities or side effects were observed, except for pain after

TABLE 14   Intravenous Copper Salicylate Therapy for Inflammatory Joint Diseases[a]

Disease	n	Clinical Results			
		Symptom-free	Improved	Slightly Improved	Unchanged
Rheumatoid arthritis	620	403 (65%)	143 (23%)		74 (12%)
Sciatica (± lumbar involvement)	320	171 (53%)	77 (24%)	16 (5%)	16 (5%)
Cervical and lumbar spine syndromes	162	95 (57%)	52 (32%)		18 (11%)
Acute rheumatic fever	78	78 (100%)			
Arthritis deformans	5		3 (60%)		2 (40%)
Total	1148	747 (65%)	275 (24%)	16 (1%)	110 (10%)

[a]   Data from References 940 and 941. Permalon (7.5–10 mg Cu as copper chloride-salicylic acid complex) was administered intravenously with saline and novocaine in a slow infusion 6–8 times at intervals of 2–4 days. 1148/1185 subjects were evaluated.

occasional extravasation. After 1954, 3 to 4 vials of Permalon (7.5 to 10 mg Cu) were administered with 500 ml of saline and 0.4 mg of novocaine in a single, slow infusion 6 to 8 times at intervals of 2 to 4 days.[940,941] These higher doses were found to be effective for all stages of rheumatoid arthritis, acute rheumatic fever, sciatica, and other spinal syndromes in 1140 subjects (see Table 14).[940,941] Improvements progressed in stages. First, rapid (1 to 2 d) relief of pain and improved mobility were seen, even in severe deformities. Second, cessation of fever and regression of articular swellings and exudations were seen. An average duration of remission was 3 years. Sedimentation rate values and Rheumatoid Factor tests slowly returned to normal after several months. No toxicities, except for occasional nausea or tinnitus, were encountered, and no gastrointestinal, liver, kidney, cerebral, respiratory, or circulatory disturbances were noted. Based on later work, total doses of copper were well within the range of tolerability.[808] After Dr. Hangarter, the sole user of Permalon, retired, its manufacture was discontinued for "economic reasons."[941] As such, more rigorous and modern clinical trials with intravenous copper salicylate have not been conducted.

Another line of evidence for the ability of copper to reduce clinical symptoms of rheumatoid arthritis is the use of D-penicillamine (β-mercaptovaline) as treatment. D-Penicillamine, a known chelator of copper, has the ability to remove copper bound to albumin (which has no antiinflammatory action) and "free" copper to exert antiinflammatory effects as low molecular weight complexes.[929] This may explain why penicillamine has therapeutic effectiveness for rheumatoid arthritis and ankylosing spondylitis (high circulating copper levels), but not osteoarthritis (normal circulating copper levels). Also, the effect of penicillamine on copper may explain why some patients fail to respond to penicillamine. When excess copper is depleted by penicillamine, then the low molecular weight complexes are no longer formed, and symptoms return. Indeed, some patients may not respond to penicillamine at all because of their depleted copper status.[929]

Recently, Pullar and others, of the University of Leeds and Royal Bath Hospital in England, studied the effects of copper sulfate supplementation on rheumatoid arthritis patients who relapsed after penicillamine treatment.[951] Copper sulfate (7.9 mg Cu, n = 13) or placebo (n = 8) was given to 21 patients with rheumatoid arthritis, along with 1000 mg/d of D-penicillamine, for 16 weeks. Urinary copper excretion was increased significantly from baseline and placebo values by 12 weeks (12.2 vs. 4.8 and 5.4 μmol Cu per 24 h, respectively). However, no significant changes from baseline or placebo values were found for articular index, plasma viscosity, C-reactive protein, ceruloplasmin, hemoglobin, grip strength, morning stiffness, and visual analog pain score. Thus, supplementation of rheumatoid arthritis patients after relapse on long-term (2 to 14 years) penicillamine therapy with 8 mg Cu per day was not successful while penicillamine was continued. These results correlate with failure of cupric oxide supplementation to affect rheumatoid arthritis patients in early research.[941] Both cupric oxide and copper sulfate are inorganic salts and possess different properties than organic copper chelates.

Copper may play two roles as adjunct therapy for inflammatory conditions. The first is to replete tissue stores and return physiological functions of cuproenzymes to normal. The second is as pharmaceutical agents to reduce inflammation. A vast amount of research has investigated the possibility of using over 140 simple copper salts and compounds as antiinflammatory agents.[810,926] While the scope of this chapter does not include the pharmaceutical aspects of copper complexes, many are derived from simple organic molecules, such as acetate, anthranilate, salicylate, penicillamine, amino acids, small peptides, and nonsteroidal antiinflammatory drugs. Most must be injected to reach sufficient levels *in vivo* to exhibit antiinflammatory properties in animal models, which would limit their clinical usefulness. At the very least, the antiinflammatory activity of copper complexes supports the notion that elevation of bloodborne copper is a physiologic response in an attempt to mediate inflammation.

At this time, there is sufficient information to justify continued clinical studies on organic copper supplements for autoimmune and inflammatory joint diseases. However, lack of discrete knowledge on which forms may be safe and useful as oral supplements and dose-response information means that therapeutic use of copper for arthritis is still largely untested.

Severe trauma and burns greatly increased the loss of copper from the body.[952] The effects of less severe injuries on copper status in humans is still lacking.

2. Osteoporosis

The section on copper deficiency symptoms described many reports of osteoporosis in premature infants, infants on prolonged TPN, and persons with Menke's disease (usually children). These situations are not normally encountered in a sports medicine or orthopedic practice, and copper deficiency symptoms were quickly reversed after addition of copper supplements. Currently, TPN contains sufficient copper to replete most individuals and thus prevent copper-deficiency-induced bone loss. Of more interest is the hypothesis that a lifelong marginal intake of copper may be associated with bone loss in adults.[902] Animal data supports the finding of bone loss with long-term, low copper intakes,[922-924] and epidemiological evidence suggests that copper intakes may not be adequate for many women (see Table 11).[779,819,953-955] For example, Krishnamachari reported that in villages in India with higher incidences of osteoporosis, lower levels of copper in the drinking water, bone, and breast milk were measured.[902] Thus, several lines of evidence support the role of long-term, marginal copper deficiency as a contributor of unknown impact to osteoporosis.

Serum copper levels in osteoporotic patients were not different from healthy elderly controls (22.6 ± 3.78 vs. 21.84 ± 4.39 µmol/l), although the elderly in general have higher serum copper levels than younger adults (16.5 ± 2.7 µmol/l).[956] However, serum ceruloplasmin levels were significantly increased in osteoporotic patients (0.42 ± 0.09 vs. 0.36 ± 0.07 g/l) compared to healthy elderly subjects. Thus, redistribution of copper to forms less available to cells was seen in human bone loss. However, there was no difference in bone copper levels found between 88 healthy elderly controls and 50 osteoporotic subjects.[957] To date, only static, quantitative levels of copper have been determined in humans with bone loss. Unfortunately, functional status of copper and copper-dependent enzymes (especially lysyl oxidase in osteoid) has not been elucidated in situations of bone loss in humans. Thus, the known insensitivity of serum and tissue levels of copper to identify deficient copper function cannot rule out a possible role of functional copper deficiency as a contributor to bone loss.

At present, there is insufficient information to determine whether increased copper intake during recovery from fractures in young, healthy athletes would speed healing. In addition, there is insufficient information to determine whether copper status is adversely affected in amenorrheic women with premenopausal bone loss. In addition, the requirements for copper in athletes have not been fully elucidated.

I. SAFETY

Ingestion of copper from foods or simple salts appears to be relatively safe in humans. Estimates of safe intakes for indefinite time periods range from 10 to 35 mg Cu per d.[808] Even 200 mg/d appears to be safe for short time periods.[808] Acute copper toxicity may be more feasible. As little as 10 mg of copper (as a salt) may produce nausea, and 64 mg copper as 250 mg copper sulfate produces vomiting.[808] Lethal doses in humans are thought to be 3.5 to 35 g. Acute toxicity symptoms are nausea, vomiting, jaundice, intravascular hemolysis, gastric hemorrhage, and hepatic necrosis. Situations where copper supplements should not be given are (1) Wilson's disease (rare congenital disorder of excess tissue copper), (2) Indian childhood cirrhosis, (3) biliary atresia, (4) α_1-antitrypsin deficiency, and (5) primary biliary cirrhosis.[958] These conditions all cause copper to accumulate in tissues.

J. SUMMARY

The exact mechanism of inflammatory and antiinflammatory actions of copper is not yet completely understood. Because of copper chemistry, both a deficiency and excess are harmful to humans. This fact severely limits therapeutic applications, although copper supplementation appears to have a wide margin of safety. The homeostatic sequestration and transport of copper also renders therapeutic applications difficult. Nevertheless, there are two ways in which copper can be used therapeutically. First, modest doses of copper (2 to 5 mg/d) as organic chelates can be used to replete potential or documented copper deficiencies in order to maintain physiological levels and functions of cuproenzymes important to connective tissues. Second, use of synthetic copper complexes (such as copper-penicillamine or copper-salicylate complexes) may mimic endogenous copper compounds and be used in a pharmacological manner.

For the field of sports medicine and orthopedics, the primary concern of copper nutrition is to maintain functional activities of lysyl oxidase and CuZnSOD in connective tissues. In this way, copper deficiencies will not delay resolution of inflammation or delay healing. The concept of accelerating resolution of inflammation or healing with copper supplements has been given almost no clinical testing, except in cases of inflammatory joint diseases (rheumatoid arthritis). While there is some evidence that intravenous administration of exogenous copper may alleviate symptoms, use of inorganic oral copper supplements for inflammatory joint conditions has been unsuccessful. Whether oral organic copper chelates would be useful for inflammatory or noninflammatory joint conditions is unknown. Likewise, the concept of using copper to accelerate bone healing or bone accretion is still hypothetical, but based on some epidemiological evidence. Table 15 lists some suggested usages for copper.

K. GUIDELINES FOR USE

Copper doses of 2 to 5 mg/d as organic chelates appear to be safe and also adequate for repletion of physiological levels of tissue copper, in the absence of malabsorption or chronic diarrhea. Organic chelates seem to possess less local irritant possibilities than inorganic copper salts and are recommended. Examples of organic chelates of copper are as gluconate, glycinate, histidinate, lysinate, and sebacate.

IV. MANGANESE

A. ROLES AND FUNCTIONS

Manganese was named after the Greek word for magic because of its marked ability to form colored compounds. Manganese was shown to be essential for animals in 1931.[959] The roles and functions of manganese salient to musculoskeletal tissues are listed in Table 16. Reviews on manganese nutriture are becoming more common.[959-968] Divalent manganese (Mn^{2+}) is an essential trace element because of its role in activating glycosyltransferase enzymes that attach modified sugars to proteins (collagen) and each other.[969] Glycosylation is a vital step in collagen synthesis that is believed to account for proper orientation of polypeptide chains in order to form triple helices and later cross-linking.[93] Synthesis of glycosaminoglycans (GAGs) and resulting proteoglycans is dependent upon glycosyltransferases that require manganese for optimum activity. Sulfotransferases that attach sulfate groups to GAGs also

**TABLE 15   Clinical Conditions with Potential
Benefit from Copper Repletion**

Inflammatory joint conditions
Rheumatoid arthritis
Psoriatic arthritis
Ankylosing spondylitis
Reiter's Syndrome
Sciatica
Chronic polyarticular synovitis
Cervical and lumbar spine syndromes
Osteoporosis, osteopenia, bone loss (?)
Wound healing (postsurgery) (?)
Degenerative joint diseases (?)

require manganese.[969] Thus, manganese is extremely important for synthesis of proteoglycans, a seminal event in the synthesis of every connective tissue.

In addition, manganese is a component of the metalloenzyme manganese-superoxide dismutase (MnSOD), a form of SOD present inside mitochondria which is substantially different from cytosolic CuZnSOD.[970,971] Thus, manganese possesses antioxidant properties by forming the active site of MnSOD. Manganese is a component of the metalloenzyme pyruvate carboxylase, necessary for gluconeogenesis and carbohydrate metabolism.[972] Thus, manganese has a role in energy production during stress situations, a function that has not been specifically investigated in situations of musculo-skeletal distress or healing. Manganese is also a component of the metalloenzyme arginase, responsible for urea production.[973] Other enzymes appear to have manganese-specific requirements for activation: phosphoenolpyruvate carboxykinase and glutamine synthetase.

B.   DEFICIENCY SYMPTOMS

From a host of animal studies, manganese deficiency has been shown to cause skeletal and cartilage abnormalities (perosis and slipped tendons in poultry),[969,974] impaired wound healing, osteoarthritis, osteoporosis, postural defects from impaired otolith development, and poor overall growth (see Table 17).[959-961,963,965,968,969] Both bone and cartilage are repaired by initiating GAG and proteoglycan synthesis, followed by collagen synthesis and deposition to form osteoids (organic matrix) in bone and cartilage in articular joint surfaces. Thus, it is not surprising that deficits in manganese function would impair growth and healing of these connective tissues in particular. It is of interest that during dietary manganese deficiency, feeding of GAG precursors (glucosamine, galactose, glucuronic acid, and ascorbic acid) did not affect manganese deficiency symptoms.[974] This little-known finding brings out the possibility that bone and joint disorders previously thought to be untreatable are actually due to an easily correctable manganese deficiency. While it is clear that experimentally induced manganese deficiencies manifest as connective tissue disorders, documentation of a link between manganese

TABLE 16   Functions of Manganese Pertinent to Musculoskeletal Tissues

Role	Functions
Specific activation of glycosyltransferases	Glycosaminoglycan synthesis
	Proteoglycan synthesis
	Collagen synthesis
	Glycoprotein synthesis
	Cell–cell interactions
Specific activation of sulfotransferases	Glycosaminoglycan synthesis
Component of manganese-superoxide dismutase	Antioxidant functions
Component of pyruvate carboxylase	Gluconeogenesis and carbohydrate metabolism during periods of stress
Component of arginase	Removal of ammonia

TABLE 17 Musculoskeletal Symptoms from Long-Term Manganese Deficiencies

Skeletal

Osteoporosis
Osteopenia
Shortened, thickened bone development
Chondrodystrophy
Perosis
Kyphosis
Scoliosis
Slipped tendons
Abnormal serum calcium, phosphorus, and alkaline phosphatase
Decreased osteoblastic activity
Increased lability of bone matrix
Increased resorption of bone
Decreased osteoclastic activity
Decreased glycosaminoglycan and proteoglycan synthesis

Cartilage

Osteoarthritis
Hip dislocation
Swollen, enlarged joints
Decreased glycosaminoglycan and proteoglycan synthesis

deficiency and human connective tissue disorders such as osteoporosis, osteoarthritis, and chronic degenerative joint diseases has only very recently been attempted.

C. ASSESSMENT

Assessment of manganese status in humans is still difficult and is not routine for most clinical testing facilities. At present, determination of manganese levels in serum or whole blood is accepted as an indicator of manganese status in humans. Values below reference ranges for the particular test methodology and equipment are presumed to be indicative of a deficient manganese status. Hair mineral analysis may also be a useful indicator of manganese status when levels are decreased in comparison to reference ranges.[959,975] At present, there is no widely accepted test for functional status of manganese, rather than measurement of static levels. Thus, inadequate data on manganese status has hampered recognition, identification, acceptance, and therapeutic intervention of manganese deficiencies.

D. INTAKES

The 1989 ESADDI for manganese is currently 2.0 to 5.0 mg/d for adults, based on results of balance studies.[976] The Selected Minerals in Foods Survey of the U.S. FDA's Total Diet Study measured manganese intakes for infants, children, teenagers, adults, and elderly for females and males.[779] Manganese intakes for female teenagers (1.76 mg/d), adults (2.05 mg/d), and elderly (2.12 mg/d) were consistently rated as low, while intake for the same age groups of males ranged from 2.57 to 2.74 mg/d, which is very close to the lower limit of the ESADDI for manganese at that time, which was 2.5 to 5.0 mg/d.[779] Another dietary survey found manganese intakes of high school girls (<0.24 to 1.53 mg/d) and college women students taking courses in nutrition (<0.38 to 1.38 mg/d) to be consistently and substantially below ESADDI limits.[953] Furthermore, analysis of hospital diets found that the daily manganese content of all types of diets analyzed ranged from <0.38 to 1.78 mg/d.[955] Thus, in hospital situations, many of which require musculoskeletal healing, the supplied diets, even if eaten in their entirety, are definitely deficient in manganese content.

Other surveys found somewhat higher intakes of manganese in smaller groups of subjects. Patterson found manganese intakes of 3.0 mg/d in 28 adults, but 30% of women consumed less than 2.5 mg manganese per day.[819] Even at 3.0 mg/d intakes, balance of manganese was negative for their subjects. Other surveys of manganese intakes in women from New Zealand and Canada found manganese intakes of 2.4 to 2.6 mg/d.[819,977]

Thus, several well-designed, thorough, and fairly accurate dietary intake surveys found that U.S. women consume a diet low or marginal in manganese intake throughout their entire lifetimes, especially during periods of bone mass accretion (teenage and young adult years) as well as periods of known bone loss (60 to 65 years). This finding strongly argues for close attention to manganese intake at all ages for all women, and also for males, since their intakes were close to the lower limit of the ESADDI for manganese. Thus, occult manganese deficiency appears to be a likely factor in bone loss and degenerative joint conditions for even well-fed Americans.

E. DIETARY SOURCES AND INFLUENCES

Foods rich in manganese include tea, coffee, chocolate, whole grains (except corn), nuts, seeds, liver, legumes, vegetables, and fruits (see Table 18).[788] Foods low in manganese include all meats (except liver), dairy products, eggs, sugar, water, corn, citrus fruits, and vegetables grown in manganese-poor soils. Fortunately, with the prevalence of food transportation, dependence on local produce has decreased, and the chance for exclusively eating foods low in manganese has lessened. However, manganese intake frequently does not correlate with manganese uptake, due to the interactions of dietary components. For example, tea, a very rich source of manganese, has polyphenols (tannins) that make the manganese in tea virtually unavailable.[978] Once again, eating a wide variety of foods in whole forms instead of processed forms will greatly improve manganese intake, in addition to many other essential nutrients.

Manganese is chemically similar to iron and seems to share intestinal uptake mechanisms with iron.[979] Thus, simultaneous intake of inorganic manganese salts with ascorbic acid improves uptake of manganese into blood and tissues.[978,979] Again, like iron, ingestion of meat (containing heme proteins) with plant sources rich in manganese improves uptake over consumption of plant foods only.[978,979] Since manganese shares serum binding proteins (transferrin) with iron,[980] it is not surprising to find that dietary heme groups found in meats improve manganese uptake.[977] Conversely, excess iron,[978,979,981,982] calcium,[983] phosphate, oxalate, and fiber (cellulose, pectin, and phytate)[977,984] can depress manganese uptake. Alkalinity decreases manganese uptake by changing manganese valences to less absorbable forms.[983] These conditions can be easily reached by consumption of antacids, or by conditions of achlorhydria. In fact, ingestion of only 500 mg of calcium as calcium carbonate turned a positive manganese balance into a negative manganese balance, at a manganese intake of 6 mg/d.[983] Calcium from milk, gluconate, or lactate sources did not influence manganese uptake as strongly as alkalinizing calcium carbonate. Taking these recently discovered factors into account, the ESADDI for manganese (2.0 to 5.0 mg/d) is being regarded as insufficient for optimum manganese status by some researchers. A new ESADDI for manganese of 3.5 to 7.0 mg/d has been proposed.[985] If the new ESADDI becomes accepted, then most Americans would automatically have a deficient intake of manganese, a situation which is politically unfavorable.

Groups at risk for manganese deficiencies include those with low caloric intakes (dieters, many elderly, anorexics), some types of strict vegetarians based on religious beliefs, those with absorption defects (inflammatory bowel diseases), Down's Syndrome, Lupus erythematosus, epileptics, and, possibly, those with excess intake of antacids, especially calcium-based antacids.

F. ANIMAL STUDIES
1. Manganese and Bone

Bones contain 25% of total body manganese.[959] Dietary deficiencies of manganese have long been recognized by veterinarians, especially in poultry and livestock.[959,965] Swollen and enlarged joints, shortened and thickened limbs, curvature of the spine, perosis, and slipped tendons are hallmarks of manganese deficiencies.

Strause and others, of the University of California–San Diego in La Jolla, studied the effects of long-term deficiencies of manganese on skeletal health in weanling rats.[922] Female rats were divided into

TABLE 18 Relative Abundance of Manganese from Food Sources[a]

High Levels (0.2–4.7 mg/100 g)	Medium Levels (0.05–0.2 mg/100 g)	Low Levels (<0.05 mg/100 g)
Nuts	Onion	Coffee
Whole grains (wheat, rye, oats)	Avocado	Meats
Whole-grain cereals, breads, flours	Hamburgers	Fish
Pineapple	Spaghetti	Dairy products
Chocolate powder	Lettuce	Eggs
Spinach	Carrot	Citrus fruits
Sweet potato	Squash	Watermelon
Legumes	Cabbage	Melons
Green beans	Tomato	Mushrooms
Strawberry	Wine	Dill pickles
Banana	Peach	Beer
Potato	Corn	Processed fruit juices
Tea, brewed	Cakes	Gelatin dessert
Chocolate chip cookies		Sodas
Cake doughnuts		Oils
Cheese pizza		Sugar, refined
		Water

[a] Sources are References 779, 788, and 955.

three groups: (1) normal manganese (66 ppm in diet) and copper (5 ppm); (2) low manganese (2.5 ppm) and copper (0.5 ppm); and (3) depleted manganese (0 ppm) and normal copper (5 ppm). Weight gain, food intake, blood hemoglobin concentrations, and mortality were not different between groups for the entire 1-year study period. Serum calcium levels did not show significant changes in both the deficient groups until fed for 6 months, and the changes persisted for another 6 months (Table 19). Both levels of manganese deficiency caused increases in serum calcium and phosphorus and decreases in femur calcium and manganese. Zinc levels in serum and bone were unaffected by manganese or manganese/copper deficiencies. Serum and bone copper levels were decreased in the manganese/copper-deficient group. Manganese levels in serum decreased in both deficient groups, although statistical significance was not reached. Manganese levels in liver and intestine were decreased in both deficient groups, and copper levels were decreased only in the manganese/copper group. Radiographic examination of femurs found that 25% of manganese and manganese/copper-deficient rats showed bone density loss. Serum levels of parathyroid hormone, calcitonin, and 1,25-dihydroxyvitamin D were unchanged after 12 months among groups.

GAG levels from humeral epiphyses of rats fed the diet devoid in manganese for 6 months were severely decreased compared to control rats (0.12 vs. 2.19 μg/mg, respectively).[923] Bone-specific proteoglycan was also severely decreased in humeral epiphyses from rats fed diets devoid in manganese (0.02 vs. 1.43 μg/mg). Fetal calvarial cultures from control and manganese-depleted rats showed greatly decreased osteoblastic cell numbers (6.8×10^5 and 2.3×10^5 cells, respectively). Cell growth rate was slower in manganese-deficient cells, as evidenced by an accumulation of osteonectin.

Thus, adverse changes in bone health were associated with diets of marginal and deficient manganese status. Combined deficiency of manganese and copper also was detrimental to bone health. This study suggests that chronic marginal intake of manganese can lead to osteopenia, even when other indicators of bone mass are normal, and even when calcium intake is normal.

Andon and others, from the Miami Valley Laboratories of Proctor & Gamble Company in Cincinnati, OH, fed weanling rats diets deficient in manganese (0.3 ppm) and manganese plus copper (0.3 and 2.0 ppm, respectively) for 12 weeks.[986] Compared to control rats fed 37 ppm manganese and 5.8 ppm copper, manganese-deficient rats exhibited a steady decrease in serum calcium levels although serum manganese was unaffected. Bone mineral density of manganese + copper-deficient rats increased slower than control rats ($p < 0.05$). This study suggests that suboptimal manganese and copper intakes combined may increase the risk of bone loss later in life by preventing the accretion of optimal bone mass in adolescence and young adulthood.

TABLE 19 Biochemical Changes Caused by Long-Term Manganese Deficiency in Rats[a]

Measured Parameter	Control (66 ppm Mn)	Low Mn (2.5 ppm Mn)	Depleted Mn (0.0 ppm Mn)
Weight gain (g)	330	369	353
Serum calcium (mg/dl) 6 months	0.91 ± 1.3	14.2 ± 1.5[b]	13.8 ± 1.4[b]
Serum calcium (mg/dl)	10.3 ± 1.5	11.9 ± 1.6	13.4 ± 1.5[b]
Serum phosphorus (mg/dl)	3.9 ± 0.1	6.3 ± 0.4[b]	5.0 ± 0.3[b]
Serum manganese (mg/l)	0.08 ± 0.05	0.03 ± 0.02	0.03 ± 0.02
Femur calcium (mg/g) 6 months	333 ± 111	200 ± 30[b]	208 ± 37[b]
Femur calcium (mg/g)	272 ± 60	221 ± 30	180 ± 16[b]
Femur phosphorus (mg/g)	167 ± 14	156 ± 9	155 ± 20
Femur manganese (µg/g)	2.70 ± 1.5	1.03 ± 0.14	0.95 ± 0.80[b]
Epiphyseal GAG levels (µg/mg)	2.19	—	0.12[b]
Bone-specific proteoglycan levels humeral epiphysis (µg/mg)	1.43	—	0.02[b]
Induction Index from implanted demineralized bone powder — 2 weeks	12.7 cartilage	0.0	0.0
Induction index from implanted demineralized bone powder — 17 weeks	31.3 bone	20.0 bone, cartilage	0.0
Resorption of implanted bone particles (% resorbed)	46.2	15.4[b]	12.4[b]
Resorption rate of implanted bone powder from experimental animals into normal animals (%)	100	121	123

[a] Data obtained from References 922 to 924.
[b] Data are significantly different ($p < 0.05$) from control values.

Strause et al. utilized the previously described diets low in manganese and copper and depleted in manganese on osteoinduction and bone resorption in the rat.[923,924] *In vivo* osteoblastic activity can be measured by subcutaneous implantation of devitalized, demineralized bone powder (DBP), consisting of connective cell tissue mesenchyme. Once implanted, DBP is converted into cartilage by 2 weeks, and calcification, vascularization, and bone formation ensues. Activity of bone resorption can be assayed by implantation of bone powder (BP), containing bone mineral. After implantation of BP, osteoclastic cells appear at the implant and within 4 weeks, there is complete resorption of bone powder. After implantation of DBP in control rats, cartilage induction was seen in 2 weeks, followed by bone induction at 6 and 17 weeks. After 6 months on a diet low in manganese and copper, no cartilage induction was seen at 2 weeks after implantation of DBP. Some induced cartilage and bone was seen at 6 and 17 weeks, although less than control rats. In rats fed a diet devoid in manganese, no cartilage and no bone induction was seen at any time interval after implantation of DBP. Osteoclastic induction was measured by implantation of BP and subsequent percentage of BP resorbed per microscopic field 14 d after implantation in rats maintained on diets for 12 months. Control rats showed 46.3% resorption of BP, while manganese/copper-deficient rats showed 15.4% resorption (33% of control) and rats fed diets devoid of manganese for 12 months showed 12.4% resorption (27% of control). Thus, long-term deficiency of manganese drastically delays osteoblastic functions and osteoclastic functions. Thus, it is possible that the osteopenia seen in rats fed the manganese/copper deficient diets is due to an imbalance of bone synthesis and resorption.

Furthermore, bones from animals fed for 12 months on diets low in manganese/copper and devoid of manganese were used to prepare BPs implanted into normal rats.[923] BP from bones deficient in manganese/copper were resorbed at 121% the rate of control BP. Likewise, BP from rats fed diets devoid of manganese was resorbed at a rate 123% greater than control BP. Resorption rates from BP of both deficient diets were significantly different from control BP, indicating increased lability of bone matrix from animals deficient in manganese. This study suggests that bone from individuals with deficient status of manganese could be more easily resorbed than normal bone.

Martin, of the Division of Orthopedic Surgery at West Virginia University Medical Center, studied the effect of two commercial feeds (Wayne Lab Blox and Purina Laboratory Chow) with different manganese contents (210 and 50 ppm, respectively) on disuse osteoporosis in rats with plaster cast immobilization.[987] Adverse changes in femurs were seen with the diet lower in manganese, but not with the diet higher in manganese. These results suggest that manganese levels sufficient for "normal" animal growth are insufficient during periods of stress, such as musculoskeletal healing.

Bolze and others studied the effect of manganese deficiency on growth, somatomedin, and GAG metabolism in young chicks.[988] It was found that when manganese deficiency had resulted in perosis and decreased growth rate, serum somatomedin activity, insulin, and glucose levels were not altered from control values. Thus, the decreased GAG synthesis and overall growth decrease resulting from manganese deficiency is not mediated by somatomedins.

Stern measured the effect of manganese concentrations on fetal rat limb bones.[989] Low manganese concentrations (0.01 to 0.3 mM) stimulated resorption, but concentrations >0.3 mM inhibited resorption. This finding offers further evidence that a deficiency of manganese may enhance bone loss.

G. HUMAN STUDIES
1. Bone Health
Strause and Saltman, of the Department of Biology at the University of California–San Diego in La Jolla, illustrated the importance of manganese in a clinical orthopedic setting by the n = 1 case study of the professional basketball player Bill Walton.[924] The career of Bill Walton was constantly plagued by musculoskeletal injuries (frequent broken bones, bone spurs, joint pain) and poor healing. After a sometimes dominating and successful career, injuries forced an early retirement. At this time, analysis of his serum showed no detectable manganese, and also low levels of copper and zinc. The low serum levels were hypothesized to have been acquired by consuming a long-term strict and very limited vegetarian diet based on religious beliefs. Dietary supplementation with trace minerals and calcium was initiated, and after several months, bone healing was complete, and Bill Walton returned to professional basketball for several more years. The therapeutic success of manganese supplementation (and other minerals) was dramatically and unknowingly viewed by millions watching Bill Walton on television.

Analysis of other patients exhibiting slow bone healing also found abnormally low serum levels of manganese, zinc, and copper. These anecdotal case studies spurred a collaborative effort with Dr. Reginster at the Medical School of the University of Liege in Belgium to examine serum and bone levels of trace minerals in postmenopausal osteoporotic women.[924] Serum manganese in osteoporotic women was 0.01 ± 0.004 mg/l, whereas age-matched normal women exhibited serum manganese levels of 0.04 ± 0.03 mg/l, a significant difference. As expected, bone calcium, trabecular bone volume, bone mineral content, and bone mineral density were all significantly and substantially lower in the osteoporotic group. Interestingly, no differences between groups were found for serum levels of copper, zinc, bone Gla protein, and 1,25-dihydroxyvitamin D. While this study does not prove that manganese deficiency caused osteoporosis, it does provide further support along with other observations in animals and humans that a deficiency of manganese contributes to induction and progression of osteoporosis in humans.

2. Degenerative Joint Disease
Manganese levels in human rib cartilage decrease with advancing age.[990] This finding suggests that ability to synthesize cartilage matrix may be impaired with age. Perhaps there is a connection between the appearance of osteoporosis and osteoarthritis in the elderly and declining manganese levels in aging cartilage.

In 1981, Fincham and others, of the Division of Nutritional Pathology of the National Research Institute for Nutritional Diseases in Parowvallei, South Africa, proposed that Mseleni hip disease was actually a manganese deficiency.[991] Mseleni disease occurs sporadically (39% of females and 11% of males) in the KwaZulu area of South Africa, especially near Lake Sibaya. Symptoms include osteoarthritis of multiple joints which progresses to a crippling hip dislocation. Most adults in the region are smaller than usual in stature, suggesting mild dwarfism (shortened and thickened bones). Epiphyseal dysplasia and disturbances of bone mineralization are evident upon closer examination of Mseleni disease subjects. An early finding is an increase in serum alkaline phosphatase,[991] similar to findings in animals. All these symptoms are identical to manganese deficiency symptoms in animals. Fish from Lake Sibaya are severely and uniformly stunted, unlike their counterparts in other nearby lakes.[992] However, the few livestock in the region range freely and eat selectively, and exhibit few signs of manganese deficiency.

Analysis of food (predominantly maize and peanuts) and water mineral contents of the Lake Sibaya region showed no manganese and low levels of magnesium, along with elevated levels of calcium.[991,992] Due to the lack of movement, dietary habits (dependence exclusively on local crops), and poverty of the inhabitants around Lake Sibaya, manganese deficiency from inadequate dietary intake seems likely to cause Mseleni disease. In addition, certain isolated areas in France (southern Finistere), the U.S. (Many Farms Indians in Arizona), and Canada (Island Lake and Red Sucker Lake) exhibited high incidences of congenital hip dislocation (similar to Mseleni disease).[993] All these areas exhibit high soil alkalinity and greatly decreased local plant food levels of manganese (0.01 to 0.05 µg/g compared to worldwide average of 0.21 µg/g). Incidence of hip dislocations has decreased as these areas become less isolated and local inhabitants consume more foods produced in manganese-repleted areas. These observations indicate that manganese deficiencies do cause joint, skeletal, and growth abnormalities in humans similar to those seen in animals under controlled conditions. Manganese deficiencies in humans do occur, do affect joint and bone health adversely, and should be considered in bone and cartilage degenerative conditions.

Fortunately, repletion of manganese status appears to be relatively simple. Again, based on relatively few human data, supplementation with divalent manganese salts is inexpensive, safe, and able to improve manganese levels in blood.[984] For supplementation purposes, many organic forms of manganese chelates with organic acids or amino acids have become available recently. Although data on relative uptakes are unavailable, organic chelates mimic forms found in whole foodstuffs. In limited testing, organic chelates (such as manganese gluconate) show superior absorption and uptake compared to inorganic manganese salts (manganese sulfate, oxide). Thus, organic chelates of manganese are preferred for oral supplementation.

H. SAFETY

Very high intakes of inorganic manganese salts (2% of dietary intake or >100 mg/kg of diet) can lead to manganese rickets by binding to phosphate in the intestinal lumen and forming unabsorbable manganese phosphates.[994,995] These conditions are almost impossible to reach in practical settings with humans. Hypothetically, since manganese and iron share chemical and biological attributes, high manganese intakes coupled with low iron intakes may aggravate iron deficiency.[965] The amount of dietary manganese intake necessary to decrease iron status in humans is not known, but appears to be over 50 mg/d. Inorganic manganese salts may imbalance iron uptake more easily than organic chelates.

Manganese toxicity symptoms include neurological symptoms and behavioral changes (schizophrenia).[996,997] However, these findings are based on toxicity from manganese ores, inhaled manganese, or well water contaminated with inorganic manganese salts that were all sources of nondivalent manganese. One report described a 55-year-old man with symptoms of presenile dementia and other brain disorders.[998] Brain, blood, and other tissue levels of manganese were elevated. The authors concluded, without presentation of any data or examination of environmental factors, that perhaps the "large doses" of multiple vitamin–mineral supplements the patient had ingested accounted for elevated levels of manganese. Thus, no substantiated cases of toxicity from manganese supplements exists. Overall, divalent manganese appears safe in doses ranging from 5 to 50 mg/d.

I. SUMMARY

Manganese plays unique and vital roles for synthesis of seminal macromolecular components of connective tissues, especially for bone and cartilage. Since acute, severe deficiencies of manganese are exceedingly rare,[959,968] defects of manganese status appear as a result of life-long, chronic, intermittent, or marginal deficiencies. Thus, acute deficiency symptoms are usually not encountered, but rather, as is the case with copper and zinc, decreased synthesis of connective tissues leads to loss of integrity for joints and bones.

From the available evidence, which includes the unique and well-known biological roles of manganese, animal studies with deficient intakes and implanted bone powders, epidemiological data on marginal manganese intakes, and the scarce human data on deficient intakes affecting bone and joint health, it appears that adequate manganese status is essential for proper bone and joint health. Also apparent is the matter of degree of manganese deficiency and severity of bone and joint disorders. Based on animal research, the likely effects of long-term, marginal manganese status are bone loss and increased joint degeneration. Osteoporosis, osteoarthritis, and invertebral disc disease are thus postulated to be likely sequelae of insufficient manganese status in humans. The common prevalence of these conditions argues that manganese deficiencies may play a role in the initiation, progression, and/or inability to rectify these major medical problems.

Assessment of manganese status is difficult and lacking in a database. Manganese nutriture is only now being understood. Therapeutic use of manganese in humans with musculoskeletal disorders has been limited to a few anecdotal cases, although veterinarians have long understood the effects of manganese deficits and commonly employ manganese salts as supplements. When supplementation with organic chelates of divalent manganese falls in the range of 3 to 50 mg/d, no toxicity has been observed. Manganese supplementation is speculated to be helpful in chronic degenerative joint diseases and osteoporosis, but no direct evidence exists to substantiate this attractive hypothesis at this time. However, the potential benefits and safety argue in favor of manganese supplementation.

J. GUIDELINES FOR USE

Guidelines for improving manganese intake include replacing refined, processed foodstuffs with whole grain products, whole nuts, legumes, fresh vegetables, and fresh fruits. Meats should be ingested simultaneously with plant foodstuffs rich in manganese, and ascorbic acid (from citrus fruits, green leafy vegetables, or supplements) ingestion may also improve manganese uptake. Manganese supplements should be organic chelates such as gluconate, ascorbate, citric acid cycle acids, or amino acids rather than inorganic salts such as sulfate, oxide, or chloride. Doses of manganese should range from 5 to 50 mg/d, which is equivalent to the range of daily manganese intakes of humans throughout the world.[977] Doses of manganese exceeding 50 mg/d for more than several months are not well studied, but have the theoretical potential to eventually imbalance uptake of other trace minerals, including iron. Table 20 lists guidelines where increased manganese intake may be clinically helpful.

TABLE 20   Conditions for Use of Manganese[a]

Osteoarthritis
Osteoporosis
Degenerative joint disease
Invertebral disc disease
Slow or improper healing of bone fractures

[a]   Dosage of manganese ranges from 5–50 mg/d as organic chelate forms (ascorbate, aspartate, citrate, gluconate, picolinate). At this time, suggested usage of manganese is based on strong hypothetical grounds, but not on actual clinical trials.

Chapter 10

ULTRATRACE MINERALS

I. BORON

A. INTRODUCTION

The element boron (B), atomic number 4, is widely distributed in the earth's crust, but is present in living organisms in ultratrace amounts. Boron is essential for dicotyledon plants (fruits, vegetables, legumes, tubers), which take up boron from the soil.[999,1000] Boron compounds complex with hydroxyl groups, facilitating flavonoid synthesis.[1000] Monocotyledon plants, which include grass grains such as rice, corn, wheat, and barley do not require boron and, thus, exhibit much lower amounts of boron (<0.2 mg B/kg).[1001] However, levels of boron in plants vary widely in different geographic areas, depending upon boron levels in water, levels in soil, length of growing time, rate of transpiration, use of fertilizers, crop rotation practices, and other agricultural practices.[1002]

The most common boron compounds are boric acid and sodium borate ($Na_2B_4O_7 \cdot 10\,H_2O$ or borax). Boric acid and borates were widely used as food preservatives from the 1870s to the 1920s and greatly contributed to preventing even worse famines during World War I.[1003] However, a study from the USDA in 1904 in which 500 mg B per day (as borax) was fed to humans reported disturbances in appetite and digestion.[1003] This finding, coupled with known toxicity of borates when applied as an antibiotic to large areas of broken skin (from burns and open wounds), led to a worldwide ban on borates as a food preservative in the 1920s.[1003] World War II saw a resurgence of boric acid used as a plentiful and inexpensive food preservative, as well as studies of effects of feeding large amounts of boron to animals, which exhibited toxicity. Once again, use of boron was banned in the 1950s.[1003] Recently, boric acid powder has found widespread acceptance as a household insecticide.[1004] In addition, the U.S. Department of the Interior has set an upper limit for boron in public water supplies at 1 μg/ml.[1005]

B. ROLES AND FUNCTIONS

In plants, boron is thought to play multiple roles in membrane transport of nutrients, hydroxylation of phenolic rings (bioflavonoids), complexing with hydroxyl groups on furanoids, steroid, sterol, and phenolic ring structures, regulation of plant hormones by membrane effects and second messenger activations, and regulation of enzyme activities.[1000-1002] A consensus of research in animals and plants indicates that boron plays a role in regulation of metabolism similar to regulatory actions of calcium. Thus, boron will exhibit many diverse and indirect actions in biological systems, which is what research to date has uncovered (Table 1).

Borates and other organoboron compounds inhibit two major classes of enzymes — oxidoreductases and serine proteases.[1001,1006] In oxidoreductases, boron competes with pyridine or flavin nucleotide cofactors (NADH, NADPH, and FAD).[1001] Examples include alcohol dehydrogenase, xanthine oxidase, glyceraldehyde-3-phosphate dehydrogenase, 6-phosphogluconate dehydrogenase, and cytochrome b_5 reductase.[1002] Thrombin, chymotrypsin, and subtilisin are known to be inhibited by borate.[1001] Other serine proteases are important mediators of inflammation and resulting tissue damage.[150] Thus, boron may possess potential antiinflammatory actions by inhibition of enzymes used to promote inflammation, tissue degradation, and leukocyte respiratory burst (free radical formation). However, before any conclusions about the antiinflammatory nature of boron can be made, concentrations for *in vitro* effects must be matched to localized *in vivo* levels. The possible antiinflammatory effects of boron compounds deserve further attention.

**TABLE 1   Potential Roles of Boron
in Biological Systems**

Membrane transport of nutrients
Regulator of secondary messengers used by hormones
Facilitation of hydroxylation of steroid, sterol, or phenolic rings
(estrogen, testosterone, activated vitamin D metabolites)
Regulation of enzyme activity
(oxidoreductases and serine proteases)

C. ANIMAL STUDIES

After a hiatus since 1947, animal studies of boron effects initiated in 1981 to trace poor growth in chicks fed a supposedly complete diet[1006] eventually led to many studies on boron and indicators of bone metabolism. Boron supplementation to vitamin D-deficient chicks improved growth, but had no effect on chicks with normal vitamin D status.[1001,1006,1007] Because vitamin D affects calcium and magnesium metabolism, interactions of boron with these minerals was explored. Growth of chicks deficient in magnesium was improved by boron supplementation, independent of vitamin D status.[1001]

Qin and Klandrof of the Division of Animal and Veterinary Sciences of West Virginia University in Morgantown studied the effect of boron supplementation on calcium metabolism with aged breeder hens.[1008] Dietary boron supplements of 60 to 100 ppm in feed with low (1.5%) or high (3.5%) calcium intakes found that supplemental boron significantly increased tibial bone ash percentage, but did not affect egg quality. Thus, boron did not greatly affect chicken calcium metabolism, but did support bone formation.

The interaction of boron and vitamin D (cholecalciferol) was studied in vitamin D-deficient chicken embryos by King and others from the U.S. Army Research Institute of Environmental Medicine in College Station, TX, in 1991.[1009] Boron (0.5 mg per egg), boron and vitamin D (0.5 mg and 0.3 µg, respectively), or vitamin D were injected into eggs of 8-day-old vitamin D-deficient embryos. Both boron and vitamin D increased bone ash and decreased epiphyseal growth plate indicators of vitamin D deficiency, suggesting more rapid bone formation with boron supplementation. From these results, an interaction of boron with vitamin D on bone formation of chicks was inferred.

King and others, using the same experimental model, except that chicks had normal vitamin D status, found that 1.0 mg of boron injected in ovo actually reduced bone organic matrix, had unfavorable effects on bone elongation, and reduced hatchability.[1010] Lower boron doses (0.1 and 0.5 mg per egg) did not show adverse effects. Thus, there is a limit to beneficial effects of boron on bone metabolism in situations without a vitamin D deficiency.

In 1989, Pardue and others injected turkey eggs with 250 or 500 µg of boron as sodium tetraborate.[1011] Tibial weight, tibial length, tibial calcium content, and bone ash were all significantly increased by boron addition. In 1992, Elliot and Edwards from the Department of Poultry Science of the University of Georgia reported on the interaction of different levels of dietary boron with calcium and vitamin D (cholecalciferol) in broiler cockerels fed tibial dyschondroplasia-inducing basal diets.[1012] Dietary boron at intakes of 0, 5, 10, 20, 40, and 80 mg/kg had no influence on weight gain, feed efficiency, or plasma mineral levels. Boron intakes of 5 and 10 mg/kg were associated with increased bone ash. However, varying dietary calcium and vitamin D intakes along with boron intakes of 0, 3, or 40 mg/kg did not show any obvious interactions.

Nielsen and others, of the USDA Grand Forks Human Nutrition Research Center in North Dakota, conducted a series of experiments to examine the essentiality of boron by its effects on major mineral metabolism.[1013] By altering the diets of weanling rats with respect to magnesium, manganese, and methionine, it was found that boron supplementation (0 or 3 µg/g of feed) manifested interactions when deficiencies of other nutrients were significant. Dietary boron deprivation depressed growth and decreased bone magnesium contents. Effects of boron deprivation were magnified by marginal magnesium or methionine intake. Since the boron supplement approximated normal dietary levels of boron, results were surmised to be physiological and not pharmacological, lending evidence that boron is essential to animals.

**TABLE 2 Effects of Boron Deficiency
in Animals**

Decreased bone calcium content
Decreased bone magnesium contents
Depressed growth

Hegsted and others, of the Louisiana State University Agricultural Center in Baton Rouge, LA, reported on the effect of two different dietary boron intakes on rats made deficient in vitamin D.[1014] Weanling rats were fed a diet deficient in vitamin D and containing either 0.16 or 2.72 µg/g boron for 11 weeks. Higher dietary boron was associated with higher absorption and balances of calcium and phosphorus, although few differences were seen in bone parameters, organ weight, and body weight. Thus, boron affected mineral balance in vitamin D-deficient rats, but did not substitute for vitamin D function.

McCoy and others fed male weanling rats standard diets with low or normal calcium contents.[1015] Boron was added at levels of 0, 3, 6, and 12 µg/g diet for 6 weeks. Femurs were removed and subjected to a 3-point flexure test, and vertebrae were subjected to a compression test to measure bone strength. Boron deficiency (0 µg B/g diet) exhibited significantly lower femur length (30.8 vs. 31.7 to 32.0 mm), vertebrae bone strength (6.1 vs. 8.6 to 8.8 kg), and bone calcium (7.5 vs. 8.2 to 8.4 mg) than boron-supplemented diets when calcium intake was low. Addition of boron to a low calcium diet did not normalize femur strength, vertebrae strength, or bone calcium. In conclusion, bone strength was shown to be adversely affected by boron deficiency.

In 1990, Bock and others fed normal or oophorectomized female rats diets containing 0 or 12 µg B/100 g.[1016] Urinary calcium and magnesium loss was greater in normal rats fed a boron-deficient diet.

Nielsen and Shuler conducted two experiments on rats to study the interaction of boron with calcium.[1017] They confirmed that boron deprivation exerted similar effects as calcium deprivation (decreased femur calcium concentration). Thus, boron and calcium metabolism were interrelated in an indirect and complex manner involving magnesium, potassium, phosphorus, copper, and zinc.

Effects of boron supplements (75 or 200 mg B per d from sodium borate) added to a basal diet containing 30 mg B per day of potassium, calcium, phosphorus, and magnesium status were measured in 18 sheep for 11 d by Brown and others.[1018] Both boron supplements significantly improved calcium absorption and retention, and the highest boron dose improved magnesium retention. No effects on potassium or phosphorus status was observed.

Studies of adjuvant-induced or formaldehyde-induced arthritis in animals showed that administration of borate or synthetic boron analogs of amino acids inhibited development of arthritis.[1019-1021]

Overall, animal studies with boron indicated that boron exerts indirect effects on mineral and bone metabolism, probably by modifying hormonal responses to vitamin D and other hormones involved in calcium and magnesium metabolism (Table 2). Interactions with other minerals known to be important for bone metabolism were also indicated. However, effects of boron were indirect and complicated, and multiple mechanisms were postulated, perhaps due to a regulatory mechanism similar to calcium. Deficiencies of boron were associated with suboptimal bone formation, and suboptimal mineral metabolism, indicating boron meets the criteria for an essential nutrient for animals.

D. HUMAN STUDIES
1. Dietary Intakes of Boron

Relatively few studies of boron intake in humans exist, due to difficulties in the technical aspects of boron analysis. A recent survey of boron levels in foods and personal care items by Hunt and others from the U.S. Department of Agriculture, Grand Forks Human Nutrition Research Center in Grand Forks, ND, has estimated that an average daily intake of boron for adolescent or postmenopausal women ranges between 0.3 and 0.6 mg/d.[1005] Schlettwein-Gsell and Mommsen-Straub of the Institute for Experimental Gerontology in Basel, Switzerland estimated daily boron intakes worldwide ranging from 0.3 to 41 mg/d, mostly depending upon local water supplies.[1022] Hospital diets in the U.S. were reported to contain 1.2 to 1.6 mg B per day for normal diets and intakes less than 1.0 mg B per d for calorie-restricted diets.[955] Murphy and others reported that boron contents from 300 lunches of schoolchildren averaged 0.5 mg B per day.[956] Diets of 33 women in college ranged from 0.5 to 2.6 mg B per day and 0.5 to 2.4 mg B per day for 15 high school girls.[853]

From the available studies, it is clear that a diet low in fruits and vegetables (common in the U.S.) will lead to low boron intakes. Meats, dairy products, eggs, and grain all contain levels of boron from negligible to low (<0.5 µg B/g wet weight).[1005,1022] Fruits, seeds, stalks, leaves, and barks from dicotyledonous plants contained high levels of boron (1.0 to 30.0 µg B/g wet weight).[1005,1022] However, the dicotyledons citrus fruits, pineapples, and berries seem to have low levels of boron.[1005,1022]

2. Boron and Bone Metabolism

In a landmark study, Nielsen and others at the Grand Forks Human Nutrition Research Center in North Dakota, of the U.S. Department of Agriculture, first reported the effects of boron supplementation on parameters of bone metabolism in humans by measuring parameters of bone metabolism.[1023] Of particular interest is the use of a proper target population — 12 postmenopausal women aged 48 to 82 — and a metabolic unit setting, where dietary intakes were carefully monitored.

All women were fed a diet low in boron for 119 d. Boron intake was 0.25 mg/d, less than the projected average intake of 1.0 to 1.5 mg B per day. Calcium intake was 600 mg/d/2000 kcal, magnesium intake varied from 116 to 316 mg/d (from low to adequate, according to the USRDA), and phosphorus intake was 870 mg/d/2000 kcal. Potassium, iron copper, vitamin D_3 (cholecalciferol), and folic acid supplements were given to ensure adequate intake of these nutrients. During the 119-d period of low boron intake, dietary aluminum (±1000 mg/d) and/or magnesium (±200 mg/d) intakes were varied, with no effects on measures of calcium metabolism. Only one subject was on estrogen replacement therapy, and data from this person was excluded from hormonal measurements.

Following the period of low boron intake, all subjects were given 3 mg/d of boron as sodium borate for 48 additional days. There were 7 subjects given 1000 mg aluminum per day for 24 d, and the five other subjects were supplemented with 200 mg/d of magnesium for 48 d, and an additional 1000 mg of aluminum for 24 d. Measurements of bone mineral metabolism included (1) urinary excretion of calcium, magnesium, and phosphorus, and (2) serum levels of 17β-estradiol and testosterone.

Figures 1 and 2 synopsize the results according to boron intakes over time. Low boron intakes reduced serum levels of 17β-estradiol and testosterone, which returned to and exceeded initial values after boron intake of 3.25 mg/d.[1023] On the other hand, urinary excretion of calcium, magnesium, and phosphorus remained unchanged by low boron intakes, but increased dietary boron intake (3.25 mg/d) led to significant decreases in urinary losses of calcium and magnesium.

These findings offer strong evidence that boron deprivation in humans leads to biochemical changes considered to be detrimental to bone health. Results suggested that boron prevented urinary loss of calcium and magnesium by an endocrine mechanism. Of great practical importance is that the dietary intake during the boron supplement period was 3.25 mg/d, which is attainable by a diet rich in fruits and vegetables.[1005,1023] Thus, higher boron intakes may be another reason that vegetarian diets are associated with less risk for development of osteoporosis.[1024,1025] Diets low in boron (including the typical Western diet rich in meat and refined grains) may contribute to osteoporosis and other bone loss disorders in humans.

In order to further study the effect of boron on calcium metabolism in humans, Nielsen and others fed a diet similar to the previous study to five men, four postmenopausal women, five postmenopausal women on estrogen therapy, and one premenopausal woman (n = 15), all over 45 years in age.[1026-1029] A dietary depletion phase lasting 63 d was low in boron (0.23 mg/2000 kcal), magnesium (115 mg/2000 kcal) and copper (1.6 mg/2000 kcal). A boron supplement of 3.0 mg/d (as sodium borate) was given for 49 d while the low magnesium and copper diet was continued.

For all 15 subjects, boron repletion significantly increased serum levels of calcitonin, 25-hydroxycholecalciferol and ceruloplasmin, plasma copper, and erythrocyte superoxide dismutase activity. Serum levels of glucose, creatinine, and urea nitrogen were significantly decreased by boron

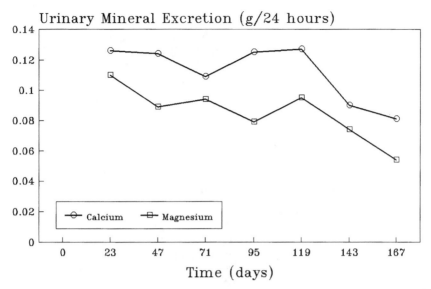

FIGURE 1. Changes in urinary mineral excretion during periods of low and high boron intakes (adapted from Reference 1023).

[1] Mean values from 13 subjects. Low boron intake (0.25 mg/d) started on day 0. High boron intake (boron supplement of 3.0 mg/d) started on day 119.

[2] Urinary mineral excretion values for calcium and magnesium were significantly different from previous values at 143 and 167 day ($p < 0.05$).

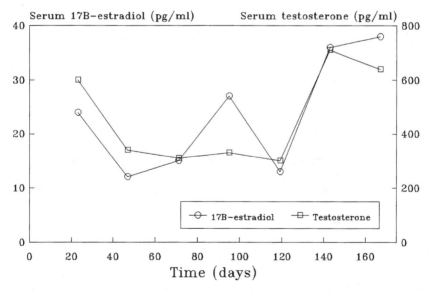

FIGURE 2. Changes in serum levels of 17β-estradiol and testosterone during periods of low and high boron intakes (adapted from Reference 1023).

[1] Mean values from 12 subjects (none were taking estrogen replacement therapy). Low boron intake (0.25 mg/d) started on day 0. High boron intake (boron supplement of 3.0 mg/d) started on day 119.

[2] Serum levels of 17β-estradiol and testosterone were significantly different from previous values at 143 and 167 day ($p < 0.05$).

TABLE 3   Effects of Boron Repletion After Boron
Deprivation During a Low-Magnesium,
Low-Copper Diet in Fifteen Humans[a]

All subjects (n = 15)

Boron Intake (mg/d)	Serum 17β-Estradiol (pg/ml)	Serum Glucose (mg/dl)	Plasma Copper (µg/dl)	Erythrocyte SOD Activity (U/g Hgb)[b]
0	52 ± 12	93	117 ± 8	2257
3	64 ± 9	88	122 ± 8	2578
p value	0.13	0.0004	0.03	0.03

Postmenopausal Women on Estrogen Therapy (n = 5)

Boron Intake (mg/d)	Serum 17β-Estradiol (pg/ml)	Serum Glucose (mg/dl)	Plasma Copper (µg/dl)	Erythrocyte SOD Activity (U/g Hgb)[b]
0	107 ± 22	91	141 ± 10	2160
3	145 ± 36	86	152 ± 9	2736
p value	0.09	0.009	0.03	0.04

[a]   Data from References 1028–1030. A diet low in boron
(0.23 mg/2000 kcal), magnesium (115 mg/2000 kcal), and copper
(1.6 mg/2000 kcal) was fed for 63 d, followed by 49 d of the same
diet with a boron supplement of 3.0 mg/d (as sodium borate).
Averages of each time period are presented.

[b]   SOD = superoxide dismutase, presented in units per gram of
hemoglobin.

repletion. Serum 17β-estradiol levels in postmenopausal women on estrogen therapy tended to increase during boron repletion (107 ± 22 to 145 ± 36 pg/ml, *p* <0.09). Thus, in diets low in magnesium and copper (not uncommon in the U.S.[779]), boron caused beneficial changes similar to estrogen and enhanced effects of estrogen therapy (Table 3).

In an additional study on the effects of boron nutriture on human physiology related to bone health, Nielsen and others studied four men, four postmenopausal women, five postmenopausal women on estrogen therapy, and one premenopausal woman (n = 14), all aged 50 to 62 years.[1028-1030] The study objective was to determine if boron behaves similarly to estrogen in humans fed an adequate diet (except for boron intake). Each subject was fed the previously mentioned diet low in boron (0.23 mg/2000 kcal) for 63 d, followed by 49 d of the same diet with a boron supplement of 3.0 mg/d. Measurements of hematological parameters and indices of bone mineral metabolism were performed.

This study is important because it showed that boron intake at physiological amounts in a diet adequate in all known nutrients has beneficial effects on indices of bone metabolism (Table 4). Thus, results of this study are attributable only to boron, and not to interactions with other mineral intakes. While urinary calcium excretion was unchanged, serum levels of 17β-estradiol in the subjects taking estrogen were increased significantly after boron repletion, but other subjects showed no effects of boron on estradiol levels. Levels of copper, ceruloplasmin, erythrocyte superoxide dismutase activity, 25-hydroxycholecalciferol, triglycerides, and urinary excretion of hydroxyproline were increased significantly in all subjects (Table 4). Triglyceride levels increased in women, but not men. Some hematological parameters showed very small, but statistically significant, changes (Table 4). Serum calcitonin and osteocalcin levels were also increased in all subjects.[1028]

Of interest are the changes in hormones known to affect bone metabolism (vitamin D and estrogen), and increased urinary hydroxyproline excretion. Increased urinary hydroxyproline excretion suggests increased collagen turnover and has been used as a nonspecific marker for bone loss or destruction.[1031,1032] However, deposition of newly synthesized collagen also elevates urinary hydroxyproline.[1033]

TABLE 4 Effects of Boron Deprivation and Repletion on Parameters Related to Bone Metabolism in Humans Fed an Otherwise Adequate Diet[a]

All Subjects (n = 14)

Boron Intake (mg/d)	Serum Estradiol (pg/ml)	Serum 25-OHD$_3$ (ng/ml)	Plasma Copper (µg/dl)	Serum Cerulo. (mg/dl)	Serum Trig. (mg/dl)	RBC SOD (U/g Hgb)	Urinary Calcium (g/d)	Urinary HP (mmol/d)	HP/ Creatinine Ratio
0	48 ± 13	18 ± 1	115 ± 9	33 ± 2	125 ± 5	2735	0.198	0.0495	0.0069
3	69 ± 22	25 ± 3	121 ± 10	38 ± 3	142 ± 18	3243	0.205	0.0601	0.0082
p value	0.06	0.04	0.02	0.002	0.004	0.04	0.36	0.001	0.006

Women on Estrogen Therapy (n = 5)

Boron Intake (mg/d)	Serum Estradiol (pg/ml)	Serum 25-OHD$_3$ (ng/ml)	Plasma Copper (µg/dl)	Serum Cerulo. (mg/dl)	Serum Trig. (mg/dl)	RBC SOD (U/g Hgb)	Urinary Calcium (g/d)	Urinary HP (mmol/d)	HP/ Creatinine Ratio
0	99 ± 15	18 ± 2	146 ± 9	42 ± 2	143 ± 25	2520	0.162	0.0520	0.0077
3	157 ± 27	30 ± 4	159 ± 11	50 ± 5	175 ± 32	3327	0.163	0.0609	0.0092
p value	0.02	0.06	0.04	0.05	0.02	0.03	0.94	0.05	0.16

[a] Data from references. 1028–1030, 1043. A diet low in boron (0.23 mg/2000 kcal), magnesium (115 mg/2000 kcal), and copper (1.6 mg/2000 kcal) was fed for 63 d, followed by 49 d of the same diet with a boron supplement of 3.0 mg/d (as sodium borate). Averages of each time period are presented.

[b] Abbreviations are 25OHD$_3$ = 25-hydroxycholecalciferol; Cerulo. = ceruloplasmin; Trig. = triglycerides; RBC SOD = erythrocyte superoxide dismutase; HP = hydroxyproline.

Since boron repletion increased urinary hydroxyproline while decreasing or not changing urinary calcium excretion, and elevated levels of activated vitamin D and estrogen, it is more likely that boron resulted in improved collagen synthesis or deposition, possibly indicating bone formation.

Combined results from the three human studies on boron deprivation and repletion and bone metabolism suggest that boron repletion caused beneficial changes in bone and mineral metabolism similar to estrogen therapy (Table 5). Boron also improved levels of other hormones known to improve bone mass, including activated vitamin D, calcitonin, and osteocalcin. Other effects of boron repletion appeared similar to regulatory effects of calcium on cell membranes, which may explain the multitude of effects on hematological and blood clinical chemistry parameters. The lack of the second and third studies by Nielsen to replicate his initial finding that boron repletion increased serum 17β-estradiol and decreased urinary calcium loss in postmenopausal women not taking estrogen may be due to the shorter depletion period (63 vs. 119 d) or smaller number of subjects (4 vs. 13) in the later studies.

Thus, boron can indirectly affect bone metabolism in a beneficial manner when dietary levels are over 3.0 mg/d and adversely affect bone metabolism when dietary levels are low (<0.5 mg/d). Modification of hormone actions and regulation of cell membrane events are postulated as mechanisms of boron action.

TABLE 5 Beneficial Effects of Adequate Boron Intake on Indices of Bone Metabolism in Postmenopausal Women

1. ↓ Urinary excretion of calcium (reduction of calcium loss)
2. ↓ Urinary excretion of magnesium (reduction of magnesium loss)
3. ↑ Urinary excretion of hydroxyproline (improvement in collagen synthesis)
4. ↑ Serum 25-hydroxycholecalciferol (activated vitamin D) (improved absorption and bone retention of calcium)
5. ↑ Serum 17β-estradiol (with or without estrogen therapy) (improved retention of bone mass)
6. ↑ Serum testosterone (improved retention of bone mass)
7. ↑ Serum calcitonin (improved retention of bone mass)
8. ↑ Serum osteocalcin (improved retention of bone mass)

Baslé and others from the Central University Hospital in Angers Cédex, France measured iliac cortical and trabecular bone concentrations of boron and other elements from 12 normal subjects (41 to 87 years) and 21 subjects with severe, untreated osteoporosis with at least one collapsed vertebra (31 to 79 years).[1034] Concentrations of boron, expressed as mg/kg dry weight of cortical bone, did not differ between normal and osteoporotic individuals (1.08 vs. 0.91 mg/kg), although trabecular bone volume was halved in osteoporotic subjects (15.7 vs. 8.2%). Other minerals, except for an increase in iron from osteoporotic subjects, showed no differences between groups. A positive correlation between magnesium and boron concentrations was seen for normal subjects (0.5594, p <0.03), but not for osteoporotic subjects (0.0311).

Children on long-term total parenteral nutrition (TPN) exhibit an osteopenia of unknown etiology.[1035] Serum boron levels from 28 children receiving TPN for an average of 9 years were found to be significantly increased compared to healthy children (11.6 ± 1.5 vs. 8.8 ± 2.8 mM, p <0.02).[1035] Children receiving TPN had an intake of 9.4 to 30 mg boron daily, which is much higher than usual dietary intakes of 1.5 mg daily. Thus, osteopenia of TPN is not likely due to a boron deficiency.

Darnton and others from Virginia Polytechnic Institute studied the effects of boron supplementation on serum levels of calcium, magnesium, and phosphorus in both sedentary college women and female college athletes.[1036] Boron supplementation was associated with increased serum magnesium levels and decreased phosphorus levels. Other interactions with bone mineral density and urinary excretion of calcium, magnesium, and phosphorus were found, but no clear-cut trend was reported.

Ferrando and Green, of the Department of Nutrition at Florida State University, administered a boron supplement (2.5 mg B per day for 7 weeks) or a placebo to 19 bodybuilders.[1037] Although plasma boron increased after supplementation, serum testosterone levels, lean body mass, and muscular strength increased in both groups and were not affected by boron supplementation. This study suggests that supplemental boron is not an anabolic steroid alternative for weightlifters at the dosage studied.

3. Boron and Arthritis

In 1982, Newnham from Thornsbury, Australia reported on the association of boron deficiency with arthritis, based on personal reversal of osteoarthritis symptoms by a boron supplement and anecdotal reports of others using boron supplements.[1038] In Australia, less arthritis in the population was found in areas highest in water and soil boron content. Human femur heads from arthritic subjects averaged 30 μg B/g compared to 56 μg B/g for a normal subject. Decreasing soil and water boron availability was blamed on excessive use of potash and phosphate fertilizers in Western countries.

Later, Newnham illustrated epidemiological evidence that suggests dietary intakes of boron are inversely correlated with incidence of arthritis in the general population.[1019] Areas with soil boron levels less than 1 ppm are associated with a prevalence of arthritis from 20 to 70% (Table 6). Areas of high boron levels in soil and water exhibited much less arthritis. From this data, Newnham advocated ingestion of 6 mg B per day, along with additional magnesium (250 mg/d) and other trace minerals for therapy of arthritis in humans. Anecdotal reports and testimonials from individuals and animals ingesting dietary boron supplements claimed relief from arthritis pain and improvement in joint range of motion. Also quoted were unpublished studies on adjuvant-induced arthritis in rats and other animals given 50 mg/kg boric acid from Adelaide University and the University of Perth. Boron supplementation also seemed to alleviate arthritis incidence and symptoms in anecdotal case reports from animal owners.

These enticing observations spurred a randomized, double-blind pilot study of boron supplementation in 20 humans (50 to 75 years) with radiographically confirmed osteoarthritis by Travers and Rennie of the Royal Melbourne Hospital in Australia.[1039] Half of the subjects (n = 10) were given placebo, and the other half were given 6 mg/d of boron from 25 mg borax (sodium tetraborate decahydrate) for 8 weeks. Pretreatment values for length of arthritis, number of joints affected, severity of arthritis, joint pain on movement, joint swelling, restricted joint movement, and analgesic ingestion (paracetamol) were comparable between groups.

After 8 weeks, 5/7 subjects on boron and 1/8 subjects on placebo showed improvement, a significant finding. Accounting for dropouts, 5/10 boron subjects and 1/10 placebo subjects showed

TABLE 6 Association of Boron Intakes with Arthritis Incidence

Geographic Area	Estimated Boron Intake (mg/d)	Arthritis Incidence (%)
Jamaica	<1	70
Mauritius	<1	50
Brazil	1	30
U.S., Great Britain, South Africa, Australia, New Zealand	1–2	20
Transkei, South Africa	3–5	4
Carnarvon, Australia	4–6	1
Israel	8–10	<1
Ngawha, New Zealand	12–15	<1

Note: Data from References 1019 and 1038.

improvements, which was not statistically significant. The "average condition" (1 = completely cured to 6 = far worse) for all joints was significantly improved for the boron group (Table 7). The boron group showed significantly less pain on passive movement and did not change their analgesic usage, while the placebo group increased analgesic usage (Table 7).

No side effects were observed, and there was no change in routine clinical measurements (weight, pulse rate, blood pressure, temperature, blood cell counts, erythrocyte sedimentation rate, clinical chemistry values). Five subjects (three boron, two placebo) dropped out of the study.

Thus, in a pilot study, boron supplementation improved some symptoms of osteoarthritis compared to a placebo. This study employed very low numbers of subjects, had a high dropout rate (25%), and a low placebo response (1/8 or 12.5% compared to an anticipated 30%). However, even with small numbers, statistical significance was reached in a relatively short time period for a chronic disease of long-standing duration (6.4 years per subject) by a single agent. Given the low cost of boron supplements, these preliminary results are encouraging enough to strongly indicate that boron supplementation (or boron status) deserves further study in osteoarthritis and, perhaps, other degenerative joint diseases.

E. SAFETY

Dietary levels of boron (as boric acid or sodium borate) ranging from 1 to 40 mg B per day have not been associated with toxicity in humans. However, boron intakes over 50 mg/d are not recommended, as this level equates to boron intakes known to cause adverse effects in animals.[1003] Ingestion of 5 g boric acid (1 teaspoon) in children, or 10 to 15 g boric acid (1 tablespoon) in adults, is a sufficient dose to cause acute gastrointestinal distress, blue-green diarrhea, and a rash in the inguinal, axillary, and facial regions.[1004] Higher doses may cause CNS irritability, seizures, shock, and renal failure.[1004] Lethal doses of boric acid in humans are 1 to 3 g for newborns, 5 g for infants, and 15 to 20 g for adults.[1004] Proposed safe maximum levels of boron in drinking water have ranged from 0.5 to 20 mg B/l.[1040]

TABLE 7 Results of Boron Supplementation (6 mg/d) on Osteoarthritis[a]

Measurement	Boron Group Pretreatment	Boron Group Posttreatment	Placebo Group Pretreatment	Placebo Group Posttreatment
Number of joints affected	4.2	4.0	5.1	5.8
Average condition of joints	3.7	3.0[b]	3.5	3.9
% Joints with pain on movement	50	27[b]	69	70
% Joints with swelling	50	46	69	57
% Joints with restricted movement	64	54	69	70
Analgesics per day	0.9	0.8	1.8	2.5

[a] Data from Reference 1039. Subjects (n = 10 for each group) were given a placebo or boron supplement (6 mg B as sodium borate) for 8 weeks. Data represents 7 subjects for the boron group and 8 subjects for placebo group.

[b] Significant difference from pretreatment value (*p* <0.05).

**TABLE 8   Guidelines for Use of
Boron Supplements**

Bone Loss Disorders
  Osteoporosis
  Osteomalacia
  Osteopenia
  Fracture healing?
Arthritis
  Osteoarthritis
  Rheumatoid arthritis?
Postmenopausal Women
Athletic Amenorrhea?

However, at doses obtainable in foods and dietary supplements, boron does not pose a hazard. Of greater concern is the increasing use of boric acid powder as an insecticide, with potential for accidental ingestion.

F. SUMMARY

Although a biochemical mechanism is still unclear, boron appears essential for animals and humans.[1041-1044] Boron deprivation leads to detrimental changes in factors affecting bone metabolism and may be associated with increased incidence of degenerative bone and joint disease. It is important to note that *physiological* intakes of boron (approximating levels easily reached by diet), and not pharmacological (high) doses, accounted for observed beneficial effects in both animals and humans. For humans, a physiological amount of boron appears to be greater than 1 mg/d,[1003] and perhaps greater than 3 mg/d. This latter value can be easily reached by an abundant consumption of fruits, vegetables, legumes, and root vegetables (tubers).[1003,1005,1022] Vegetarian diets are associated with a lower incidence of osteoporosis[1024,1025] and are also high in boron, among other factors. Thus, adequate dietary boron may be necessary to prevent osteoporosis and other bone loss disorders, and perhaps some arthritis.

G. GUIDELINES FOR USE

Table 8 lists the conditions which may show potential benefit by instituting adequate boron intake. Of chief interest is osteoporosis, for which supportive evidence in humans is available. Other conditions, including arthritis, are still speculative at this time with respect to boron status, but preliminary evidence indicates that boron may be helpful and is most likely not harmful. One interesting possibility that has yet to be explored is the effect of boron on fracture healing, an important event in sports medicine as well as hip, spinal, and wrist fractures common in osteoporosis. Another interesting possibility would be the effect of boron on amenorrheic female athletes. Combinations of boron with other nutrients (such as calcium or magnesium) may offer additional advantages over boron alone.

A diet rich in fresh fruits and vegetables will supply what appears to be an adequate intake of boron (Table 9). However, this advice may be faulty if the geographic areas from which an individual consumes fruit and vegetables are low in soil and water boron. Without comprehensive surveys of boron levels in foods and geographic areas, one cannot be completely ensured that boron intake will be adequate from increased consumption of fresh fruits and vegetables. This raises the issue of boron supplementation. Certainly boron supplements are now widely available and accessible to the public (mostly as a result of the study by Nielsen reported in 1987).[1023] Doses range from 1 to 3 mg B per unit dose (tablet or capsule). At supplemental boron intakes of 3 to 6 mg/d, no untoward effects have been reported or are anticipated, based on safety studies of boron, even if dietary boron intakes are on the high end of those reported (41 mg/d).[1022] Certainly, potential benefits of ensuring adequate boron nutriture outweigh the risk of no effects from boron. It is not yet known if short-term, higher doses of boron would accelerate intended boron effects. Excess boron intake (>50 mg/d) is to be avoided, since intakes of 500 mg B per d are definitely associated with disturbances in appetite, digestion, and skin health in humans.[1003]

TABLE 9   Foods Rich in Boron (Partial List)

Food	Boron Content (µg/g wet weight)
Apple cider, apple juice, avocado, beef bouillon, broccoli, carrots, celery, frozen cherries, grape jelly, grape juice, canned peaches, canned pears, tea	1–2
Applesauce, beets, chicory, cocoa powder, garlic, herb spices, radishes, spinach	2–5
Dates, dried onion flakes, wine	5–10
Alfalfa, almonds, ground cinnamon, hazelnuts, honey, parsley flakes, peanuts, prunes, raisins	>10

In conclusion, maintenance of boron intakes between 3 to 6 mg/d by dietary manipulation (increasing consumption of fresh fruits and vegetables) or supplements is recommended for bone loss conditions (especially osteoporosis), postmenopausal women (regardless of estrogen replacement therapy status), and degenerative joint diseases.

II. FLUORIDE

A. BACKGROUND

The major role of fluoride in connective tissue healing is maintenance of bone mass. Fluoride replaces hydroxy ions in hydroxyapatite crystals and is incorporated into bone and teeth. Fluoride has been recognized since the 1930s as an ultratrace element necessary for reduction of dental caries during formation of teeth during growth and development.[1045-1047] The Estimated Safe and Adequate Daily Dietary Intake (ESADDI) is 1.5 to 4.0 mg/d for adults.[1046] Actual intakes of fluoride for adults have shown a median of 1.4 mg/d worldwide.[1048] In the U.S., best estimates of average fluoride intake are within the ESADDI.[1046]

Because most fluoride intake is derived from water intake, local geographic influences and addition of fluoride to municipal supplies of tap water largely determine fluoride intake. As a result, fluoride deficiencies severe enough to affect dental enamel and bone density appear to be isolated and uncommon. However, fluoride toxicity is an increasing concern.[1046] Acute lethal doses of fluoride in man are 32 to 64 mg/kg, an extremely high dose. Nevertheless, accidental acute fluoride poisoning has resulted in at least 45 deaths (43 from an accidental poisoning in a single hospital in the early 1940s).[1046] Of more practical concern is chronic fluoride toxicity, manifested as dental and skeletal fluorosis.[1046] Dental fluorosis (ranging in severity from white spots on teeth to hypomineralization with staining and pitting of enamel) is increasing in frequency in the U.S. but, overall, is usually mild with no aesthetic changes. Skeletal fluorosis results from chronic ingestion of 10 to 25 mg of fluoride per day for years. Skeletal hypermineralization, soft tissue calcification (especially tendons and ligaments), and exostosis formation are apparent and may progress to crippling.[1046] Thus, fluoride exhibits a narrow window of safe and adequate intake. Bone defects are manifested during both deficiency and toxicity of fluoride.

B. HUMAN STUDIES

Correlation with bone density and fluoride intakes from water led to the extensive study of fluoride supplements for therapy of postmenopausal osteoporosis.[1049] Over 30 years of clinical research has revealed that high fluoride doses increase bone density and mass, but bone quality is questionable, and adverse side effects were common (see Table 10).[439,1049]

C. SUMMARY

For the reasons listed in Table 10, supplemental fluoride does not appear to be safe or effective for possible repletion of lowered bone mass in younger athletic populations. Likewise, fluoride supplementation

TABLE 10 Summation of Clinical Findings in Fluoride Therapy for Osteoporosis

1. ↑ Bone mineral density in 70% of osteoporotic subjects
2. Dose-dependent increase in bone density (2–9%/year) after 30–75 mg/d of sodium fluoride
3. Product formulation (plain, enteric-coated, time-released) made no difference in effects on bone mass
4. Supplemental calcium (1000–1500 mg/d) was required
5. Conflicting findings between study results were common
6. Fluoride therapy did not promote positive calcium balance
7. Fluoride therapy did not reduce vertebral fracture rate in osteoporotics
8. Fluoride therapy may increase peripheral (hip) fractures
9. High rate of Painful Lower Extremity Syndrome (osteoarticular pains and stress fractures)
10. May increase skeletal fragility regardless of bone mass changes
11. High rate of gastric mucosal damage

does not appear to be beneficial in healing of fractures. Although controlled studies of fluoride supplementation in athletic populations are not found, a sufficient rationale to justify further studies or clinical use of high-dose fluoride supplementation does not exist. Fluoride supplementation over ESADDI amounts (4 mg/d) is not recommended.

III. SELENIUM

A. ROLES AND FUNCTIONS

Selenium is an essential ultratrace dietary nutrient.[1050-1054] Selenium exerts most of its biological roles by forming selenocysteine residues at the active site of glutathione peroxidase (GPx) enzymes.[1050-1054] GPx is the major quantitative cellular antioxidant and is active against hydrogen peroxide, hydroperoxides, and phospholipid hydroperoxides. GPx utilizes glutathione (GSH) as a rechargeable intermediate. Reduction (recharging) of other antioxidants (tocopherols, ascorbate, thioredoxin) is accomplished directly or indirectly via GPx activity and GSH. Selenium is also involved in biological transformation of xenobiotics, protection against heavy metal toxicity, and regulation of GPx and hydroperoxide metabolism.[1050-1054] Roles in cancer prevention, cardiovascular disease prevention, immune function, and other free radical-mediated pathologies have been postulated.[1050-1054]

B. DEFICIENCY SYMPTOMS

The major deficiency symptoms of selenium in humans have been documented in certain regions of China and eastern Siberia. Of interest to connective tissue healing is Kashin-Beck disease, and endemic osteoarthropathy in China.[1051,1055-1057] Kashin-Beck disease is a chronic, disabling, degenerative osteoarthrosis that affects mainly children and adolescents. Kashin-Beck disease occurs in areas with very low soil and food selenium levels, but other factors are thought to be involved. Therefore, one manifestation of a selenium deficiency in humans may be degenerative joint disease. Kashin-Beck disease has been reversed by sodium selenite supplementation (0.5 to 2.0 mg sodium selenite per week).[1051,1055-1057] Other deficiency syndromes may be hyperlipidemia, cardiovascular disease, and increased risk for cancers, but a clear cause and effect is difficult to prove.

Selenium-deficient mice (adult third-generation deficient animals) exhibited deformities and aberrant joint cartilage anatomy.[1058] Knee joint cartilage exhibited more cell layers than normal and no tidemark. Clusters of hypertrophic chondrocytes, necrotic chondrocytes, fewer, thinner, and shorter collagen fibrils, and disorganized arrangement of fibrils were found in selenium-deficient mice. These findings resembled chondronecrosis, which was almost identical to human Kashin-Beck disease findings.

Long-term TPN in humans without selenium intake has frequently resulted in lowered serum levels of selenium and depressed activity of blood GPx activity.[1054] Some patients exhibited cardiomyopathy and muscle weakness (two signs of selenium deficiency in animals), but those findings could not conclusively be attributed to selenium deficiency. Overall, selenium deficiency symptoms are not well defined in humans and may manifest as vague muscular complaints.[1057] Perhaps a selenium deficiency predisposes to symptoms that manifest when other conditions are met.

C. ASSESSMENT

Plasma (serum), erythrocyte, or whole blood levels of selenium are in primary use as indicators of selenium status in humans.[1050-1052,1054,1057] Plasma levels tend to reflect short-term selenium status, and erythrocytes tend to reflect long-term status. Hair selenium levels also indicate long-term status if selenium-containing shampoos are not used. More functional assays of selenium status are determinations of GPx activity in erythrocytes or platelets. In general, these methods of selenium status are believed to accurately reflect selenium status.

D. INTAKES

The 1989 RDA for selenium was 55 μg for females and 70 μg for males,[976] a change from the 50 to 200 μg/d previously suggested as the ESADDI. The 1989 RDAs reflect selenium intakes that were adequate to raise GPx activity to plateau levels, with a built-in safety factor. Actual selenium intakes are difficult to determine since a wide variation exists in foods. Analysis of U.S. and Canadian diets ranged from 81 to 224 μg/d.[1051] Thus, there does not appear to be problems with deficient intakes of selenium in the U.S., although regional differences may be present.

E. DIETARY SOURCES

Selenium is found in two basic forms — inorganic and organic. Inorganic selenium is encountered as water-soluble selenites (SO_3^{2-}) and selenates (SO_4^{2-}) found in water supplies.[1054] Organic selenium is found as selenomethionine and selenocysteine in plant and animal foods. Selenomethionine is the major organic form of selenium in the diet. Selenomethionine is the major storage form of selenium in the body and is converted to selenocysteine in a highly regulated manner for inclusion into GPx enzymes. Selenocysteine can also be produced from inorganic sources. At present, supplemental forms of selenium include sodium selenite, sodium selenate, selenomethionine, and selenium-enriched yeast.

Food sources of selenium show a wide variation in content based on soil selenium levels. Thus, tables of selenium contents of foods are not accurate. In general, inorganic selenium is ingested from water supplies, and less from foods, while organic selenium is ingested from plant and animal foodstuffs.

F. HUMAN STUDIES

1. Inflammation

Selenium supplementation with inorganic or organic sources reproducibly leads to increased plasma, erythrocyte, and tissue selenium levels and, usually, increased plasma and tissue GPx activities. *In vitro*, selenium salts increased phagocytosis and bactericidal capacity of human neutrophils at 100 to 200 ng/ml (physiological concentrations), but had variable effects on lymphocyte functions.[1059] Oral selenium supplementation to healthy humans increased NK cell activity, but had no effect on neutrophil chemotaxis or phagocytosis, except for a slight increase in intracellular *S. aureus* killing.[1059] However, animal studies showed that the inflammatory process itself did not clearly modify selenium status. Selenium deficiency prolonged inflammation, and selenium supplementation decreased inflammation in animal models. On the other hand, species differences were seen among animal species in terms of selenium effects. Thus, even though selenium is an important antioxidant, and free radicals are involved in inflammation, direct effects of selenium on inflammation were minor.

2. Rheumatoid Arthritis

Numerous studies have found reduced serum levels of selenium in patients with rheumatoid arthritis.[1060-1071] Usually, serum selenium levels in patients with rheumatoid arthritis were reduced to 67 to 75% of normal control or other joint disease control patient levels. GPx activity in serum or cells was slightly reduced in some studies, but not all, leaving the impression that lowered serum selenium was not correlated with lowered tissue GPx activity. Nevertheless, selenium supplementation to rheumatoid arthritis patients (up to 256 μg/d for up to 6 months) led only to slight improvements in some clinical signs in about half of the studies reported.[1067,1070,1072,1073] After selenium supplementation, serum levels rose to normal levels, and tissue GPx activities were increased. Thus, failure to find clinical benefits after selenium supplementation was not due to inability to affect GPx activity. In fact, gold salts and D-penicillamine are known to specifically inhibit GPx activity in patients with rheumatoid arthritis.[1070] Thus, GPx activity may not be directly related to disease status in rheumatoid arthritis. However, upon closer examination, one study found that neutrophil GPx activity was decreased in rheumatoid arthritis patients, and neutrophil GPx activity was not increased after selenium supplementation, unlike other tissues and cells.[1067] Since neutrophils are involved in production of free radicals at joint sites in rheumatoid arthritis, perhaps the lack of clinical results was due to the unresponsiveness of neutrophils to the protective effects of selenium on GPx activity.

3. Degenerative Joint Diseases

Several reports found decreased levels of serum selenium in osteoarthritis patients (143 ± 23 vs. 160 ± 25 μg/l).[1071,1074] Jameson and colleagues found that administration of 140 μg/d selenium as sodium selenite and 100 mg/d tocopherol raised whole blood GPx activity in 75% of subjects.[1074] The subjects with increased GPx activity also exhibited significantly reduced pain scores for longer time periods than subjects who did not exhibit increased GPx activity. However, the overall reduction in pain score when compared between placebo and supplemented groups was not quite significant. Of course, considering the effects of vitamin E already mentioned in Chapter 5,[546-548] the effects seen in this study could be attributable to tocopherol rather than selenium. As previously mentioned,[546] an individual case study found relief from knee pain after supplementation with tocopherol and selenium.

One report studied the effect of long-term (6 months) supplementation with a commercially available product from Europe containing selenium and vitamins A, C, and E.[1075] Hill and Bird, from the Clinical Pharmacology Unit of the Royal Bath Hospital in Harrogate, England, administered one tablet of selenium-ACE (with 144 μg selenium and unspecified amounts and forms of vitamins A, C, and E) to 14 subjects with osteoarthritis and placebo tablets to 16 subjects with osteoarthritis. After 6 months, there were no significant differences between groups in pain score, stiffness, or well-being score. Since the amounts of additional vitamins were not specified, it is difficult to estimate effects from these ingredients. However, if only one tablet was ingested, then amounts of A, C, and E would have to be low, compared to other studies. Thus, this study suggests further that selenium alone is without effect in human inflammation and joint damage. The effects of selenium supplementation (and GPx activity) on degenerative joint diseases are not fully understood, but merit further work, based on results of all studies combined.

G. SUMMARY AND GUIDELINES FOR USE

Research on the use of selenium for connective tissue disorders is very recent, with initial reports in 1985. Therefore, insufficient data has been collected on the clinical responses to selenium supplementation. Preliminary work suggests that selenium alone does not greatly affect inflammatory processes or joint degeneration in humans. However, since antioxidants have interactions, selenium may depend on other antioxidants such as tocopherol or ascorbate to exert effects. If functional status of these antioxidants in appropriate cells and sites is not considered, then a beneficial effect may not be apparent. Therefore, it is logical to administer selenium along with other antioxidants. As the study by Hill and Bird showed, minimal levels of antioxidants are not effective at modifying osteoarthritic symptoms. This clearly illustrates the need for high but rationally safe doses of each antioxidant to be tested.

There are some differences between the inorganic and organic forms of selenium in terms of affecting serum and tissue levels of selenium and GPx. In short, both forms are effective, and both forms have unique advantages and disadvantages over the other. It is likely that a 1:1 combination of each form

TABLE 11   Guidelines for Use of Selenium

Chronic Inflammatory Conditions
   Rheumatoid arthritis and other inflammatory joint conditions
   Bursitis, tendinitis, tenosynovitis, stress fractures
Degenerative Joint Conditions
   Osteoarthritis
   Chondromalacia
Low back pain, invertebral disc disease

mimics food sources of selenium, and the inclusion of both forms in future research is encouraged. Usual supplemental sources of selenium are sodium selenite and selenomethionine.

Safety of selenium is an issue.[1050-1054] Signs of human toxicity from naturally occurring food and/or water from areas with very high selenium levels in the environment, or accidental overdose from selenium supplements containing 182 times the label claim for selenium, have found symptoms of garlic body odor, loss of hair, nail problems, nausea, vomiting, irritability, fatigue, and peripheral neuropathy.[1054] A consensus of findings suggests that toxicity symptoms are not seen until several mg of selenium are consumed daily for long time periods. Thus, daily doses of 1000 µg selenium or less appear to be safe for extended time periods, if kidney function is normal. Doses of 200 µg daily appear to be completely safe for very long time periods. Even though human studies of selenium supplementation have found improvements in selenium status (both normal controls and diseased individuals), daily doses were never greater than 250 µg/d. The effects of higher doses for short time periods tapered down to known safe levels have not been examined.

Guidelines for selenium supplementation are based on its role in the human antioxidant defense system and results of trials for other conditions (hyperlipidemia, cancer). Although the specific effects of selenium are still being studied, it is suggested that selenium be considered equally important as the other nutrient antioxidants (β-carotene, tocopherol, ascorbate). Thus, doses of selenium of 100 to 200 µg/d are considered safe and are able to improve GPx activity and other indicators of selenium status. Use of higher doses (500 to 1000 µg/d) for short time periods (2 to 3 months) may be investigated in inflammatory conditions of long duration. Since the pharmacokinetics of selenium effect on GPx activity indicates that several weeks are required before activity increases, selenium supplementation for acute inflammatory events does not appear likely to show clinical benefits, although there is no relevant human research on this topic. Guidelines for use of selenium are listed in Table 11.

IV. SILICON

Relevance of silicon to injury rehabilitation revolves around its recent roles in metabolism of connective tissue cells and structural roles in cartilage and bone.[1041-1044,1076-1079] Silicon probably forms silanolate ester-like linkages with organic molecules (glycosaminoglycans or cellular matrix proteins?) in connective tissues.[1080] Silicon is concentrated in connective tissues of the body (cartilage, bone, skin, tendons, trachea, aorta), which suggests a role in homeostasis of these tissues.[1076] Silicon appears to be intimately involved with calcification of cartilage and osteoid in bone formation.[1043,1076,1079] Possible associations with osteonectin have been proposed.[1043] Silicon is necessary for optimal activity of bone prolylhydroxylase and prolyl-4-hydroxylase, galactosyl-hydroxylysyl glucosyltransferase, and lysyl oxidase.[1076] Also, silicon is a major intracellular ion of osteogenic cells, especially during periods of metabolic activation.[1079] In osteoblast culture, silicon enhanced DNA synthesis, an anabolic event.[1081] Thus, by virtue of enzyme activation, structural cross-linkings, or interactions with calcification proteins, silicon appears helpful for formation of connective tissues, especially bone and cartilage.

Deficiencies of silicon in animals are difficult to produce, but involve defective metabolism and formation of bone and connective tissue (joints).[1043,1076] Detailed studies of bone metabolism in silicon-deficient rats found decreased activity of acid and alkaline phosphatase, and decreased uptake of calcium into ectopic bone.[1082]

The role of silicon in maintenance of bone mass was assessed by measurement of serum silicon levels in healthy controls and children receiving total parenteral nutrition containing 0.6 to 1.2 mg/d silicon for approximately 9 years.[1035] Children on TPN showed osteopenia compared to healthy children (77.5 ± 17.3% trabecular bone mass as measured by computerized tomography of the lumbar spine). Serum silicon was significantly lower in TPN children (207 ± 68 vs. 547 ± 390 ng/ml, p <0.001). Longer duration of TPN was associated with a higher degree of osteopenia. Thus, low intakes of silicon in humans are associated with osteopenia.

Deficiencies of silicon have been linked to osteoporosis, osteoarthritis, atherosclerosis, and hypertension, but no firm connections have been documented.[1076] The human requirement for silicon is estimated at 5 to 20 mg/d, which is at or below usual dietary intakes of approximately 31 mg/d.[1043,1076] Richest food sources of silicon are unrefined grains with high fiber content, cereal products, root vegetables, and apples (pectin).[1076] Animal foodstuffs have very low levels of silicon. Doubtless, humans that do not possess sanitary living conditions (unwashed, whole raw foods) derive a larger intake of silicon from dirt. Food silicon is mostly in the form of silicates, which is also the major form in blood and urine.[1076] Oral consumption of silicates has proven to be nontoxic (at least for the silicate moiety) at high intake levels. Silicates are common antacids and food additives.

Animal studies with silatranes (synthetic organic silicon compounds) have found preliminary suggestions of enhancement of wound healing, but data on humans are lacking.[1083-1085] No literature has reported on silicon supplementation for human connective tissue disorders, but Ayurvedic and Chinese herbal medicine texts describe the use of Tabashir (joints of specific female bamboo plants very rich in silicates) for bone pains. This was apparently due to the similarity in appearance between joints in bamboo stalks and the human spine. Thus, there is no research on the effects of silicon for disorders of cartilage or bone tissues. Further research into the therapeutic effects of silicates in humans with osteoarthritis and osteoporosis seems worthy of attention.

V. OTHER ULTRATRACE ELEMENTS

Other ultratrace elements possess insufficient data on their possible roles in connective tissues or healing processes to make any specific suggestions or conclusions. Some are essential, and should not be ignored, but no specific information is available to show effects on musculoskeletal healing. These ultratrace elements are arsenic, chromium, germanium, molybdenum, nickel, strontium, and vanadium.

Chapter 11

NORMAL CELLULAR COMPONENTS: PROTEASES, NUCLEIC ACIDS, AND ANTIOXIDANT ENZYMES

I. PROTEASES (PROTEOLYTIC ENZYMES)

A. ROLES AND FUNCTIONS

Proteases (proteolytic enzymes) are ubiquitous in living organisms. Proteases fulfill a wide variety of regulatory and functional roles in almost every cellular process. Repair and healing processes are no exception. As soon as proteases were available commercially in purified forms, and their roles in the inflammatory process were beginning to be ascertained, a logical step was to administer proteases from exogenous sources to accelerate or enhance healing. During the 1950s, a large number of clinical trials were conducted with intravenous or intramuscular injections of proteases, usually trypsin, chymotrypsin, or crude preparations of pancreatic proteases.[1086,1087] However, many adverse reactions to repeated injections of proteinaceous material were encountered, and injectable use of proteases was virtually abandoned. Oral use soon followed, and a very large database of several hundred articles on human subjects accumulated on the mechanisms, bioavailability, and clinical effects of oral proteases as therapeutic agents. Table 1 lists the various medical uses of proteases, including those not pertinent to healing of injuries.[1087] This section will be mostly concerned with the antiinflammatory effects of proteases.

A large number of studies have found multiple mechanisms of effect for orally administered proteases, consistent with the large number of roles endogenous proteases fulfill *in vivo*.[1086-1093] Table 2 lists some of the documented mechanisms of antiinflammatory effects for proteases. All proteases sever peptide bonds in proteins with varying degrees of specificity for amino acid residues and conditions of activity. Since inflammation is amplified by a cascade effect, ablation of the initial cascade events can prevent progression of excess inflammation. Repair and proliferative phases can begin sooner, resulting in enhanced healing rates. Inhibition of proinflammatory events leads to reductions in clinical symptoms of inflammation — heat, pain, swelling, redness, and loss of function. Since inhibition is never total, enough proinflammatory processes remain to stimulate progression of inflammation to repair and remodeling phases of healing (unlike high-dose corticosteroids). Thus, unlike standard analgesic (aspirin) agents or NSAIDs, proteases can prevent prolongation or enhance or accelerate the healing process.

B. DIETARY SOURCES AND INFLUENCES

Table 3 lists the more common, commercially available proteases used in research studies, clinical practices, and in pharmaceutical agents. The pancreases of pork and beef animals slaughtered for meat are processed by defatting and controlled drying into an enriched fraction with different grades of crudity called pancreatin. Pancreatin possesses trypsin, chymotrypsin, carboxypeptidase, elastase, and other peptidase activities.[1087] Further purification of pancreatin yields a trypsin/chymotrypsin mixture (heavily in favor of trypsin). Purified trypsin hydrolyzes peptide bonds, mostly at lysine and arginine residues. Purified chymotrypsin is specific for hydrolysis of peptide bonds around carboxyl groups. Bromelain is a group of enzymes with proteolytic and other activities isolated from pineapple stems and fruit

TABLE 1 Medical Uses of Proteases

1. Digestive enzyme replacement
   (digestive aids, cystic fibrosis)
2. Debridement (topical uses)
   (wounds, skin ulcers, burns, gangrene, acne, skin cleansing)
3. Mucus or exudate liquefaction
   (bronchial asthma, chronic bronchitis, chronic chest infection, pleural effusions, respiratory diseases, otitis media, sinusitis)
4. Ophthalmology
   (cataract surgery, vitreous hemorrhages)
5. Fibrinolysis
   (thrombophlebitis, dissolution of thrombi, coronary artery occlusion, pulmonary embolism, artery or venous occlusions in general)
6. Potentiation of drug effects (especially antibiotics)
7. Antiinflammatory effects

TABLE 2 Antiinflammatory Mechanisms of Proteases

1. Destroy or inactivate cell surface enzymes involved in formation of eicosanoids
   (thromboxane synthetase, not cyclooxygenase)
   (decreased proinflammatory eicosanoids, increased antiinflammatory eicosanoids)
2. Destroy or inactivate bradykinins
   (reduction in pain, prevention of progression of inflammation)
3. Reduction in viscosity of extracellular fluid
   (increased nutrient and waste transport to and from injured site; reduces edema)
4. Activation of endogenous proteases (plasmin)
   (prevention of excess thrombin clot formation)
5. Induction of antiproteases
   (antiproteases mediate inflammation, inhibit progression of inflammation; reduction of acute phase reactants)
6. Substitute for endogenous proteases
   (activation of endogenous systems for resolution of inflammation; formation of regulatory peptides)
7. Molecular debridement
   (removal of necrotic tissue, proteins; aids phagocyte functions; reduces edema)

TABLE 3 Identity of Proteases Found in Products

Pancreatin (pancreas powders)
Trypsin/chymotrypsin
Trypsin
Chymotrypsin
Bromelain
Papain
Chymopapain
Fungal proteases
Subtilins
Ficins
Streptokinase–streptodornase

(*Ananus comosus*). Bromelain exhibits broad spectrum lytic activity for peptide bonds. Papain and chymopapain are isolated from the latex of green papaya fruit (*Carica papaya*) and exhibit similar actions as bromelain. Fungal proteases (Brinolase) are usually produced by fermentation of *Aspergillus oryzae* fungi, and they exhibit broad spectrum peptide specificity. Subtilins are isolated from fermentation of selected *Bacillus subtilis* bacteria. Subtilins are a group of proteases with wide specificity for peptide bonds. Ficin is isolated from the sap of the South American fig tree (*Ficus glabrata* or *Ficus laurifolia*). Ficin, chymopapain, and subtilins are not usually used for preparation of oral products. Streptokinase-streptodornase was used in some studies, and consisted of bacterial protease (*Haemolyticum streptococcus*) with DNAse activity. Pepsin is not used as an antiinflammatory agent since its activity is only manifested at pHs encountered in the acidic stomach environment. Most research has been reported on proprietary products consisting of either trypsin/chymotrypsin, chymotrypsin, bromelain, or papain.

In order for oral protease products to exert systemic effects on inflamed sites, their activity must be present at the inflamed site. This means that clinical utility of oral proteases depends on their ability to enter circulation intact. Since proteases are proteins themselves, how are they able to resist degradation in the stomach and small intestine? Assuming they resist degradation, how do proteases enter circulation? The prevailing dogma is that ingested proteins are broken down into single amino acids, dipeptides, tripeptides, and a few larger peptides, and absorbed into gut enterocytes, where complete hydrolysis to single amino acids occurs. The single amino acids enter portal circulation for transport to the liver and the rest of the body. Proteases are small proteins, usually in the range of 20,000 to 350,000 Da.[1087] However, small size is no guarantee of being able to resist digestion and pass into circulation. Furthermore, even if proteases enter circulation, have they been damaged by digestive processes enough to lose their enzymatic activity and, therefore, their function? The absorption of proteases after oral administration to animals and humans has been extensively studied by major pharmaceutical companies. The prevailing findings of most of these bioavailability studies is that proteases can be absorbed intact, with activity preserved, into the circulation in measurable amounts.[1086,1087,1094-1103] Most studies followed specific measurements of enzyme proteolytic activity, but some actually used radioactive tracer methodology, electrophoretic separation, and antibody identification to show that activity of absorbed enzymes was intact. In general, percent of total protease activity absorbed into circulation was from 1 to 40%. Protease activity was shown to concentrate somewhat at inflamed sites. Thus, oral proteases have been repeatedly documented to be absorbed intact with activity retained and to localize at inflamed sites. Furthermore, evidence of oral absorption is supported (but not proven) by the antiinflammatory effects seen after oral administration of proteases.

C. HUMAN STUDIES
1. Sports Injuries

Since proteases were shown to exert antiinflammatory activities, oral administration of proteases in sports injuries was studied in over 20 reports.[1087,1104-1124] The results of several studies will be presented. Blonstein, the Senior Medical Officer of the Amateur Boxing Association, authored two studies of oral protease administration to boxers. Blonstein's first report utilized a streptokinase–streptodornase product that was slowly dissolved in the mouth (buccal or sublingual delivery).[1104] There were 494 boxers divided into two equal groups — one group (n = 247) received two tablets 30 to 60 min before boxing. The other group (n = 247) was given placebo tablets. Although the number of hand sprains and cuts were the same for each group, the protease-supplemented group exhibited fewer hematomas (7 vs. 18) and general bruising and superficial laceration (14 vs. 21). In a second study, 88 boxers were given four protease tablets daily for 3 days following a boxing match, while 34 were given placebo tablets. Supplemented boxers resumed boxing in 1 week, compared to 2 to 3 weeks for the placebo boxers to resume competition. Cuts took half the time to heal in the supplemented group, compared to the placebo group. By coincidence, identical twins were in each group. The supplemented twin resolved shoulder bruises in 5 d; the placebo twin took 2 weeks to resolve two black eyes. Thus, prophylactic supplementation with protease tablets reduced incidence and recovery time for boxing injuries. Administration of protease tablets after boxing for 3 d reduced healing time of injuries by 50%.

In a second report, Blonstein studied the effect of trypsin/chymotrypsin (Chymoral®) tablets or placebo given as prophylaxis before boxing to two groups of boxers (n = 225 for each group).[1105] Significant reductions in hematoma (3.1 vs. 8.0%) and general bruising (6.2 vs. 9.3%) incidence were seen for the supplemented group. Another 88 injured boxers were given protease tablets (8 per day for 3 d, n = 55) or placebo (n = 34). Again, supplemented boxers healed in half the time required for placebo boxers.

Boyne and Medhurst, of the Chelsea Football Club in England, administered eight Chymoral tablets daily (in divided doses on empty stomachs) immediately after injury to soccer players with significant injuries for an entire season.[1107] Results were compared to the previous season, which utilized the same players. The number of man/games lost was reduced during the supplemented year (from 131 to 90, $p < 0.01$), even though more games were played and more injuries were suffered in the supplemented year. Average days lost per injury were reduced from 15 to 11 (not significant), but recovery from soft-tissue injuries (bruises, hematomas, effusions) was significantly reduced from 12 to 7 d ($p < 0.001$). However, recovery time from tendon and ligament injuries was only reduced by 15.5%, a nonsignificant difference. Thus, outcome results were that oral protease supplementation reduced recovery time from soft-tissue (muscular) injuries, resulting in fewer players lost for less time.

Matta and Mouzas, of the Accident and Emergency Department of North Middlesex Hospital in London, administered four tablets daily for 5 d of streptokinase–streptodornase to 60 patients with hematomas, ecchymoses, sprains, or contusions or placebo to 60 patients with similar injuries.[1119] Improvement after 1 week was greater in the supplemented group compared to the placebo group (82 vs. 28%), and unchanged patients were greatly reduced in the supplemented group (12 vs. 72%).

Oral administration of fungal protease (Asperkinase®) or Chymoral in athletic injuries was reported by Donaho and Rylander of the University of Delaware.[1114] For severe and moderate injuries of football players, the two protease supplements were compared to historical controls of the previous year. Supplementation with either enzyme resulted in recovery periods of 5.1 d, compared to 8.4 d the previous year ($p < 0.05$). The fungal protease group exhibited the fastest recovery (3.9 d). Findings of reduced swelling, immobility, inflammation, tenderness, and pain along with reduced recovery time were observed.

A double-blind study with the University of Pittsburgh football team was conducted by Deitrich in 1965.[1113] Randomly, 29 injured players were assigned to placebo (n = 18) or Orenzyme® (trypsin/chymotrypsin mixture, n = 11) tablets, and took eight tablets daily for 3 to 21 d. The percentage of actual vs. predicted days disabled for each player was plotted. Of the 11 supplemented players, 7 recovered in less than half the time predicted. Only 2/18 placebo players recovered in less than half the time predicted. The median percentage of actual to predicted disability time was 33% for supplemented and 73% for placebo players ($p < 0.01$). Injuries consisted of sprains, contusions, strains, and one fracture. Thus, oral protease treatment produced a significantly reduced disability time compared to placebo, for healing of minor football injuries.

Holt, from Wayne State University in Detroit, MI, studied the effects of Papase® (papain) tablets on healing of injured athletic team members.[1118] Contusions, sprains, and strains were treated with Papase in 65 athletes and compared to 60 athletes who were untreated. Nearly 70% of Papase-supplemented athletes showed a better than expected recovery, whereas only 20% of nonsupplemented athletes showed a better than expected recovery.

Buck and Phillips studied the effect of Chymoral or placebo tablets on 91 injuries to soccer players in South Africa in a double-blind study.[1109] The difference between placebo and protease groups for recovery time (time to return to action) favored the protease group. At 3 and 4 d postinjury, the protease group showed 26 and 38% more players recovered than the placebo group. The healing of hematomas was significantly better in the protease group, while enhancement of healing of sprains approached significance. Again, protease administration resulted in faster recovery times after minor soft-tissue injuries.

Trickett, from Tulane University in New Orleans, LA, measured time to recovery after administration of papain tablets to 40 athletic injuries.[1123] One tablet every 2 h was given the first day immediately after injury, followed by four tablets daily thereafter. Marked or moderate improvement (compared to predicted values) was found in 85% of treated athletes. Sprains, contusions, pulled muscles, and fractures showed excellent results in terms of expected recovery time and reduction of expected symptoms. When protease supplementation was started one or more days after injury, results were not as good as when supplementation was started immediately after injury.

Rathbeger reported on administration of Chymoral tablets to soft-tissue athletic injuries.[1120] Eight tablets of Chymoral were ingested daily by 26 subjects, and 20 subjects were given placebo in a randomized, double-blind fashion. Significant benefits were seen for the Chymoral group for reduction of bruising, time of return to full function, and time deemed fit to play. Reductions in swelling favored the protease group, but significance was not reached ($p < 0.16$). All protease subjects (100%) were fit to play after 12 d, when only 55% of placebo subjects were fit. Protease supplementation significantly reduced recovery time and accelerated time for athletes to resume play.

Sixty patients with moderate to severe injuries to head or face were randomly allocated to either placebo or Chymoral treatment by Tsomides and Goldberg, from Marblehead, MA.[1125] Injuries were generally contusions with lacerations, abrasions, or fractures from automobile accidents, sports injuries, falls, or flying objects. Injury scores of edema and ecchymoses were graded for 7 d. Protease supplementation (2 tablets 4 times daily) led to highly significant ($p < 0.001$) reduction in overall scores sooner than the placebo group. The rate of resolution of edema and ecchymoses was significantly faster after protease supplementation. On the seventh day postinjury, only 4/30 protease subjects had injury scores greater than zero, while 23/30 placebo subjects had scores greater than zero. Protease supplementation clearly was effective at reducing signs of swelling and bruising in moderate to severe traumatic facial injuries.

The studies mentioned above date from the 1960s. Very little published research has occurred since then on proteases and sports injuries. However, three reports from Germany were published in 1990.[1126-1128] Kleine studied the effects of Wobenzym®, a mixture of pancreatin, papain, bromelain, trypsin, and chymotrypsin, on experimental hematoma formation.[1126] Healthy volunteers (12 in each group) had 2 ml of their own blood injected subcutaneously into the forearm. This model was shown to simulate normal traumatic hematomas in pain course, color, and speed of recovery. Tenderness (pain) was measured by a standardized tonometer that applied pressure to the hematoma. There were 10 tablets of either placebo or Wobenzym administered, and tenderness was measured nine times over the next 6 h. Compared to placebo, protease supplementation led to a significantly greater improvement in pain reduction (both values were compared to nonhematoma tenderness as a control). A second trial by Kleine administered either placebo or Wobenzym to two groups of 50 subjects each. Tablets were given for 14 d, and pain was measured after application of a standard pressure (3.42 kp/cm^2) daily. The protease group exhibited a quicker return to no pain (3.8 vs. 7.0 d), and lower tenderness scores (5.7 vs. 10.5) than the placebo group, indicating significant benefits from the protease supplement.

Rahn studied the effects of Wobenzym supplementation on recovery from surgical treatment of meniscus sports injuries.[1127] Placebo or protease tablets were administered in randomized, double-blind fashion to two groups of 40 subjects each for 7 d postsurgery. A marked reduction of edema and improvement in mobility and flexibility were seen for the protease group compared to the placebo group. On the average, protease group subjects were able to bend the knee joint to 90° on the 7th postoperative day, while placebo group subjects could not do so until the 9th postoperative day. A second trial by Rahn studied the effects of placebo or Wobenzym on surgical treatment of fractures in 120 patients. There were significant reductions in postoperative edema, pain, and hospital stay. Protease group subjects left the hospital in 17.7 d, compared to 24.1 d for placebo group subjects. Best effects were seen when protease supplementation preceded and followed surgery, rather than only preceding or only following surgery.

Baumüller studied the effects of Wobenzym on ankle sprains in 44 patients in a randomized, placebo-controlled, double-blind study.[1128] Subjects received one teaspoonful of enzyme or placebo granules three times daily for 10 d, starting 1 d after injury. The protease group exhibited less swelling, less pain, more flexion of the ankle joint, and quicker return to work (1.7 vs. 4.4 d) and training (9.4 vs. 15.9 d) than the placebo group. Thus, in each recent study on protease supplementation for sports injuries, significant antiinflammatory effects were found that also translated into significant benefits in outcome of therapy — quicker return to recovery, work, or training.

It must be kept in mind that for each reported study, standard care was also given, and usually consisted of rest, ice, and physical therapy to varying degrees among studies. Thus, protease results were seen in addition to regular care of injured athletes. This means that protease supplementation exhibited practical benefits that can be applied to any clinical practice for rehabilitation of sports injuries.

2. Postsurgery

The use of proteases to reduce swelling, bruising, and inflammation associated with surgical procedures has been well-studied. Many types of surgeries have been examined, and for purposes of illustration, a nonexhaustive review of episiotomy surgery repair will be considered, along with several reports on hand fractures. Episiotomy surgery is well defined and its recovery course is routine. Thus, episiotomy surgery repair is suited for experimental investigations. Pollack studied 69 episiotomy patients given either placebo or papain in a double-blind study.[1129] The protease group showed significantly greater incidence of marked and moderate responses for pain, itching, edema, and erythema (86 vs. 39%). At time of discharge after 6 days, 59% of protease patients were completely recovered, compared to 21% of placebo patients.

Schmitz and Pavlic reported that in a blinded study of 500 episiotomy patients, Chymoral supplementation resulted in significantly less pain on walking, fewer analgesics used, and less frequent catheterizations.[1130] Bumgardner and Zatuchni reported that administration of chymotrypsin led to significant reductions in pain, edema, and inflammation compared to placebo in 301 patients.[1131] Another randomized, double-blind study by Soule and others found that Chymoral supplementation significantly reduced edema, ecchymosis, and pain on sitting compared to placebo in 204 total episiotomy patients.[1132] Zatuchni and Colombi administered placebo or bromelain to 160 episiotomy patients in another randomized, double-blind study.[1133] Again, significant decreases in edema, pain, and inflammation were found for the protease group. Howat and Lewis conducted yet another double-blind study of episiotomy patients and oral bromelain.[1134] Although reduction of edema and bruising was more rapid after bromelain, results did not reach statistical significance. Albright found that 395 patients given oral chymotrypsin after episiotomy required fewer analgesics and exhibited less pain than untreated controls.[1135] Another 494 patients given intramuscular chymotrypsin had equivalent results to oral administration. Thus, 1788 patients given either placebo or oral proteases for episiotomy pain and inflammation showed clear-cut benefits after protease administration, usually in double-blind studies. Thus, oral protease administration appears to be effective at reducing inflammation, pain, edema, and swelling in most subjects, compared to no protease administration in a simple surgical model.

Likewise, use of oral proteases for treatment of vasectomies,[1136] hand fractures,[1137,1138] and a wide range of traumatic injuries, cutaneous infections, and postsurgery cases (n >700)[1139] all showed significant benefits after oral protease supplementation. However, favorable results were not universal. Two studies by Morrison on arthrotomies and facial injuries did not find significant benefits after oral bromelain.[1140] However, number of subjects per group was considerably smaller (n = 4, n = 12) than other studies, and dosage of protease was given every 6 h, instead of every 2 to 4 h as in other studies. Papain prevented the occurrence of experimental peritoneal adhesions in monkeys.[1141] Other literature reports on use of proteases included effects on plastic surgery, dental surgery, vein stripping, and general surgery. Since results for each field appeared similar, focus on a narrow condition — episiotomy — was chosen as an example of effects of oral protease supplementation after surgical trauma in humans. Overall, results were positive, with clinical benefits found for most studies. Results were accelerated recovery to complete healing, and less pain, edema, and inflammation than control groups.

3. Degenerative Joint Conditions

Cohen and Goldman studied the effects of oral bromelain (Ananase) on joint status of 29 patients with rheumatoid arthritis previously treated with corticosteroids.[1142] All patients had finished corticosteroid treatment with success, but all exhibited residual joint swelling and stiffness that was not affected by maintenance doses of corticosteroids. Each person ingested 1 to 2 tablets every 3 to 4 h of bromelain for 3 weeks to 13 months. Joint circumferences (knees, wrists, ankles, fingers) were measured periodically. Excellent and good responses were classified as complete or almost complete reduction in swelling. After bromelain supplementation, excellent or good results were measured in 72.4% of subjects, a significant improvement. Thus, bromelain was shown to be effective in reducing joint swelling seen in rheumatoid arthritis patients after corticosteroid therapy.

Hingorani administered a randomized, double-blind study of placebo or Chymoral supplementation to 50 consecutive patients admitted for severe low back pain to Newcastle General Hospital.[1143] Most subjects had lumbar spondylarthrosis. Subjects ingested two tablets four times daily for 2 d followed by one tablet four times daily for 8 d. The study ended after 10 d. No differences in percentage of patients improved for pain, tenderness, and mobility were found between groups. However, straight-leg raising was significantly improved in the Chymoral group. This measurement is an expression of nerve compression and indicates that protease supplementation reduced local inflammation and edema, relieving nerve compression. Thus, protease supplementation accelerated resolution of severe low back pain. Other conditions would not be expected to differ since bed rest usually corrects pain, tenderness, and mobility.

Gaspardy and others administered two tablets of Chymoral four times daily for 7 d to patients with sciatica.[1144] Significant reductions in pain and inflammation were recorded. Gibson and others administered Chymoral or placebo in the same manner as Gaspardy to 93 patients admitted to Guy's Hospital Arthritis Research Unit in London with lumbar disc prolapse of less than 6 months in duration.[1145] No differences between groups was found for percentage of subjects who needed treatment, percentage of subjects who needed surgery, mean time in bed, mean hospital time, mean time off work, percentage of subjects showing improvement in pain, total neurological signs improved, spinal flexion improvement, or spinal extension improvement. However, there were significant differences in favor of Chymoral for reduction of analgesic dosage (-1.1 vs. +0.07 units/d) and for improvement in straight-leg raising (+13 vs. +7.6°). Thus, protease therapy did reduce edema and inflammation sufficiently to improve physical function in lumbar disc prolapse patients, but not sufficiently to affect overall outcome. However, chronic conditions of disc prolapse have deteriorated to the point where the body can no longer return disc anatomy to normal, and, thus, outcome would not be expected to differ between protease and placebo groups. Also, hospitalized patients reflect worst case scenarios of lumbar disc prolapse. Perhaps the reduction of inflammation around joints with less severe symptoms would lead to additional advantages for protease supplementation. Therefore, in four separate studies, reduction of inflammation surrounding joints was seen in degenerative joint conditions. Sometimes, clinical response was sufficient to reduce analgesic need and usually improve physical function of the joint. These findings strongly indicate that longer time periods or higher doses of protease administration should be considered in chronic degenerative joint conditions. Protease supplementation seemed to reduce inflammation during acute symptom flareups of low back pain.

D. SAFETY

Every study quoted reported on the absolute lack of side effects attributable to oral protease therapy. Indeed, there were more frequent side effects from the placebos than from proteases. In many thousands of subjects, oral protease supplementation has not been associated with any side effects.

E. SUMMARY AND GUIDELINES FOR USE

Protease supplementation appears to be useful for reduction of inflammation in acute traumatic conditions. The known mechanisms of action, the proven bioavailability, and preponderance of positive clinical studies strongly argue in favor of protease supplementation for acute injuries. If the results of so many studies were so successful, then why is protease therapy not utilized more often today? Most of the research using proteases was performed during the 1960s. At that time, corticosteroids were entrenched as first-line agents for reduction of pain and inflammation for chronic conditions. NSAIDs also were introduced shortly after the same time period, and exhibited very successful clinical amelioration of pain with antiinflammatory effects in both acute and chronic conditions. Since compliance and dosing of proteases was more difficult than NSAIDs or corticosteroids, since prevailing dogma wrongly cast suspicion on oral use of proteins, and since other medications were highly effective at reducing pain

TABLE 4   Guidelines for Proper Use of Oral Protease Supplements

1. Prophylaxis is ideal; otherwise, initiate supplementation as soon as possible after injury occurs
2. Ingest 2–8 tablets 3–5 times daily on an empty stomach; water or juice preferred to take tablets
3. Enteric coating preferred (not needed for bromelain)
4. Multiple proteases preferred (combinations of trypsin, chymotrypsin, bromelain, and papain)
5. Continue supplementation for 1 week or until improvement is noticed

(and thus improving patient satisfaction), the use of proteases fell out of favor before it had the chance to become fully integrated into medical practices.

Nevertheless, protease administration offers a safe option to reduce some or most symptoms of inflammation and also to accelerate or enhance healing (which is generally not encountered with NSAIDs). Overall, for acute traumatic injuries, proper protease administration can result in a 50% reduction in time to heal. Usually, symptoms of inflammation (pain, swelling, heat, and redness) are much reduced. However, these results can only be achieved if certain criteria are met. Table 4 lists the proper way to administer oral protease supplements for maximum clinical effect.[1108] First and foremost, supplementation must be initiated as soon as possible after an injury occurs. Based on the mechanisms of protease actions, proteases will be most effective during the inflammatory healing phase, which occurs from the first hour after injury to several days postinjury. Prevention of inflammatory cascade initiation by exogenous proteases is a treatment goal. Prophylaxis would be ideal, with supplementation beginning 1 to 2 h ahead of potential time of injury. This is especially useful before games or events (football, soccer, basketball, hockey, lacrosse, boxing, martial arts, rugby, rodeo, wrestling).

Ingestion of protease supplements must be accomplished on an empty stomach. Proteases will be slowed in their serum uptake if food is present in the stomach or proximal small intestine. Peak serum levels may be below thresholds needed to saturate inflamed sites if proteases are not ingested on an empty stomach. Enteric coating of tablets to resist stomach acidity has been shown to be helpful for achieving highest serum levels. However, due to the wide range of pH stability for bromelain, this enzyme does not necessarily need to be enteric coated. Also, animal research has indicated that multiple proteases are more effective at reducing inflammation than a like amount of a single protease. Thus, combination of animal proteases with plant proteases offers a wider spectrum of action than a single protease. Preferred combinations would include trypsin and chymotrypsin with bromelain and papain. Fungal proteases have not been studied as extensively as trypsin, chymotrypsin, bromelain, or papain, but would be expected to be more similar to plant proteases in spectrum of action.

Another consideration is label potency claims. A bewildering and incomparable variety of units is used to express protease activity. Different units of protease activity have been developed over the years, but each is more or less specific to a particular enzyme. Thus, assays for trypsin activity will show low activity for bromelain, and vice versa. Typical units encountered are USP, NF, MCU (milk-clotting units), GDU (gelatin digestion units), Armour units, Rorer units, and weights (mg, µg). This author has found that units of activity listed on product labels have no relationship to actual product potencies (unpublished results). Shelf life of proteases is limited to about 1 year. In general, if a practitioner finds a product that produces visible clinical results, then that product is likely to be potent. If no clinical effects are apparent, switch to another product.

One final factor to consider is a patient's religious preference. Pancreatin, trypsin, and chymotrypsin are derived from beef or pork (usually pork) and, thus, may not be acceptable to Orthodox Jews and strict vegetarians. Bromelain, papain, and fungal proteases are all derived from vegetable sources and should be compatible for most persons.

Table 5 lists conditions which are applicable to protease supplementation. Acute, traumatic injuries, especially bruises, hematomas, contusions, ecchymoses, sprains, strains, lacerations, abrasions, fractures, and surgery are all conditions which have shown clinical benefits from oral protease supplementation in clinical trials. In this author's personal experience as a martial arts student and instructor, time to heal is considerably and noticeably accelerated when proper supplementation is followed (see Table 4). After direct observation of several anecdotal cases where no or almost no swelling and bruising was

**TABLE 5   Indications for Oral Protease
Supplementation**

Acute, traumatic injuries
    Bruises, hematomas, contusions, ecchymoses
    Sprains
    Strains, muscle pulls
    Lacerations, abrasions, wounds
    Fractures
Surgical procedures of all kinds
Sciatica and acute lower back pain
Chronic joint conditions?
    Rheumatoid arthritis
    Osteoarthritis
    Bursitis
    Tendinitis, tenosynovitis, metatarsalgia

apparent after various surgical procedures, this author remains convinced of the usefulness of proper protease supplementation.

Expected results of oral protease supplementation are reduction in inflammation (pain, swelling, redness, heat) and quicker return to function after traumatic injuries. Time to complete recovery is accelerated. Proteases represent a viable adjunct or option for resolution of acute trauma commonly encountered in athletes and sports medicine practices. Protease products are available at pharmacies and also at mail order companies that specialize in selling to health care professionals. Some health food stores may have protease products that are not primarily digestive aids.

II. NUCLEOTIDES (RNA)

Identification of purine nucleotides as cellular growth regulators, based on receptor studies, has shed new light on the role of RNA components.[1146] Nucleosides and nucleotides appear to be an ancient means of intercellular regulatory signals, affecting cell proliferation and differentiation. Nucleotides and nucleosides are released by damaged or hypoxic cells and possess stimulatory effects on cell proliferation. Nucleotides are required by proliferating cells, both as a stimulatory signal and a precursor for nucleic acids.[138,139,180,1146] Also, stimulatory effects on immune function of injured animals have been attributed to nucleotide supplementation.[138,139,180] The implications for the healing process are obvious — provision of exogenous nucleotides or nucleosides may stimulate proliferative and repair phases of inflammation during healing, leading to faster recovery.

Tissues that show greatest response to nucleotides are lymphocytes and gut enterocytes.[138,139,180] Healing of severe traumatic injuries or major surgery is dependent upon prevention of infection (preservation of immune functions) and adequate nutriture during healing (via gut enterocytes). Thus, effects of nucleotides have been studied on human subjects with severe metabolic stress, trauma, or surgery.[216,223,1147] Two recent studies on effects of nucleotides (RNA) on human healing are available. However, provision of exogenous RNA was not the primary variable. RNA was administered as part of a modified enteral feeding program containing supplemental arginine and ω3 fatty acids. Compared to standard enteral diets, RNA-containing diets were associated with fewer infections and significant reduction in hospital stay.[1147] Another trial compared standard enteral feeding with a similarly modified enteral diet (additional arginine, RNA, and ω3 fatty acids) for 8–10 d in 20 ICU patients with sepsis after multiple trauma or major surgery.[223] Both enteral diets improved nitrogen retention and protein status, but the modified diet led to improved lymphocyte functions and 3-methylhistidine balance. Long-term followup (6 and 12 months) showed no adverse effects from diets and no clear-cut differences in outcome.

Thus, prevailing evidence points to the need for further study of oral administration of nucleotides (RNA) to injured patients. A possible mechanism of action has been established, and commercial sources are available. However, no specific studies of necessary doses for effects and no specific studies of effects in injured athletes have been reported. RNA and nucleotide supplementation to enhance healing is a topic for further research.

III. ANTIOXIDANT ENZYMES

Another normal cellular component that has found therapeutic uses for musculoskeletal healing is exogenous administration of endogenous antioxidant enzymes superoxide dismutase (SOD) and catalase. Since the oral absorption of these enzymes has not been documented in animals (or in man),[1148,1149] the use of SOD and catalase falls into nonnutritional categories of injectable or topical administrations. SOD is currently marketed as Orgotein® for the human market, and as Palosein® for the veterinary market for injectable modes of administration. Numerous studies have found significant and potent antiinflammatory effects for injections of SOD in osteoarthritis, rheumatoid arthritis, and other chronic degenerative diseases in humans.[1150-1153] Use of topical catalase on burns, wounds, and skin ulcers has found some clinical benefits.[1154-1157] Since the clinical applications of these antioxidant enzymes fall outside of nutritional practice, their properties will not be considered further in this chapter.

Oral dietary supplements containing SOD and catalase have been marketed to health care professionals since the late 1970s. The actual SOD and catalase activities of a cross-section of antioxidant enzyme products showed that label claims were met for some, while others had absolutely no enzyme activity.[1158] Thus, a wide range of potencies exists for products currently on the market. One quick and convenient way to check for catalase activity of such products is to crush a tablet and place the powder in a glass or test tube containing 3% hydrogen peroxide. Generation of bubbles indicates formation of oxygen by catalase activity. Absence of bubble equates to absence of catalase activity. It was found that SOD and catalase activities paralleled each other in dietary supplement products.[1158] Thus, practical application of antioxidant enzymes as nutrients for musculoskeletal healing does not appear promising.

Chapter 12

GLYCOSAMINOGLYCANS

I. INTRODUCTION

Glycosaminoglycans (GAGs), formerly named mucopolysaccharides, are an integral component of all connective tissues.[67-86,1159] Table 1 lists the various GAGs, their molecular constitution, and tissue predominance. GAGs are long-chain, high-molecular-weight polymers of repeating units of an aminosugar (sometimes sulfated) and an organic acid or sugar.[67-86,1159] In cartilage, most GAGs are attached in large numbers to a core protein, resembling a bottlebrush in three-dimensional structure.[67-86,1159] The resulting proteoglycan (PG) subunits are attached to a very long hyaluronic acid molecule (about 2 million Da) via link proteins to form aggregating proteoglycan.[67-87,1159] In cartilage, the predominant PG is termed aggrecan and consists of chondroitin sulfate GAGs and keratan sulfate GAGs attached to a glycosylated core protein, many subunits of which are attached to hyaluronic acid (an unsulfated GAG) to form PGs.[87] PGs, by virtue of their dense negative charge from sulfates, attract and hold large amounts of water, forming a stiff gel. In cartilage, PG gel is not saturated with water and exerts a swelling effect which is held in place by collagen fibers. PGs are linked to collagen fibers to help form connective tissues, and PGs provide resiliency, load distribution, shock-absorbing, compressive, and lubricating properties to connective tissues and joints. Small PGs (decorin, biglycan, and fibromodulin) are present at 5% of total PGs in cartilage and are found in all other tissues.[79-83] Small PGs consist of a single polypeptide chain with one GAG chain attached (decorin, biglycan) or four chains attached (fibromodulin). In addition, membrane-associated PGs comprise around 1% of total PGs in cartilage, are ubiquitous to all cells, and are involved in cell–cell and cell–matrix interactions, as well as specific binding of growth factors.[79-83]

GAGs and PGs are continuously, albeit slowly, remodeled in connective tissues, including articular cartilage, with turnover half-lives of approximately 700 d in healthy human joints.[42,79] Turnover of GAGs is accelerated in wound healing, arthritic joints, and burns.[68,121,1159] Although GAGs are a component of all connective tissues, their deposition and/or turnover achieves clinical significance in skin during wound healing, ulcers, or burns; in bone during fracture repair and osteoporosis; and in joints during osteoarthritis, autoimmune inflammatory joint diseases, chronic degenerative joint diseases, and traumatic injuries. In these instances, GAG synthesis is necessary for healing, and enhancement of GAG and PG deposition may enhance tissue repair.

GAGs are synthesized primarily by fibroblasts (skin, tendons, ligaments), osteoblasts (bone), and chondrocytes (cartilage). Thus, enhancement of these cells' ability to manufacture GAGs and secrete PGs is a key goal during any healing or joint disease process. This chapter will be concerned with the effects of different GAGs and their components as therapeutic agents for musculoskeletal healing. Table 2 lists GAGs with experimental data.

II. GREEN-LIPPED MUSSELS (*Perna canaliculus*)

A. ROLES AND FUNCTIONS

During the mid-1970s, a health food product, Seatone, consisting of freeze-dried *Perna canaliculus* extract (from green-lipped mussels or New Zealand mussels), was promoted in Australia and New Zealand as having benefits for different types of arthritis, based on anecdotal case reports.[1160] One possible mechanism of action was the provision of GAGs, which make up approximately 20% by weight of Seatone.

TABLE 1   Identity, Composition, and Tissue Location of Glycosaminoglycans in Human Tissues

Glycosaminoglycan	Composition	Predominant Locations
Hyaluronan (HA)	N-Acetylglucosamine D-Glucuronic acid	All tissues, synovial fluid, vitreous humor, cartilage
Chondroitin sulfates (CS)	N-Acetylgalactosamine D-Glucuronic acid	Cartilage, arterial walls, skin, bone, most tissues
Keratan sulfates (KS)	2-Acetamidoglucosamine Galactose	Cartilage, arterial walls
Dermatan sulfates (DS)	N-Acetylgalactosamine Iduronic acid	Skin, skeletal tissues (cartilage, bone, invertebral disc, tendons), cornea, blood vessel walls
Heparan sulfates (HS)	N-Acetylglucosamine Iduronic acid	Arteries, lungs, cell membranes (not in skeletal tissues)
Heparin (Hep)	N-Acetylglucosamine Iduronic acid	Mast cells, lungs, liver, intestines

Note: Basic references on glycosaminoglycan chemistry and structures include 68 to 87 and 1159.

TABLE 2   Glycosaminoglycans and Derivatives Used in Clinical Studies of Musculoskeletal Healing

Green-lipped mussel powder (*Perna canaliculus*)
Cartilage powders
    Bovine trachea, shark cartilage, whale nasal septa
Cartilage extracts
    Rumalon (GPC), Catrix-S
Purified glycosaminoglycans
    Hyaluronan, chondroitin sulfates
Semisynthetic glycosaminoglycans
    Arteparon (synthetically sulfated chondroitin sulfates; glycosaminoglycan polysulfate; GAGPS)
Synthetic glycosaminoglycans
    Pentosan polysulfate (SP54)
Glucosamine and glucosamine salts (hydrochloride, hydroiodide, sulfate)

B. ANIMAL STUDIES

Adjuvant polyarthritis was induced in rats by injection of modified Freund's adjuvant into footpads by Cullen and others from the University of Auckland in New Zealand.[1160] Seatone was fed for 7 weeks to the experimental group (1 g Seatone per kg diet) starting immediately after injection. No difference in arthritic scores were seen between control and experimental rats, suggesting that Seatone was ineffective at the dosage and manner ingested for inflammatory arthritis of autoimmune or delayed hypersensitivity type.

Rainsford and Whitehouse, from the University of Tasmania Medical School and Australian National University, administered whole, freeze-dried mussels to rats or pigs along with varying doses of aspirin or indomethacin.[1161] Specific antiulcerogenic effects of oral mussel powder were seen for both species. Mussel powder did not inhibit the therapeutic effectiveness of aspirin or indomethacin. Thus, Seatone became a candidate for gastroprotection with concurrent administration of aspirin or NSAIDs.

C. HUMAN STUDIES

Highton and others from the University of Otago Medical School in Dunedin, New Zealand initiated a preliminary study on Seatone with five rheumatoid arthritis patients in a double-blind, placebo-controlled, crossover trial with 6-week periods.[1162] No dosage was given. No differences between the placebo period and Seatone period were observed for the following: Ritchie index, joint swelling scores, time to walk 10 m, grip strength, duration of morning stiffness, subjective patient assessment, number of tender or swollen joints, and erythrocyte sedimentation rates or analgesic (paracetamol) requirements.

In 1980, Gibson and others from the Victoria Infirmary and Glasgow Homeopathic Hospital in Glasgow, Scotland reported on two studies using Seatone for arthritis.[1163] A preliminary, open trial with 86 subjects (55 with rheumatoid arthritis, 31 with osteoarthritis) for 0.5–4.5 years found benefits for 67% of rheumatoid arthritis patients and 35% of osteoarthritis patients, with no toxic effects. No changes in clinical laboratory measurements (including sedimentation rates) were observed. These findings prompted a placebo-controlled, double-blind, crossover study in 28 subjects with rheumatoid arthritis and 38 with osteoarthritis. All subjects were waiting for joint surgery and had disease durations of over 12 years. A dosage of 1050 mg/d was given for 3 months of either placebo or Seatone and, after a washout period, all subjects received Seatone for an additional 3 months. Based on clinical and subjective assessments, subjects were grouped into responders and nonresponders. Responders (15/33 osteoarthritis subjects and 19/25 rheumatoid arthritis subjects) exhibited significant improvements in articular index, limbering up time, visual analog pain scores, time to walk 50 ft, and functional index.[1163] No changes were seen in responders for grip strength. No changes in any parameter were observed in nonresponders. The authors concluded Seatone was beneficial in a subset of persons with advanced arthritis.

An editorial in *Lancet* criticizing the experimental design of the study by Gibson[1164] was followed by a letter from Gibson which rearranged the data according to outcome.[1165] Significant differences between placebo and Seatone periods were seen for articular index, limbering up time, and functional index in rheumatoid arthritis patients, and for functional index, visual analog pain scale, and time to walk 50 ft for osteoarthritic patients. Another study by Huskisson and others of St. Bartholomew's Hospital in London administered 900 mg Seatone or placebo daily for 4 weeks in a randomized, placebo-controlled, crossover study.[1166] No significant effects compared to placebo period was observed for Seatone administration. This study and a critical letter[1167] prompted another letter from Gibson, in which further statistical analysis of data from the original study was published.[1168] Gibson pointed out that the study by Huskisson did not last longer than typical placebo response periods of 6 weeks, and effects of Seatone were not significant until after 3 to 6 months of treatment. Therefore, it may be concluded that short-term administration of Seatone is ineffective in rheumatoid arthritis, and Seatone therapy must be continued for at least 3 months. An additional letter by Gibson reported radiographic evidence of reversal of rheumatoid joint pathology, although without details.[1169]

Caughey and others, from various facilities in Auckland, New Zealand, conducted a placebo-controlled study with 47 rheumatoid arthritis patients.[1170] Subjects were divided into two groups, and both groups were given 750 mg/d of naproxen. One group was also given 1050 mg/d Seatone and the other group was given a placebo. After 6 weeks, naproxen was replaced by a placebo, and the dropout rate was monitored for an additional 6 weeks. Typical measurements and assessments were also performed, but did not show any significant changes during the study period both within and between groups. Remaining patients with Seatone were 7/24 compared to 4/24 for the placebo group, which was not statistically significant. Thus, small numbers of subjects and short experimental periods of administration for Seatone did not produce clinically obvious results.

Larkin and others from the Center for Rheumatic Diseases in Glasgow studied 35 patients with rheumatoid arthritis in a randomized, double-blind, placebo-controlled study of Seatone (920 to 1150 mg/d) or placebo for a 6-month period.[1171] All patients continued with NSAID therapies. After 6 months, there was no significant difference between the starting and ending values for both groups, and no significant differences between groups. Ritchie index, grip strength, limbering up time, visual analog pain scale, and laboratory blood tests were measured. After this controlled study of sufficient duration, no further research studies on Seatone and arthritis have been reported, and no confirmation of the results of Gibson has been performed.

D. SUMMARY

Seatone appears to have lost research interest as a treatment for rheumatoid arthritis. Although the study by Gibson eventually presented data in a more rigorous format than originally reported, and found significant benefits from Seatone equivalent to gold salts, no other studies found any beneficial effects from Seatone for rheumatoid arthritis. The lack of identification of "active" ingredients in mussels, and the lack of identification of a mechanism of action, has further hampered research interest in Seatone. At this time, Seatone does not appear to be a useful therapy for arthritides, but research studies have been few in number.

III. CARTILAGE POWDERS

The most basic use of GAGs is in the native form of dried cartilage. Commercial sources of cartilage powders are bovine trachea, bovine nasal septa, whale nasal septa, and shark skeletons. After an initial observation that hog gastric mucosal extracts containing mucopolysaccharides enhanced gastric ulcer healing in animals,[1172] Prudden and associates, along with other investigators, began a lengthy series of studies of cartilage powder effects on experimental wound healing in both animals and humans.[1173-1193] Usually, surgical wounds were made on rats, and cartilage powder was topically applied to the edges of the wound before closure by standard sutures.[1188] In almost every case, healing of surgical wounds, as assessed by tensiometric measurements (wound breaking strength or tensile strength), was accelerated by cartilage powders. The enhancement was achieved within the first 3 d after wounding, and then no further gains were observed. This time period corresponds to the synthesis of GAGs in healing wounds. Enhancements of 20% were routinely achieved in rats, mice, guinea pigs, and humans. A well-controlled study in humans found that cartilage increased wound tensile strength by 40% over control wounds in the same person.[1186] In addition, parenteral administration of cartilage pellets or saline extracts of cartilage powders away from the wound site led to enhancement of wound healing. The active component of cartilage was believed to be an acidic mucopolysaccharide, which is now known to be PGs or GAGs.[1183] Thus, further work on cartilage powder shifted from the crude tissue to its chief mucopolysaccharide molecular component — chondroitin sulfates.

IV. CHONDROITIN SULFATES

A. ROLES AND FUNCTIONS

Chondroitin sulfates (the plural form more closely approximates an accurate description since each individual molecule is slightly different) were extracted and purified during the 1960s. As a result, several studies were performed with the goal of acceleration of connective tissue healing, as suggested by fractionation studies of cartilage powders. Furthermore, exogenous administration of chondroitin sulfates stimulated secretion of PGs in cartilage or chondrocyte cultures.[1194-1197] These studies suggested that if sufficient chondroitin sulfates were presented to cells manufacturing PGs, matrix synthesis could be stimulated, which may, in turn, accelerate the overall healing process.

B. INTAKES AND DIETARY SOURCES

PGs and GAGs are obviously constituents of a normal, balanced diet that contains animal food-stuffs. Animal flesh, soups with bones, shark fins, tripe, gristle, and other connective tissues all contain varying amounts of PGs and GAGs. However, there are no data reported on the GAG content of common foods, since many people remove or discard gristle before ingestion of animal foodstuffs. Since PGs make up approximately 1 to 2% of dry weight of normal tissues, it can be estimated that an average daily intake of GAGs may be near 1 g from a nonvegan diet. The human gut contains specific enzymes, such as chondroitinases, which are able to digest GAGs after their release from connective tissues by acid-pepsin treatment in the stomach. Acid-pepsin treatment of connective tissues is one method of preparation for chondroitin sulfates products.[1198] Thus, normal gastric secretions are able to initiate digestion of GAGs by their release from ingested connective tissues. However, digestion of GAGs from foodstuffs may not be complete, as connective tissue fibers are normally found in fecal residues.

Uptake of purified chondroitin sulfates (CS) has been studied in animals and humans. Andermann, from the Service de Recherches Biopharmaceutiques in Kayserberg, France, administered either 100 mg CS/kg as a slurry in water or olive oil, or 250 mg CS in a capsule to anesthetized rabbits.[1199] Serum was assayed for intact CS by precipitation with cetyl pyridinium chloride, modified to detect only long-chain, high-molecular-weight CS. No uptake of CS into serum was seen after oral administration by any means. However, the possibility that CS was digested into smaller subunits was not able to be examined by this study. Rabbits are primarily herbivores; since they do not normally eat flesh, it is less likely that rabbits possess the digestive enzymes necessary to fully degrade a large bolus of mammalian PGs and GAGs, which omnivores and carnivores (humans and dogs) seem to possess.

Another study using rabbits did find uptake of long-chain, sulfated mucopolysaccharides (SP54, or pentosan polysulfate), but after administration of enteric-coated capsules, not after administration of an aqueous solution.[1200] Previous studies of heparin (a sulfated GAG) also documented uptake into serum after oral (endoduodenal) administration.[1201] Thus, in animal studies, long-chain sulfated GAGs have the ability to be absorbed after oral administration, even though results of one study with methodological flaws did not find evidence of oral uptake. The issue of biological activity and uptake is paramount since small pieces of CS (<6000 Da) are inactive in biological activity assays.[1202]

Morrison and co-workers, from the Institute for Arteriosclerosis Research in Loma Linda, found that significant amounts of CS were found in the circulation after oral administration to mice, rats, and dogs.[1202] Interestingly, CS doses of 2.0 mg/g to dogs produced a twofold higher peak serum uronic acid level than doses of 4.8 mg/g in rats. Perhaps this finding indicates that animals regularly consuming meat would have enhanced ability to digest GAGs. If so, then humans should also possess more enhanced ability for CS uptake than mice, rats, or rabbits.

Morrison and co-workers studied the uptake of purified chondroitin sulfates into humans.[1202] CS were labeled with radioactive sulfur (^{35}S) by injecting suckling rats with sodium [^{35}S] sulfate, and extracting and purifying the radioactive CS. When 50 mg of labeled CS was fed to humans along with 950 mg of cold CS, 90% of radioactivity was found in the urine by 96 h. Eight percent of total radioactivity was found in the urine in high-molecular-weight form. Thus, at least some CS was absorbed from the intestine in nearly intact form. The low-molecular-weight radioactivity in the urine could have resulted either from absorption and subsequent metabolism of ingested CS to produce sulfates, or the sulfates could have been freed by intestinal or microbial enzyme activity, followed by uptake of free sulfate into the bloodstream and urinary excretion. Regardless, evidence of absorption of intact or large fragments of CS was found after oral administration in man.

Morrison and colleagues also found further indirect evidence for absorption of CS after oral administration in their human study on atherosclerosis.[1203-1206] There were 120 patients with documented coronary heart disease (atherosclerosis) divided into two groups of 60 subjects each. One group received conventional treatments, while the other group received the same conventional treatments plus daily oral CS. Doses started at 10 g/d for the first 3 months, then shifted to 1.5 g/d for 4.5 years, then to 0.75 g/d for 1.5 more years. After 6 years, 4/60 CS-treated subjects had died, while 13/60 untreated subjects had died. Likewise, 6/60 CS-treated subjects had acute cardiac incidents, while 42/60 untreated patients had acute cardiac incidents. Both differences were highly significant. Since oral CS was shown to have lipid-clearing activity in humans, the observed results were surmised to be due to absorption of large fragments of CS into circulation after oral administration. Then, lipid-clearing and, possibly, wound healing effects were postulated to have accounted for the observed results.

Pharmacological studies of Ateroid, a standardized mixture of "sulfomucopolysaccharides" obtained from mammalian organs by extraction and purification processes, have been conducted in animals and humans by Crinos Preclinical Research Laboratories in Como, Italy.[1207] Ateroid consists of a mixture of chondroitin sulfates, heparan sulfates, dermatan sulfates, hyaluronan, and heparin.[1208] Oral administration of tritiated or fluorescein-labeled GAGs to rats found uptake into plasma, kidney, testes, spleen, small intestine, and liver.[1207-1209] Furthermore, after oral administration of Ateroid to rats, a correlation between plasma levels of Ateroid and lipoprotein lipase activity ("clearing activity") was found, indicating that ingested GAGs possessed biological activity. In large doses of 100 or 200 mg/kg to rabbits, or 500 mg/kg to rats, Ateroid showed significant antithrombotic activity, similar to intravenous doses of 5 mg/kg.[1207,1209,1210] Obviously, absorption of at least large fragments of long-chain GAGs from Ateroid was required for biological activities of lipoprotein lipase release and antithrombotic actions seen in animals after oral administration.

Human studies with the same GAGs given as an oral preparation found reduction of plasma cholesterol and triglycerides, decreased β-lipoproteins (now known as LDL particles), and increased fibrinolytic activity.[1209] These results indicate that absorption of GAGs may occur in humans. In fact, oral Ateroid is under consideration as a drug for the treatment of senile dementia by atherosclerosis in humans.[1211] Statistically significant improvements in symptom scores of mental function for 8776 subjects suggest that oral administration of Ateroid is accompanied by sufficient uptake to either change ionic surface charges of blood vessels or reduce atherosclerotic plaque. Thus, further evidence for oral uptake of GAGs in humans can be found. At this point, it is certain that CS can be absorbed intact or in large fragments in humans with sufficient concentrations to exert biological effects and enter tissues.

C. ANIMAL STUDIES

During the 1960s, studies with highly purified chondroitin sulfates implanted into animals found induction of ectopic bone formation.[1212-1214] For example, in controlled studies, purified chondroitin sulfates administered as a paste into extracted tooth sockets of dogs led to an acceleration of bone formation in the first 6 weeks of healing.[1213] After 8 weeks, control sockets were similar to chondroitin sulfate-treated sockets. These typical findings illustrated that topical application of chondroitin sulfates accelerated bone formation and socket healing, but did not alter the ultimate quantity or quality of bone formed. Results such as these led to the use of chondroitin sulfates as implant materials for refilling of bone defects, burn wounds, and plastic surgery in animals and, eventually, humans.[1216-1218] In addition, chondroitin sulfates, both singly and as a component of viscoelastic products with hyaluronic acid (such as Viscoat), applied topically to keratoconjunctivitis sicca (dry eyes) or after cataract surgery in humans, were associated with modest improvements in healing and postsurgical recovery.[1219-1222] Although these studies utilized nonnutritional routes of administration of chondroitin sulfates, they affirm the concept that if sufficient chondroitin sulfates are present in a healing tissue, then healing can be accelerated.

Another area of study for chondroitin sulfates was acceleration of wound healing, similar to studies with cartilage powders. Several investigators using animal models found that chondroitin sulfates accelerated surgical wound healing. Suyama et al., of Kanazawa University School of Medicine, found that intravenous injections of 20 mg/kg/d of purified chondroitin sulfates for 3 d improved tensile strength of rat surgical wounds at 7 d by 20%.[1223] Ashby and Nose of the Cleveland Clinic Foundation reported that intraperitoneal injections of 5 or 50 mg of purified chondroitin sulfates delayed skin graft rejection in mice from 7 to 24 d.[1224] Fialkova et al. demonstrated an acceleration of wound tensile strength in rats.[1225] Oelsner et al., from Yale University School of Medicine, administered 25 ml of 25% solutions of purified chondroitin sulfates intraperitoneally to rabbits after uterine surgery.[1226] Chondroitin sulfate infusion resulted in no adhesions in 23/26 animals, compared to 14/30 adhesion-free animals given saline (p <0.001). Lower concentrations of chondroitin sulfates were less successful.[1226-1228] A further study by the same group found that intraperitoneal injection of chondroitin sulfates was as effective as carboxymethylcellulose for prevention of postoperative adhesions in rat uterine horns.[1229]

However, instillation of Viscoat (containing hyaluronic acid and purified chondroitin sulfates) around full-thickness tendon lacerations with surgical repair did not alter adhesion strength or tensile strength of rabbit tendons after 3 weeks of immobilization, as reported by Meyers and others at Duke University Medical Center.[1230] Again, all of these studies used very high doses of chondroitin sulfates in parenteral modes of administration, which are not completely analogous to a nutritional usage of chondroitin sulfate. However, the concept that chondroitin sulfate could accelerate wound healing and reduce postoperative abdominal adhesions was confirmed. It is not known if oral doses of chondroitin sulfates would have similar effects.

Maier and Wilhelmi, from the Biological Research Laboratories of CIBA-Geigy in Basel, Switzerland, compared the ability of a number of agents, including chondroitin sulfates, on the prevention of spontaneous osteoarthrosis in C57 black mice.[1231] All agents were administered by mouth for 3 to 4 months for 5 d each week. At doses of both 50 or 150 mg/kg/d, CS supplementation led to a 25% decrease in the number of osteoarthritic knee joints compared to untreated mice, a difference which did not quite reach statistical significance. In addition, an approximate 15% reduction in severity of osteoarthritic changes was found. While the protection offered by CS administration was statistically significant, other antiinflammatory agents commonly used on humans with osteoarthritis actually caused significant increases in number of osteoarthritic knee joints (acetylsalicylic acid, ibuprofen, naproxen, prednisone). Thus, long-term oral administration of high doses of CS to mice led to modest benefits in prevention of spontaneous osteoarthritis.

D. HUMAN STUDIES

Early studies from Germany reported therapeutic effectiveness of intraarticular injections of chondroitin sulfates to subjects with osteoarthritis.[1232,1233] However, numbers were small and data mostly subjective.

In 1974, Prudden and Balassa reported on clinical observations of an injectable form of chondroitin sulfates named Catrix-S, an "activated acid-pepsin-digested bovine tracheal cartilage of calf origin".[1198] Catrix-S was injected subcutaneously in several sites for a total dose of 100 ml, with total doses of 100 to 1200 ml over a period of 3 to 8 weeks to 28 subjects with severe osteoarthritis. "Excellent" results were obtained in 19/28 (68%) subjects, who went from severe restriction of movements to only slight discomfort and virtually no disability. Another six showed "good" results, which meant a marked decrease in pain and improvement in mobility. The average period of relief was 7 months, and ranged from 6 weeks to over 1 year at the time of publication. No toxicities, other than occasional pain during injection, were noticed. This pilot study showed that administration of chondroitin sulfates deserved closer scrutiny for osteoarthritis.

Topical application of Catrix-S paste to mandibular alveolitis (dry sockets), hemorrhoids, psoriasis, fissure-in-ano, pruritus ani, and dermatitis was associated with significant clinical improvements, even in double-blind studies.[1198] Another pilot study of nine subjects with deforming or disabling rheumatoid arthritis followed the effects of Catrix-S injections. Again, excellent (3) or good (6) results were obtained in all nine subjects after about 3 months of injections. Ulcerative colitis and regional enteritis patients also showed varying degrees of improvements after injections of Catrix-S.[1198] The net result of these pilot studies is to provide further evidence that presentation of chondroitin sulfates to connective tissues can improve the healing response.

Kerzberg et al., from Ramos Mejia Hospital in Buenos Aires, Argentina, studied 17 subjects with knee osteoarthritis for 20 weeks in a randomized, double-blind, crossover schedule.[1234] All patients were given 500 mg of aspirin three times daily (1500 mg/d) as an analgesic during the entire study period. Subjects received either placebo injections or 150 mg of purified chondroitin sulfates, given as intramuscular injections three times per week for a total of 2.25 g. Treatment periods were for 6 weeks, followed by a 4-week washout period, and another 4-week period after both treatments. Chondroitin sulfates injections resulted in a significant ($p < 0.05$) improvement in articular mobility compared to placebo, pretreatment, and posttreatment values. Chondroitin sulfates treatment led to subjective improvement of articular pain in 13/17 subjects, and physician evaluation showed subjective improvement in 13/17 chondroitin sulfates-treated subjects. Placebo treatment was judged superior in 2/17 subjects. Another German-language study by Thilo, cited by Kerzberg, found increased mobility and reduced pain in 35 subjects with osteoarthritis after treatment with oral chondroitin sulfates for 3.5 months.[1235]

The use of CS for osteoarthritis was recently reviewed by Pipitone from the University of Bari in Italy.[1236] Various preparations of CS have shown absorption into the body, concentration in cartilage, remarkable safety, ability to inhibit some degradative enzymes, and good therapeutic efficacy in preliminary human trials. A multicenter clinical trial with a CS product called Matrix was reported by Oliviero and others from University of Naples.[1237] Improvements in pain scores and in mobility were found for 200 subjects. Another study by Rovetta of the University of Genoa in Italy utilized i.m. (intramuscular) injections of CS to 40 subjects with tibiofibular arthritis of the knee.[1238] Likewise, improvements in spontaneous pain, pain on loading, pain on passive movement, and changes in analgesic medications were found for each category after 25 i.m. injections of Matrix over 6 months. Both authors of these papers described the safety and efficacy of oral GAG therapy for joint diseases.

E. SAFETY

Animal studies showed that no acute oral LD_{50} was attainable, as mice showed no effects from a single dose of 15.65 g/kg, the highest possible dose of dissolved chondroitin sulfates.[1239] Likewise, no adverse effects were seen after a year of feeding chondroitin sulfates at 5% of the diet to rats, or a year of daily dosing with 500 mg to dogs.

In several large clinical trials, as well as a study on atherosclerosis lasting for 6 years, there have been no major side effects attributed to oral CS at doses of 1.5 to 10 g/d.[1206,1239] Less than 1% of patients had to cease taking CS. When injected, stomach upset and a few skin rashes were seen when side effects did occur. Oral administration of CS led to only very minor, if any, changes in coagulant profiles. Therefore, the ability of chondroitin sulfates to affect thrombus formation *in vitro* is not encountered *in vivo*. Most subjects given CS were diseased, with either atherosclerosis or degenerative joint diseases. Many of these subjects were also taking other anticoagulant therapy, including coumadin, with no apparent additive toxicity.[1204] Thus, purified chondroitin sulfates administered orally appear to have almost no adverse side effects.

F. SUMMARY

Chondroitin sulfates, when in their purified form, are absorbed by humans in various chain lengths, and incorporated into tissues. Chondroitin sulfates have the ability to inhibit degradative enzymes and stimulate further GAG and PG synthesis in connective tissue cells, especially chondrocytes. Thus, feedback from levels of chondroitin sulfates may represent one method used by our bodies to regulate the synthesis of connective tissue matrix. Chondroitin sulfates exhibit chondroprotective abilities. Certainly, oral doses of CS and other closely related GAGs have promising therapeutic benefits for degenerative joint conditions and excellent safety.

G. GUIDELINES FOR USE

At this time, there appears to be enough information to vindicate the use of chondroitin sulfates for degenerative joint diseases and repair of cartilage. Such circumstances would include osteoarthritis, other forms of arthritis, chondromalacia patellae, and almost every condition, injury, or syndrome that adversely affects joint health. Daily doses of at least 1 g are required for oral administration of CS. Attention should be paid to the purity and identity of CS products, since confusion over the identity of CS still exists, and studies routinely used purified chondroitin sulfates. In fact, suppliers of "purified chondroitin sulfates" in the U.S. sometimes possessed subpotent batches upon independent analysis (unpublished results). Enhancement of healing of other connective tissues, especially skin and bone, is also supported by the literature. However, insufficient clinical trials have been performed to quantitate clinical expectations from administration of oral chondroitin sulfates. Thus, a sound mechanism of action, availability, safety, proven bioavailability, and promising preliminary clinical results have been demonstrated for purified chondroitin sulfates and musculoskeletal tissue healing.

V. HYALURONAN (HYALURONATE, HYALURONIC ACID)

A. ROLES AND FUNCTIONS

Hyaluronan (HA) is the new term for hyaluronic acid or hyaluronate.[1240] Hyaluronan was first characterized in 1934 from bovine vitreous humor, and named for the Greek word for glass (hyalos).

TABLE 3 Mechanisms of Action for Hyaluronan in Musculoskeletal Healing

1. Stimulation of hyaluronate biosynthesis in human synoviocyte cultures by high molecular weight hyaluronan
2. Inhibition of neutrophil and macrophage migration and motility reduces joint levels of free radicals produced by these cell types
3. Decreased levels of proinflammatory prostaglandins after intraarticular injection of high molecular weight hyaluronan
4. Improved viscosity of synovial fluid, resulting in improved mechanical functions of joints, resulting in less degradation of cartilage
5. Prevention of loss of proteoglycans from cartilage by mechanical protection (coating properties)
6. Prohibition of presentation of inflammatory proteins to cartilage by acting as a molecular sieve in synovial fluid
7. Replacement of degraded low molecular weight hyaluronan in synovial fluid

HA is a very long chain (5 to 10 million Da) of repeating subunits consisting of N-acetyl-D-glucosamine and D-glucuronic acid. Hyaluronan is an unsulfated GAG, unlike most other GAGs (see Table 1). In aqueous solution at low concentrations (0.2 to 0.3%), HA forms a viscous, slimy gel that offers excellent lubricating properties, resistance to shear forces, shock absorption, and resistance to friction (viscoelastic properties). Synovial fluids in joints consist mainly of hyaluronate solutions, which provide almost frictionless surfaces for joint motions. HA also is a major component of vitreous humor in the eye, which aids in maintenance of proper hydrostatic pressure in the eye (shock-absorbing qualities to protect the retina). In cartilage and other connective tissues, HA forms the backbone of PGs, often attached to hundreds of proteoglycan subunits. HA, with fibronectin, helps anchor cells to the extracellular matrix. HA is an integral component of all connective tissues, especially cartilage. Hyaluronan is required for proper structure of connective tissues, and is usually synthesized at the beginning of connective tissue synthesis after inflammation or injury.[1241-1243]

Because of its presence in vitreous humor, rooster combs, umbilical cords, and synovial fluids, purified hyaluronan has been easy to obtain for commercial purposes since the late 1950s. One hypothesis for using HA as a treatment for degenerative joint conditions is that high-molecular-weight HA can replace degraded hyaluronan in both synovial spaces and the surface of articular cartilage. Improved lubrication of arthritic joint surfaces is another postulated mechanism of action for HA. Restoration of synovial fluid integrity may restore abnormal joint load forces to normal, allowing normal repair processes to ensue. Exogenous hyaluronan may also provide material for synthesis of hyaluronan and other GAGs during repair processes of synovium and connective tissues.[1244] Synthesis of new hyaluronan is a seminal event in deposition of proteoglycans and, subsequently, collagen fibrils.

Hyaluronan (as a high-molecular-weight species of 2 million Da.) exhibited inhibitory effects on *in vitro* cartilage degradation by activated neutrophils at levels >1.0 mg/ml.[1245] HA may also prevent attachment of inflammatory mediators or immune complexes to immune and synovial cell receptors, thus limiting inflammatory responses.[1246] HA binds acute phase reactant proteins in synovial fluid of rheumatoid arthritis subjects, which may further aid HA in resisting degradation from free radicals.[1247] HA, and one of its two components, D-glucuronic acid, possess antioxidant activity against free radicals formed by activated neutrophils.[1246] Thus, native hyaluronan possesses other properties that promote joint health in addition to viscoelastic properties. Table 3 lists some proposed mechanisms of action for the use of hyaluronan in connective tissue healing.

B. INTAKES AND DIETARY SOURCES

At present, purified hyaluronan is readily available as sodium hyaluronate, a dry powder. However, these preparations have only been used as intraarticular injections, and oral administration of HA has not been reported. Dietary intakes of HA are very low and can be considered to be insignificant. It is not known whether orally ingested HA can be digested or absorbed, but if other GAGs are any indication, at least some of oral HA could be absorbed into circulation. Since HA forms slimy, viscous solutions at low concentrations (1 to 10 mg/ml) in water, any potential oral HA products would have to be a dry powder.

C. ANIMAL STUDIES

At present, HA (as sodium hyaluronate) is an accepted and widely used therapy for osteoarthritis and degenerative joint conditions in veterinary practice. Primary use is in race horses, with applications for dogs also common. HA is usually injected intraarticularly in a series of injections until symptoms abate. Because of the rather large numbers of studies supporting the benefits of intraarticular HA for veterinary uses, only a few examples will be explored in this book. Again, presentation of data from intraarticular injection studies is not a nutritional application, but, rather, a pharmaceutical application. This data serves to illustrate the potential abilities of HA as a therapeutic agent. It remains to be confirmed in oral usage, although the extreme viscosity and slimy nature of HA solutions present some organoleptic problems for oral use.

Wiig and others from the University of California–San Diego studied the effect of HA injected at the site of the anterior cruciate ligament after a partial laceration was produced in rabbits.[1248] After 4 weeks, animals were sacrificed and anterior cruciate ligaments assessed for healing. Compared to contralateral knees treated identically without HA, 8/11 animals showed higher healing grades. Thus, HA has the potential to enhance anterior cruciate ligament healing, which is a common sports injury.

Researchers from the Fidia Research Laboratories in Abano Terme, Italy, and The Universities of Parma and Padua conducted a series of experiments with dogs made osteoarthritic by the Pond-Nuki method.[1249,1250] Intraarticular injections of sodium hyaluronate once weekly for 7 weeks were given 7 d after surgery. Hyaluronate treatment delayed the appearance of cartilage damage and prevented further deterioration, once damage was present. Treatment seemed to restore surface integrity of cartilage and preserve normal morphology of chondrocytes and synovial cells. Thus, regular intraarticular injections of hyaluronate improved the clinical response to osteoarthritis in canines.

Injections of HA into rabbit knee joints after experimental joint contracture secondary to joint immobilization was initiated led to a 50% decrease in joint stiffness and prevented the loss of GAGs normally seen.[1251] The results could be explained by increased synthesis of endogenous HA, leading to improved lubricating properties of immobilized joints. Another potential application of HA was to reduce postoperative adhesions after tendon repair. Thomas and others from Johns Hopkins University School of Medicine found better sliding properties and fewer adhesions after HA treatment of middle digit flexor profundus repair in the rabbit.[1252] HA was placed between the tendon and its sheath after tendon repair. However, the quality of tendon repair was not affected by this manner of HA administration. In another study on effect of HA on rabbit tendon repair by Meyers, a combination of HA and chondroitin sulfates (Viscoat) instilled around a full-thickness plantaris tendon laceration did not find any significant differences from control tendons for adhesion strength or tendon strength after 3 weeks.[1230]

D. HUMAN STUDIES

The effect of intraarticular injection of HA into human knee joints with osteoarthritis was studied by Namiki et al. at the Department of Orthopaedic Surgery at Tokyo Women's Medical College in Tokyo, Japan.[1253] In this study, 43 patients received between 1 and 16 injections once weekly of 2.5 ml of a 1% HA solution. Clinical evaluation included points for pain, range of motion, amount of synovial effusion, and ability to perform normal daily activities. Favorable results (improvement in clinical evaluation score) were obtained in 26/43 (57.8%) patients. It was noticed that less severe osteoarthritis led to greater improvements. Intrinsic viscosity was increased after HA injections, offering a biochemical mechanism of improved joint lubrication.

Punzi and others, from the Institute of Internal Medicine in Padova, Italy, administered HA intraarticularly (2 ml/week for 4 weeks) into knee joints of 17 patients with various arthropathies (osteoarthritis, rheumatoid arthritis, psoriatic arthritis, recurrent monoarthritis, gout, and chondrocalcinosis).[1254] Significant reductions in synovial fluid volume and articular disability (motion, spontaneous pain, articular tenderness) were noticed after 2 weeks. Likewise, a multicenter, double-blind, placebo-controlled trial of 63 patients with knee osteoarthritis was conducted by Dixon and others of the Royal National Hospital for Rheumatic Diseases, Torbay Hospital, and King's College Hospital in England.[1255] Up to 11 injections of 20 mg of sodium hyaluronate were given over a 23-week period. Statistically significant reductions in pain at rest and pain on movement were measured for the HA group. Daily activities tended to be better in the HA group, but statistical significance was not reached when compared to the placebo group. Several other studies also found benefits after intraarticular injections of HA to humans with osteoarthritis.[1256-1265]

The tympanic membrane offers an excellent model for studying wound healing. The tympanic membrane is isolated, easily observable, and easily measured. After success in healing of tympanic tears in rats with hyaluronate, effects in humans were investigated. In 1986, Stenfors, from the Department of Otolaryngology of Keski-Pohjanmaa Central Hospital in Kokkola, Finland, reported at a symposium on hyaluronan on the healing of perforated tympanic membranes (eardrums) in unselected patients.[1266] A solution of 1% sodium hyaluronate (Healon) was locally applied between 1 to 16 times on the tympanic membranes of 25 patients with tears lasting from 1 d to 10 years. Of 25 tears, 15 were completely healed, with better results on small and medium-sized tears. Scar formation was normal, and hearing was improved. Six patients required myringoplasties. The overall impression was that hyaluronate provided an alternative to myringoplasty in small and medium-sized tympanic membrane tears.

Another study by Stenfors observed the effects of local application of a solution of 1% sodium hyaluronate on very large, traumatic ruptures of the tympanic membrane in 3 patients.[1267] All patients were treated within 3 h after injury. Hyaluronate was applied to the tear, and the edges of the tear were suspended in the viscous hyaluronate. Reapplication of hyaluronate was accomplished at 3, 7, and 14 d postinjury, if closure was not seen. Closure was complete by 7 d in 2 patients, and by 14 d in the other. Posthealing hearing was normal. Hyaluronate thus assisted repair of the tympanic membrane without antibiotics and appeared to enhance healing.

Another human clinical condition which presents as an excellent model for study of antiarthritic treatments is Temporomandibular Joint Pain and Dysfunction (TMJ Syndrome). Kopp and others from the Universities of Lund and Goteborg in Sweden selected 33 patients with TMJ unresponsive to previous conservative treatment.[1268] The patients were separated into two groups, one receiving sodium hyaluronate injections, and the other receiving betamethasone, and two injections were made, 2 weeks apart, into the temporomandibular joint. Patients were assessed 4 weeks after the last injection (7 weeks total time period). Hyaluronate led to 13/18 (72%) of patients reporting improvement, and betamethasone led to 8/15 (53%) patients with improvement. Three patients on betamethasone reported a worsening of symptoms, not seen for hyaluronate. The improvements were significant for each treatment, and the treatments did not differ significantly from each other. Thus, intraarticular injections of sodium hyaluronate are as effective as a corticosteroid (betamethasone) for subjective and clinical relief of short-term TMJ Syndrome.

In vitro cultures of synoviocytes from human osteoarthritic synovium with different concentrations of HA found that production of prostaglandin E_2 was inhibited by HA.[1269] Likewise, intraarticular injection of HA to 8 subjects with various arthropathies found a significant reduction in synovial prostaglandin E_2.[1270] These results offer an additional biochemical mechanism whereby exogenous HA may reduce pain in osteoarthritis by reduction of proinflammatory prostaglandins, and decreased response to other inflammatory mediators, especially interleukin-1.

However, preliminary evidence suggests that hyaluronate byproducts, including formate, formed by free radical attack on synovial hyaluronan during inflammatory joint diseases or exercise, may enact a positive feedback loop to perpetuate joint inflammation.[1271] Thus, in circumstances where free radical damage in joints is apparent, exogenous HA may exacerbate joint pain under certain conditions. These conditions (synovitis) have been seen in very few patients in HA clinical trials, suggesting that attention should be paid to antioxidant status of patients with joint inflammation before HA treatment.

E. SUMMARY

A large number of reproducible studies have found modest to dramatic benefits in pain reduction and improvement of daily activities in patients with osteoarthritis and other degenerative joint conditions after intraarticular administration of hyaluronan. In addition, HA treatments for veterinary uses have become widely accepted and utilized. However, almost all of these studies utilized intraarticular injections of HA, in order to deliver high molecular weight HA into synovial joints for almost immediate effects. It is unlikely that significant amounts of high molecular weight HA can be transferred to joint spaces after oral ingestion of HA, although this hypothesis remains untested. Thus, although HA is a naturally occurring component of foodstuffs, similar to chondroitin sulfates, it is not a candidate at this time for oral supplementation to enhance musculoskeletal healing. Thus, HA has distinct pharmacological applications, which cannot be duplicated by simply ingesting HA as an oral supplement. Inclusion of an overview of HA therapies serves to illustrate the concept and utility of glycosaminoglycans as therapeutic agents for degenerative joint conditions. However, other sections of this chapter will explore the use of HA components (especially glucosamine salts) to accomplish the same results as injectable HA therapy, by enhancement of hyaluronan synthesis.

VI. RUMALON® AND ARTEPARON®

A. INTRODUCTION

Rumalon and Arteparon represent other pharmaceutical preparations derived entirely from proteoglycans or glycosaminoglycans. These two agents were recently termed chondroprotective agents because of their actions in promoting cartilage anabolism and decreasing cartilage catabolism.[1272] Their primary clinical usage in humans has been for degenerative joint conditions, especially osteoarthritis. Both are routinely administered as subcutaneous injections and, like hyaluronan, almost no data is available on oral applications of Rumalon or Arteparon. However, like hyaluronan, these agents have been extensively studied in Europe for many years in long-term studies involving large numbers of subjects.[1273] Both are considered viable treatment options for osteoarthritis in some European countries. Because each is composed of PGs or GAGs, a brief review of their therapeutic benefits will be given in order to further support the concept of GAGs as useful treatments for degenerative joint conditions. The number of studies on each agent is large, and the thorough review of such studies is beyond the scope of this book, since both are commonly administered as intramuscular or intraarticular injections, which is not a nutritional mode of administration. However, because research has indicated that levels of Arteparon and Rumalon are significant in joint tissues and synovial fluids, then results from studies of Arteparon and Rumalon have direct bearing to oral administration of GAGs that also produces measurable blood and tissue levels of exogenous GAGs. For this reason, a brief review of the effects of Arteparon and Rumalon will be presented.

B. ROLES AND FUNCTIONS

Rumalon is a glycosaminoglycan-peptide complex (GPC) extracted from bovine cartilage and bone marrow by Robapharm in Basel, Switzerland.[1272] It is commonly supplied in vials containing 2.5 mg of GPC, along with buffers and cresol as a preservative. Each batch is standardized by an elastase inhibition assay and guinea pig anaphylaxis test. Recent reviews have synopsized the attributes of GPC, which are listed in Table 4.[1272-1280] GPC has distinct anabolic and anticatabolic effects on cartilage, especially osteoarthritic cartilage. Importantly, GPC has the ability to partially counteract the deleterious side effects to cartilage of pharmaceutical analgesic agents, including corticosteroids and aspirin.

Arteparon, or glycosaminoglycan polysulfate (GAGPS), is a semisynthetic mixture of glycosaminoglycans originally prepared from bovine trachea and lungs by Luitpold-Werk in Munich, Germany.[1272] After isolation of GAGs from bovine trachea (consisting mostly of chondroitin sulfates), sulfate groups were esterified to isolate CS to increase the number of sulfate groups per disaccharide unit from one to three. The size of commercial GAGPS chains is 2,000 to 16,000 Da. Arteparon was initially produced over 35 years ago as a synthetic heparinoid, and has been one of the most widely studied GAGs for arthritis in humans. In the U.S., Arteparon is marketed under the trade name of Adequan® for veterinary use in equines and small animals (dogs and cats). Like Rumalon, Arteparon has been studied extensively in Europe and has been the subject of a number of review articles.[1272-1280]

TABLE 4 Chondroprotective Attributes of Rumalon® (GPC)

Anabolic Effects

Maintain cartilaginous phenotype of chick embryonic chondrocytes in culture (instead of conversion to fibroblastic morphology)

↑ Sulfate incorporation into cartilage, chondrocyte, and fibroblast cultures (both normal and osteoarthritic)

↑ Synthesis of sulfated proteoglycans by cartilage and chondrocyte cultures and *in vivo* in animals (both normal and osteoarthritic)

↑ Collagen synthesis (proline incorporation) of cartilage (osteoarthritic only) and *in vivo* in animals

↑ Synthesis of proteoglycan link proteins (osteoarthritic cartilage)

↑ Wound healing by enhancing formation of granulation tissue

Anticatabolic Effects

Inhibition of endogenous autolysis of cartilage cultures

Inhibition of degradative enzymes (hyaluronidase, collagenase, β-glucuronidase, human granulocytic elastase)

Preservation of normal morphology of chondrocytes after corticosteroid treatment (*in vitro* and *in vivo*)

Prevention of progression to arthritis induced by sodium iodo-acetate, indomethacin, phenylbutazone, dexamethasone

Inhibition of degenerative changes in subcellular organelles (mitochondria, endoplasmic reticuli, etc.) caused by corticosteroids

Antiarthritic Effects (Animal Studies)

↓ Cartilage surface changes

↓ Loss of proteoglycans from cartilage

Maintenance of cartilage thickness

↓ Period of lameness after experimental arthropathy

Improvement in walking ability, acceleration, and vertical forces after experimental arthropathy

↓ Development of cartilage fissures in patellar contusion models

Improvement and acceleration of repair of experimental cartilage lesions

↓ Incidence and severity of spontaneous arthritis in C57 black mice

TABLE 5 Chondroprotective Attributes of Arteparon® (GAGPS)

Anabolic Effects

Increase in synthesis of hyaluronan and proteoglycans from cultured human articular cartilage, chondrocytes, and synoviocytes

Increase in collagen, noncollagen protein, proteoglycan, and glycosaminoglycan synthesis in human osteoarthritic cartilage cultures

Stimulation of hyaluronan synthesis by synoviocytes (both *in vitro* and *ex vivo*)

Increase in synthesis of mRNA in chondrocyte cultures

Anticatabolic Effects

Inhibition of degradative enzymes (lysosomal enzymes, hyaluronidase, keratan sulfate glycanohydrolase, keratan sulfate sulfohydrolase, β-*N*-acetylglucosaminidase, chondroitin sulfotransferase, neutral proteases, myeloperoxidase, β-glucuronidase, β-galactosidase, α-glucosidase, α-mannosidase, cathepsins, human granulocyte elastase)

Inhibition of activation of plasmin and plasminogen activators by inhibition of serine proteases (inhibition of interleukin-1 activation)

Inhibition of prostaglandin E_2 synthesis and leukotriene B_4 synthesis (antiinflammatory action)

Inhibition of hemolytic complement activity and formation of C3a and C5a

Attainment of concentrations in human osteoarthritic joints and synovial fluid (1 to 2 μg/ml) after intramuscular injection of 50 mg Arteparon were identical to *in vitro* concentrations showing degradative enzyme inhibition

Antiarthritic Effects (Animal Studies)

Prevention of degenerative changes in rabbit knee joints after immobilization (atrophy)

Enhancement of healing of artificially induced cartilage lesions in rabbits and dogs

Reduction of iodoacetate-induced osteoarthritis in chickens and rats

Reduction of corticosteroid- or NSAID-induced osteoarthritis in chickens and rats

Slight reduction in spontaneous osteoarthritis of C57 black mice

Reduction of arthritis changes in knee joints of rabbits and dogs after meniscectomy (both prophylactic and therapeutic effects)

Table 5 lists some attributes of Arteparon as a chondroprotective agent. A brief description of some studies on humans with Rumalon or Arteparon will be presented.

C. HUMAN STUDIES

1. Rumalon (GPC)

Wagenhäuser led a team of investigators in a multicenter trial of Rumalon given to 1704 osteoarthritis patients from departments of rheumatology and orthopedics in Milan, Helsinki, Marburg, Madrid, and Zurich.[1281] After 4 months of intramuscular injections (separated by a 2-month interval), Rumalon was judged to be effective in 70% of knee, 64% of finger, 60% of hip, and 61% of spinal osteoarthritis cases.

Adler and others, from the Department of Physical Medicine and Rehabilitation of the Hadassah Medical School in Jerusalem, Israel, conducted a double-blind study of Rumalon on 106 patients with bilateral osteoarthrosis of the knees.[1282] A total of 20 intramuscular injections (3 per week for 6 weeks) of Rumalon was given, and patient progress followed for 12 months. Rumalon treatment exhibited improvement of symptoms and reduction in severity in 64% of osteoarthritic patients, while placebo treatment resulted in improvements in 29% of patients. Rumalon-treated patients showed six "excellent" results (remission) compared to no placebo patients with excellent results. The differences between treatment were statistically significant.

Schiavetti and others, from the Center for Rheumatology of San Camillo Hospital in Rome, Italy, studied the effects of Rumalon therapy for 5 years to 250 patients treated with conventional therapies and compared results to 250 patients treated similarly, but without Rumalon.[1283] After 5 years, significant differences in the Rumalon group were fewer painful exacerbations, less functional incapacity, and less radiological progression.

Another study reported by Denko, from Case Western Reserve University in Cleveland, OH, followed the progress of 20 patients with long-term osteoarthritis of the hip.[1284] In addition to standard analgesics (aspirin and indomethacin), injections of Rumalon were given once weekly for 1 to 68 months. Results were monitored by radiographic examination of hip joint space, an objective measure. Of the subjects, 5/20 exhibited recovery of joint space with clinical improvement, 11/20 improved clinically with no change in joint space (although 6 later worsened), 1/20 showed no clinical benefits or joint space change, and 3/20 worsened. Eventually, 5/20 subjects received hip prostheses. A dose response was observed, with patients receiving higher doses for longer periods of time exhibiting greater improvements.

Rejholec and Králová, from the Internal Medicine/Rheumatology Polyclinic of Charles University in Prague, Czechoslovakia, studied the clinical response to Rumalon therapy in a long-term, blind-observer study lasting 10 years (1965 to 1975).[1273,1285] Almost 400 patients with hip osteoarthritis were narrowed down into two closely comparable groups of 112 subjects each. Both groups received physiotherapy and analgesics and were measured for radiographic changes, joint mobility, functional capacity, analgesic drug requirement, frequency of surgical interventions, disability rate, and loss of working days. One group received a series of 25 intramuscular injections twice per year, while the other group received injections of vitamin B_{12}, which has no known antiarthritic effects. Radiographic changes showed a slower progression for the Rumalon-treated group (see Table 6). Analgesic usage decreased significantly from 5.5 to 4.0 acetylsalicylic units per day in the Rumalon group, but did not change in the control group. Likewise, total hip replacement was significantly less in the Rumalon group (6 vs. 17 subjects). Other measurements, such as time to ascend and descend a 15-step staircase, joint mobility, and symptomatology scores, all showed significant benefits in the Rumalon group. Importantly, the control group eventually lost 191 working days out of 250 per year, while the Rumalon group only lost 34 working days per year. The control group contained six times more invalids after 10 years than the Rumalon group (Table 6).

The resulting cost savings to society from Rumalon treatment were analyzed in a companion paper by Dinkel.[1286] Calculating the cost savings in reduced analgesic usage, reduced total hip replacements, lost working days, and prevention of total disability, a savings of 1.5 billion DM (in 1984) could be realized if Rumalon was accepted for widespread use in then West Germany alone. Thus, a natural

TABLE 6   Synopsis of Results from a Long-Term Study of Rumalon® (GPC) on Hip Osteoarthritis

Measurement	Control Group 1965–1975	Rumalon Group 1965–1975
Radiographic staging (Kellgren)		
Stages I+II (n)	52/112–15/83	52/112–31/83
(% of n at time point)	46–18	46–37
Stages III+IV (n)	60/112–68/83	60/112–52/83
(% of n at time point)	54–82	54–63
Walking ability (time in s for ascending and descending 15 steps)	38–85	41–63
Symptoms of secondary inflammation (week/year)	16.7–16.1	17.5–6.9
Analgesic usage (acetylsalicylic units/d)	5.6–5.7	5.7–3.6
Lost working days per year	30–191	38–34
Total inability to work (n)	71/83	12/83
Decrease in hip joint space (%)	–74.5	-47.0
Total hip replacements (n)	17/83	6/83
Progression from unilateral to bilateral hip osteoarthritis (n)	39/83	28/83

Note: 224 patients with documented osteoarthritis of one hip were divided into two groups. Both groups were given physiotherapy and analgesics as standard treatments. The Rumalon group was given in two series of injections per year for 10 years. The Control group was given vitamin B_{12} injections in the same schedule. Measurements are reported at the beginning of the study period (1965) to the end (1975), or as the values at the end of the study period. Difference for each parameter between groups was statistically significant by chi-square or *t* tests ($p < 0.05$). Data is from References 1273 and 1285.

product (cartilage extract) composed of PGs and GAGs showed the ability to reduce the social economic burden as well as delay progression of osteoarthritis in a long-term, single-blind study. Of great importance was the finding that divergence between the two groups was not noticed until after 2 years of therapy. Thus, studies lasting for less than 3 years may not find significant differences between standard therapies and Rumalon therapy, which would mislead investigators into reporting that Rumalon would be ineffective.

Yet another study by Rejholec, started in 1977, followed 47 control patients and 50 patients treated with Rumalon for 5 years.[1273] All patients had carefully matched osteoarthritis of the knee (radiographic stages II to III). Again, 10 courses of Rumalon therapy were administered at 6-month intervals. Significant decreases in knee pain, compared to the placebo group, were seen for the Rumalon group after 4 months of therapy, and was continued for 60 months. Time for ascending and descending a 15-step staircase actually improved by 5 s in the Rumalon group, but worsened by 7 s in the control group. Radiographic changes were quantitated and were significantly less pronounced in the Rumalon group. Only two patients had tibial osteotomies in the Rumalon group, while 10 patients in the control group had osteotomies. Most importantly, all subjects in the control group were certified unfit for work after 5 years, while only 15% of the Rumalon group was unfit. Rumalon led to a stabilization of osteoarthritis in 40% of subjects, with only 8% of control subjects showing stabilization. Again, similar to hip osteoarthritis, long-term therapy with Rumalon led to slow but consistent delay in progression of osteoarthritis of the knee. In general, the knee study was conducted after criticism of the hip study was encountered. Additional and more specific measurements were included in the knee study, and results were quite similar to hip osteoarthritis.

In both long-term studies from Czechoslovakia, and in the other studies mentioned, no significant side effects were noted after Rumalon injections. Occasionally, some pain during injection was encountered, but this is common to any injection and was not specific to Rumalon. Thus, the safety of parenteral administration of native PGs and GAGs has been repeatedly demonstrated in humans.

Thus, long-term therapy with PGs administered as an injectable led to consistent and significant amelioration of osteoarthritis in humans. These results can be extrapolated to oral administration of GAGs by combining results of several studies. First, intramuscular administration of Rumalon, which implied presentation of increased levels of GAGs to cartilage, improved the clinical picture of osteoarthritis. Second, the injectable mode of administration limited the total amount and the time of presentation to cartilage for GAGs. Third, oral administration of chondroitin sulfates is known to produce larger areas under the curve for blood concentrations of GAGs than intramuscular injections (see the section on chondroitin sulfates). Fourth, larger absolute doses of GAGs than is possible to be administered by injection can be given orally to reach and maintain elevated serum levels of GAGs all day, every day, not intermittently. Fifth, larger quantitative amounts of GAGs presented to cartilage by oral routes should produce faster clinical responses (within the limits of cartilage turnover, which is normally 200 to 700 d) than intermittent injectable GAG therapy. These differences will be examined when glucosamine salts are considered later in this chapter. Thus, injectable studies with Rumalon provide indirect support for oral administration of GAGs to replete cartilage and joints with essential raw materials and regulatory molecules by an oral route, which can then be considered a nutritional approach.

2. Arteparon (GAGPS)

Similar to Rumalon, Arteparon has enjoyed a long history of human clinical use. Following is a presentation of selected studies, with the intent to document the chondroprotective ability of a product that is a chondroitin sulfate with additional sulfates and, thus, possesses somewhat different properties. Again, the intent is to illustrate that if sufficient levels of a GAG with therapeutic properties is presented to cartilage, then clinical improvements in degenerative joint conditions can be obtained. Oral administration offers an alternative route to parenteral administration, as indicated by studies with chondroitin sulfates. Again, selected studies provide a thorough, but not exhaustive, review of the abilities of GAGPS in human degenerative joint conditions.

In 1978, Wägenhauser, from the Universitäts-Rheumklinik in Zurich, Switzerland, reported on the effects of 6 months of treatment with intraarticular injections of Arteparon to 31 patients with knee osteoarthritis, compared to 31 control patients, in a double-blind, randomized study.[1287] Significant improvements in joint pain and mobility were found. Verbruggen and Veys, from the Department of Rheumatology, University of Ghent, Belgium, injected Arteparon into the knees of 28 osteoarthritic patients.[1288] After a single injection, synovial fluid hyaluronan concentrations rose, as did the anomalous viscosity index. Repeated injections led to a greater production of large molecular weight hyaluronan in synovial fluid.

Tsuyama and others treated 27 patients with knee osteoarthritis and 31 controls with intraarticular injections of Arteparon for 10 weeks.[1289] Significant improvements in function and overall assessment scores were found after 10 weeks, compared to placebo injections. A multicenter study at 26 orthopedic clinics throughout Japan separated 120 total patients with osteoarthritis of the knee into two groups: control (1 mg Arteparon) and treated (50 mg Arteparon).[1290] An average of nine intraarticular injections over a period of 2 months was given. Although improvement was gradual, the treated group exhibited a significantly higher overall assessment of usefulness (71 vs. 41%). Joint function, pain scores, and daily living scores were significantly improved in the treated group after 10 injections.

Anderson investigated the effects of 10 intramuscular injections of Arteparon over a 6-month period to 20 patients with knee osteoarthritis, compared to 20 controls.[1291] Significant improvements in the ability to walk and flex the knee, reduced pain, and physician evaluation of effectiveness (85 vs. 20%) were noted. Siegmuth and Radi, from Luitpold-Werk pharmaceutical company in Munich, Germany, also investigated the effects of 15 intramuscular injections of Arteparon over a 6-month period in 68 treated and 67 control patients with osteoarthritis of the knee and/or hip in a double-blind, randomized trial.[1292] After 2 months, a significant difference was seen for the Arteparon group for reduced pain, walking distance, and increased joint flexibility.

Pastinen treated half of 30 subjects with osteoarthritis of the hand with 9 local injections of Arteparon in a double-blind study.[1293] After followups for 6 months to 5 years, grip strength was significantly increased after 6 months, and restricted activity was improved after 1 year. This study points out the longer time intervals necessary for adequate studies of chondroprotective agents, since the turnover of cartilage is very slow (200 to 700 d).

In 12 patients with chondrocalcinosis, intraarticular injections of Arteparon were given for 2 to 7 weeks, followed by 1 year of observations by Sarkozi and others from the Department of Rheumatology, Central Hospital of Hungarian State Railways in Budapest.[1294] All cases were bilateral, and the less-affected joint served as a control joint. For the entire year of followup, significant reductions in pain and improvements in joint mobility were seen for injected joints, but not for untreated joints. In addition, a marked decrease in cartilage calcification accompanied by an increase in excretion of inorganic phosphate was seen. Thus, Arteparon showed clinical utility in another degenerative joint disease, chondrocalcinosis.

Arteparon therapy was examined in several sports medicine applications.[1295-1298] Hess and Thiel, of the St. Elizabeth Orthopedic Clinic in Saarlouis, Germany, studied the effects on intraarticular Arteparon injections to 212 athletes with posttraumatic cartilage damage of the knee of long standing.[1295] There were 10 total injections (2 per week) given, and results were assessed 14 d after the last injection. Overall, "freedom from symptoms" and "marked improvement" were seen in 65% of patients for reduction of pain, 73% for decrease in effusions, and 60% for improvement in joint flexibility. The authors remarked that the favorable outcomes prevented the need for surgery in many patients. Kvist and others, from the Sports Medical Research Unit of the University of Turku in Finland, compared the effects of Arteparon injections and oral indomethacin for 39 young athletes with "jumper's knee" (apicitis patellae and peritendinitis of ligamentum patellae).[1296] Arteparon injections (six total over a 2-week period) were given subcutaneously near the patella to 18 athletes. Oral indomethacin (25 mg three times daily) was given for 2 weeks to 21 athletes. The Arteparon group showed a 94% success rate (symptom-free or almost cured), while the indomethacin group showed a 43% success rate after 2 weeks. After 8 weeks, 4/18 Arteparon-treated athletes relapsed, and 8/21 indomethacin-treated patients relapsed. Then, 11 of the uncured or relapsed patients from the indomethacin group were treated with Arteparon. Of these patients, eight became symptom-free or almost cured after 2 weeks of Arteparon therapy, with three relapses after 8 weeks. In both study segments, results from Arteparon were "significantly better and of longer duration."[1296] Kvist also reported results of Arteparon used for chondromalacia patellae in then East Germany on 1607 patients. Excellent or good results were seen in 50% of patients after arthrotomy and in 65% of patients with Arteparon treatment alone. Clinical responses were seen after six to eight intraarticular injections of Arteparon, and 20 to 30 injections were typically needed.

Lysholm, from the Department of Orthopedic Surgery, University Hospital, Linkoping, Sweden, studied the effect of local injections of Arteparon to 25 young athletes (20 ± 3 years) with patella tendinitis on measurements of muscle torque by a Cybex test, and knee pain on exertion.[1297] After 5 weeks of local injections and activity modifications, subjects were assessed 3 weeks later for quadriceps muscle torque. Half of the patients showed improvements in producing greater torque with less pain. The other half showed no changes. Sprengel and others, from the Polyclinic for Orthopedics of the Medical Academy of Erfurt in East Germany, studied 75 combinations of 25 methods of treatment on 150 knees with chondromalacia patellae.[1298] Their results found that combinations of therapies were not significantly better than single therapies consisting of either Arteparon injections, iontophoresis with histamine, or short waves. In this study, Arteparon was considered as conservative, standard treatment and gave effects similar to other accepted therapies.

Finally, long-term study of Arteparon in human knee osteoarthritis was studied by Rejholec in concert with their studies on Rumalon.[1273] In an open study of 5 years duration, 50 patients with osteoarthritis of the knee were given 10 courses of intramuscular Arteparon therapy at 6-month intervals. Each course of Arteparon therapy consisted of two injections per week for 7.5 weeks of 50 mg Arteparon in 1 ml. Controls were 47 matched patients. All subjects received analgesics (NSAIDs) and physio-therapy. After 5 years, blind comparison of radiographic images at 0 and 5 years showed that the degree of narrowing in the Arteparon group was 57 to 60% that of the control group. Osteophyte development ranged from 43 to 72% of control values, and marginal erosions and bone necroses were 62% of control values. Thus, objective measurements showed that Arteparon therapy significantly delayed joint erosion compared to standard therapies (NSAIDs). Typical of standard therapies, the different pain measure-ments (arthritic pain, night pain, pain on maximum passive movement) decreased significantly for the control group during the first two years of study, then rose to greater than initial levels, even though analgesic usage increased. The Arteparon group showed a greater initial decrease in pain, followed by a slow but consistent further decrease in knee pain, concomitant with decreased analgesic usage. Analgesic usage (in acetylsalicylic units per day) in the control group rose from 3.3 to 3.6 U/d, while the Arteparon group dropped from 3.6 to 1.6 U/d. Knee joint mobility (in degrees) decreased from 116 to 110° in the control group and expanded from 116 to 123° in the Arteparon group. The time to stand and sit five times increased from 12 to 14 s in the control group and remained the same (11 s) in the Arteparon group. The time to ascend and descend a flight of 15 steps lengthened from 32 to 38 s in the control group and lessened from 32 to 29 s in the Arteparon group. The time to walk 10 m rose from 14 to 18 s in the control group and decreased from 14 to 12 s in the Arteparon group. The percentage of subjects able to work decreased from 24 to 0% in the control group, while the same parameter in the Arteparon group rose from 21 to 49%. In 5 years, 13 control patients underwent tibial osteotomies, while only two subjects on Arteparon treatment had osteotomies. Finally, the overall doctor's assessment (on a scale of 0 to 3) changed from 1.62 to 1.90 in the control group and improved significantly from 1.74 to 0.42 in the Arteparon group. Thus, many objective and subjective parameters measured over a 5-year period showed that intramuscular injections of Arteparon led to reduced symptoms of osteoarthritis and reduced NSAID consumption, reduced surgical intervention, and improved quality of life and ability to work. Of importance is the finding that differences between Arteparon and control groups took 2 years to reach significance, but after 2 years, there was clear and continual divergence of measurements between control and Arteparon groups. Thus, delivery of polysulfated chondroitin sulfates to joint tissues resulted in chondroprotective attributes that were slow acting, but clinically significant.

D. SAFETY

Since Rumalon and Arteparon have been administered as injectables, this mode of administration is strictly pharmaceutical. In over 25 years of clinical use, very few side effects have been noticed for Rumalon, with only occasional pain at the injection site reported.[1272-1277] Arteparon has about one third of the anticoagulant activity of heparin and has caused a small but significant number of side effects. Only one death out of hundreds of thousands of doses has been attributed to Arteparon, and this one fatality was an anaphylactic response.[1277] Occasionally, bleeding or hematoma formation at the injection site was encountered, but very seldom were any systemic effects observed. One patient previously treated with Arteparon demonstrated an allergic reaction to heparin, suggesting crossreactivity of the two heparinoids.[1299] Side effects were reported to occur in less than 1% of patients receiving Arteparon. Thus, injectable glycosaminoglycan derivatives posed little safety concerns, even after years of treat-ment.

E. SUMMARY

The ability of native and modified glycosaminoglycans to enhance cartilage healing has been consistently documented in both animal and human studies. Mechanisms of action have been hypoth-esized and evidence in support of those hypotheses has been reported. Compared to commonly used antirheumatic, antiinflammatory, and analgesic drugs,[1300,1301] side effects are minor or nonexistent. However, unlike analgesics or antiinflammatory drugs, Arteparon and Rumalon do not exert immediate effects. They are not analgesic, and their benefits take weeks, months, or sometimes years to become discernible. However, the changes are due to a delay in progression of joint damage, and probably due to an improvement in joint cartilage and synovium repair. One wonders what results would have been found if concomitant analgesic and antiinflammatory drugs had not been used, since some of these drugs are known to disturb chondrocyte metabolism adversely. Also, the use of intermittent injections involves a considerable number of office visits, in addition to the pharmacokinetic considerations of a cyclic nature of chondroprotector presence. Perhaps an oral mode of administration would offer adequate levels of glycosaminoglycans continuously, which would accelerate and/or intensify observed results compared to injectable modalities. Regardless, the concept of improving cartilage metabolism and repair, and preventing degradation by glycosaminoglycans, has been confirmed.

VII. GLUCOSAMINE SALTS

A. INTRODUCTION

Glucosamine is a naturally occurring aminosugar found in glycoproteins and glycosaminoglycans. Glucosamine itself constitutes half of hyaluronan, keratan sulfates, heparan sulfates, and heparin. Epimerases easily convert glucosamine into galactosamine, which constitutes half of chondroitin sulfates and dermatan sulfates (see Table 1). It is entirely logical to extend the results from studies of long-chain glycosaminoglycans to their precursors, including glucosamine. Prudden and co-workers, from Columbia University in New York, attempted to isolate the active part of their cartilage powders that conferred an acceleration of wound healing after topical application to surgical wounds.[1302] After analysis of cartilage batches that differed in ability to accelerate wound healing, the major difference was more glucosamine in the more successful batch. Therefore, glucosamine and *N*-acetylglucosamine, both topical and parenteral, were applied to rat surgical wounds, and a slight increase in wound strength (3 to 10%) was found. However, topical application of insoluble chitin — a long-chain, linear polymer of *N*-acetylglucosamine — was associated with a 30% increase in wound tensile strength, which was greater than the increase from cartilage powders. This effect was explained by the large amount of lysozyme in healing wounds, which presumably degraded chitin into *N*-acetylglucosamine *in situ* in large quantities at the wound site. Increased availability of glucosamine would then accelerate or enhance synthesis of new HA, GAGs, and PGs.

B. ROLES AND FUNCTIONS

An examination of glycosaminoglycan synthesis in chondrocytes and fibroblasts also reveals the importance of glucosamine. Normal glycosaminoglycan synthesis first involves the synthesis of a core protein pool and their transport to Golgi apparatus.[73] Next, carbohydrate residues, including glucosamines, are added to core protein, followed by rapid polymerization of a staggering number of long GAG chains, with sulfation of aminosugar residues occurring almost simultaneously. After synthesis of the proteoglycan subunits, their transport outside the cell and subsequent assembly into aggrecan (proteoglycans on hyaluronan) in extracellular matrix follows. What is remarkable about this process is the rapidity of synthesis and sulfation of proteoglycan subunits, which is on the order of 10 to 15 min or less in adult articular cartilage.[79] The availability of glucosamine is the key, rate-limiting step in GAG and PG synthesis.[88,1303] If sufficient glucosamine is available, then synthesis of PGs can proceed. Thus, one hypothesis for enhancement of cartilage repair is to provide sufficient glucosamine to ensure rapid synthesis of GAGs. Enhanced synthesis of GAGs and PGs may then be able to overcome the degradation occurring during joint diseases or after injury.

Glucose is the predominate precursor for GAG components.[88,1303] Glucose is phosphorylated by ATP to form glucose-6-phosphate, which is epimerized to fructose-6-phosphate. Donation of an amino group by glutamine, mediated by glucosamine-6-phosphate synthetase, then forms glucosamine-6-phosphate, which is subsequently acetylated, converted to *N*-acetylglucosamine-1-phosphate, and uridine diphosphate added (at the expense of uridine triphosphate) to form UDP-*N*-acetylglucosamine, which is added to growing GAG chains. An alternate pathway exists for introduction of glucosamine.[88,1303] Phosphorylation of glucosamine with ATP forms glucosamine-6-phosphate, which then enters GAG synthesis. It is probably this alternate pathway that utilizes exogenous glucosamine for matrix synthesis. Thus, two potential mechanisms for action exist for glucosamine salts — provision of precursors to GAG synthesis and a stimulatory effect on incorporation of other precursors into connective tissue matrix.

Karzel and Domenjoz, from the Institute for Pharmacology, University of Bonn, studied the effect of administration of aminosugars on GAG production by cultured embryonic mouse vertebral cartilage fibroblasts.[88] This culture system produced mostly hyaluronan. At concentrations of 100 µg/ml, glucosamine base, glucosamine·HCl, glucosamine·HI, and glucosamine sulfate all produced increased GAG production (157 to 170%). Other GAG components, such as D-glucuronic acid, *N*-acetylglucosamine, galactosamine, *N*-acetylgalactosamine, and betaine glucuronate, did not produce increased GAG synthesis. Vidal y Plana and others, from Rotta Research Laboratories, also studied the effect of glucosamine·HCl on mouse embryonic fibroblast cultures.[1303] They found that glucosamine produced a dose-dependent increase in GAG production, identical to results of Karzel. Similarly, glucosamine salts enhanced radioactive sulfur incorporation into cartilage slices *in vitro*.[1304] Adult rat femoral cartilage cultures also exhibited a steady, dose-dependent increase in GAG synthesis (radioactive sulfur incorporation) and collagen synthesis (radioactive proline incorporation) by glucosamine over a range of concentrations (0 to 200 µg/ml). In addition, the effect of several NSAIDs on synthesis of cartilage macromolecules was examined in the rat femoral cartilage culture system.[1303] Ibuprofen, sulindac, protacine, naproxen, and indomethacin all exhibited dose-dependent inhibitions of collagen and GAG synthesis at concentrations ranging from 0 to 200 µg/ml. Addition of 0.5 m*M* glucosamine (108 µg/ml) along with NSAIDs led to small but significant reversals of inhibition. Thus, exogenous glucosamine salts are able to be utilized by connective tissue cells for GAG synthesis and appear to exert a stimulatory effect on GAG, PG, collagen, and matrix synthesis. Importantly, high levels of glucosamine exhibited restorative effects on cartilage simultaneously treated with NSAIDs. This observation may mean that many human clinical trials utilizing GAG preparations along with standard NSAIDs for osteoarthritis showed lesser effects than if the NSAIDs were not present. Also, use of GAG preparations along with NSAIDs offers hope that the deleterious side effects of NSAIDs may be partially prevented, thus improving the therapeutic benefits to the arthritis patient.

C. INTAKES AND DIETARY SOURCES

Glucosamine is almost universally found in small amounts in most foods. However, no research exists to quantitate the levels of glucosamine in foodstuffs. Obviously, foods richest in cartilage and glycoproteins would be the richest food sources of glucosamine. Due to inadequacy of knowledge of glucosamine levels in foods and lack of data on bioavailability of glucosamine from foods, clinical application of glucosamine centers around oral administration in supplement form (or as a drug, depending upon the country).

Bioavailability of oral glucosamine, glucosamine sulfate, or *N*-acetylglucosamine is excellent.[1305-1307] Studies utilizing radioactive glucosamine salts found that glucosamine was absorbed intact and almost completely, with only 5% excreted in feces of rats.[1306] Glucosamine levels in plasma reached a broad peak at 1 h that continued for 10 h.[1307] After a very short time (<60 min), radioactivity in the form of glycoproteins was also encountered in plasma. Thus, glucosamine was taken up and utilized very quickly by peripheral tissues. Most of the ingested glucosamine (82%) was metabolized into carbon dioxide and expired. However, significant levels of radioactivity were found in all organs, including femoral cartilage, femurs, and sternum, which possessed the same levels as plasma 8 h after administration. Further studies in dogs showed that articular cartilage had active uptake of glucosamine from plasma. Thus, oral administration of glucosamine leads to rapid, complete absorption and uptake by all tissues, including connective tissues, in animals.

Absorption of unlabeled glucosamine sulfate in humans was determined.[1307] Glucosamine (6 g) was administered in a single dose as sugar-coated tablets to human volunteers. Intact glucosamine levels in plasma and urine were determined by ion-exchange chromatography. Plasma levels of glucosamine at all times after oral administration were <10 µg/ml, but urinary glucosamine levels were increased rapidly, so that 4 h after oral administration, 85% of the oral load was found in urine. Thus, pharmacokinetics of glucosamine in humans was not substantially different than in rats and dogs. The high absorption rate and tissue uptake of glucosamine was not surprising, given that at physiological pH, 75% of glucosamine is not ionized and, therefore, easily crosses membranes.[1307] Thus, glucosamine salts are rapidly absorbed and taken up selectively by articular cartilage.

D. ANIMAL STUDIES

Setnikar and co-workers, from Rotta Research Laboratories in Monza, Italy, studied the antiinflammatory effects of oral glucosamine sulfate compared to aspirin and indomethacin in rat models.[1308] Glucosamine had no analgesic activity and did not affect inflammation mediated by proteolytic enzymes or by prostaglandins. Several models of inflammation (rat paw edema from carrageenin, dextran, and formalin) showed inhibition by glucosamine, but edema provoked by specific inflammatory mediators (bradykinin, serotonin, and histamine) were not protected. Glucosamine did inhibit superoxide generation by macrophages *in vitro* and activity of liver lysosomal enzymes, pointing to a membrane-stabilizing effect. Glucosamine was effective only at much higher levels (10 ×) than aspirin or indomethacin, but the very much greater safety of glucosamine meant that the therapeutic benefit of glucosamine was similar to aspirin and indomethacin.

Setnikar and co-workers further studied the antiinflammatory and antiarthritic properties of oral glucosamine sulfate in rats.[1309] Effective oral doses were 50 to 800 mg/kg for prevention of kaolin-induced tibio-tarsal arthritis and adjuvant-induced arthritis in rats. Compared to indomethacin, glucosamine was 50 to 300 times less effective, on a dose basis. However, the toxicity of glucosamine was compared to indomethacin, and glucosamine was at least 1000 to 4000 times safer than indomethacin.[1308,1309] Dogs given oral doses of 2149 mg/kg/d for one year did not exhibit any adverse pathology, while dogs given 1 to 2 mg/kg/d of indomethacin eventually showed intestinal ulcers and some perforations. Thus, prolonged usage of glucosamine has a theoretical therapeutic advantage over NSAIDs for therapy of chronic degenerative joint diseases.

E. HUMAN STUDIES

Preceding many of the biochemical investigations an animal studies was one German trial by Vetter from the Auerbach Rheumatology Clinic, using injectable glucosamine sulfate and glucosamine iodide (Dona 200).[1310] Two intramuscular injections were given to 60 patients with knee or hip osteoarthritis. Glucosamine injections compared favorably with physical therapy, corticosteroids, and mucopolysaccharide treatments for pain and joint function. Results were long-lasting (3 months), which suggested a regulatory function for glucosamine. In another German study, Mund-Hoym also reported on therapeutic benefits for osteoarthritis patients after treatments with glucosamine sulfate.[1311,1312] Table 7 lists results of this and other human clinical trials of glucosamine and osteoarthritis.

Crolle and D'Este, from the 1st Medical Division of Guistinian Hospital in Venice, Italy, randomly divided 30 subjects with chronic osteoarthritis into two groups of 15 subjects each.[1313] The placebo group received one intramuscular injection daily of piperazine/chlorbutanol for 7 d, followed by 14 d of oral placebo capsules. The treated group received 1 intramuscular injection daily for 7 d, followed by 1.5 g/d of oral glucosamine sulfate for 14 d. No other antiinflammatory or analgesic drugs were given during the study period. Both treatments exhibited significant and equivalent decreases in joint pain at rest, active movement, or passive movement after 7 d. Overall symptom scores also decreased similarly after 7 d. The time to walk 20 m, walking speed over 20 m, and restrictive function symptoms were also decreased similarly in each group after 7 d. However, after 21 d, the glucosamine group continued to improve, while the placebo group returned to baseline levels for pain, restricted function, time to walk

TABLE 7 Synopsis of Human Clinical Trials of Glucosamine Salts in Osteoarthritis

Reference	n	Dosage	Study Design	Significant Results
1310	60	200 mg GS 200 mg GI im, ia	Open	Favorable comparisons to corticosteroids, physical therapy for reductions in pain, and joint function improvements
1313	15 exptl 15 ctrl	400 mg/d GS × 7d im; 1.5 g/d GS po × 14 d	rdb 21 d	↓ Pain at rest (0.21 vs. 1.71) ↓ Pain on active movement (0.67 vs. 2.53) ↓ Pain on passive movement (0.20 vs. 1.80) ↓ Restricted function (0.38 vs. 1.69) ↓ Time to walk 20 m (29 vs. 50 s) ↓ Overall symptom score (1.5 vs. 7.5)
1314	10 exptl 10 ctrl	1.5 mg/d GS po	rdb 6–8 wk	↓ Pain score (1.25 vs. 2.30) ↓ Joint tenderness (1.21 vs. 2.20) ↓ Joint swelling (1.25 vs. 2.20) ↓ Restricted movement (1.06 vs. 1.70) ↓ Time to clinical improvement (14.2 vs. 40.6 d) ↑ % Of responders (80–100 vs. 20-40%)
1315	40 exptl 40 ctrl	1.5 mg/d GS po	rdb 30 d	↓ Articular pain score (0.95 vs. 3.08) ↓ Joint tenderness (0.70 vs. 2.85) ↓ Joint swelling (0.35 vs. 1.53) ↓ Restriction of active movements (0.88 vs. 3.00) ↓ Restriction of passive movements (0.73 vs. 2.83) ↓ Time for reduction of symptoms by 50% compared to placebo (20 vs. 36 d) ↓ Sum of symptom scores (72 vs. 36%) ↑ Physician rating as excellent or good (29/40 vs. 17/40) ↑ Frequency of symptom-free patients Pain and tenderness (10/40 vs. 0/40) Restriction of movements (9/40 vs. 0/40) Overall symptoms (8/40 vs. 0/40) Normalization of cartilage ultrastructure by electron microscopy
1316	28 exptl 26 ctrl	? mg GA ia once weekly for 5 consecutive weeks; 4 weeks delay before evaluation	rdb 9 weeks	↓ Spontaneous pain score (0.18 vs. 1.61) ↓ Joint tenderness (0.29 vs. 1.71) ↓ Pain on standing (0.36 vs. 1.36) ↓ Pain on walking (0.50 vs. 1.89) ↓ Overall pain score (1.14 vs. 6.71) ↑ % Completely pain-free subjects (13/28 vs. 2/26) ↑ Flexion angle of knee (146 vs. 141°) ↑ Active mobility performance (0.58 vs. 0.39)
1317	15 exptl 15 ctrl	400 mg/d GS × 7d im, followed by 1.5 g/d po for 14 d	rsb 21 d	↓ Overall symptom score (2.4 vs. 8.3) ↓ Pain at rest (0.33 vs. 1.80) ↓ Pain at active movement (0.73 vs. 2.20) ↓ Pain at passive movement (.066 vs. 2.13) ↓ Function limitation (0.66 vs. 2.06)
1318	18 exptl 20 ctrl (ibuprofen)	1.5 g/d GS po	rdb 8 weeks	↓ Articular pain score (0.8 vs. 2.2) ↓ Articular pain score at 8 weeks compared to ibuprofen (1.2 g/d) group (0.8 vs. 1.2) ↑ % Of good efficacy by physician evaluation compared to ibuprofen (44 vs. 15%)

TABLE 7 (continued) Synopsis of Human Clinical Trials of Glucosamine Salts in Osteoarthritis

Reference	n	Dosage	Study Design	Significant Results
1319	1208 exptl	1.5 g/d po	Open, multicenter 50±14 d	58.7% physician-rated "good" therapeutic results 36.0% physician-rated "sufficient" ↓ Overall symptom score (2.5 vs. 8.7) ↓ Pain at rest (0.3 vs. 1.5) ↓ Pain on standing (0.5 vs. 1.9) ↓ Pain on exercise (0.8 vs. 2.4) ↓ Limited active movements (0.6 vs. 1.3) ↓ Limited passive movements (0.4 vs. 1.3) ↑% Responders compared to previous treatments (antiinflammatory agents, injectable cartilage extracts) (95 vs. 72 vs. 77%)
1320	68 exptl	1.5 g/d GS po	Open 20 weeks	↓ Pain at rest (0/68 vs. 42/68) ↓ Pain during movement (0/68 vs. 68/68) ↓ Rubbing noises of knee (4/68 vs. 49/68) ↓ Pain at knee displacement (0/68 vs. 48/68) ↓ Pain at pressure (0/68 vs. 45/68) ↓ Apical pressure pain (0/68 vs. 49/68) ↓ Medial/lateral side pain (0/68 vs. 59/68)

Note: Significant results indicate posttreatment values vs. pretreatment values for the glucosamine-treated group that exhibited statistical significance ($p < 0.05$), except as noted. Usually, for each measurement, the difference between experimental and control groups was statistically significant, indicating more favorable clinical results with glucosamine salts.

Abbreviations: exptl = experimental group (administered glucosamine salts); ctrl = control group (administered placebo or standard therapy); GA = Glucosamine Hydrochloride; GS = Glucosamine Sulfate; GI = Glucosamine Iodide; im = intramuscular injection; ia = intraarticular injection; po = *per os* (oral administration); rdb = randomized-order, double-blind; rsb = randomized-order, single-blind.

20 m, and walking speed for 20 m. After 21 d, differences between glucosamine and placebo groups were highly significant. The overall symptom score for the glucosamine group was reduced by 80% (7.5 to 1.5), while the placebo group showed a return to pretreatment scores (6.8 to 5.8). Four glucosamine-treated patients (27%) became symptom free after 21 d. Although most patients were "severely ill," no side effects in either group were observed. Thus, a randomized, double-blind, placebo-controlled study found large and significant therapeutic benefits from both injectable and oral glucosamine sulfate for osteoarthritis patients. The short course of study makes the results even more remarkable, considering the chronic nature of osteoarthritis.

Pujalte et al., from the National Orthopedic Hospital in Manila, Philippines, randomly divided 20 patients with knee osteoarthritis into two groups.[1314] Either placebo or 1.5 g of glucosamine sulfate (two 250-mg capsules three times daily) was given by mouth for 6 to 8 weeks in a double-blind fashion. An overall composite symptom score for pain, joint tenderness, swelling, and restricted movement was recorded, in addition to physician assessment. All scores were significantly decreased by glucosamine treatment, whereas placebo scores did not decrease significantly. In addition, the time necessary for clinical improvement was 13 to 14 d for the glucosamine group and 41 to 43 d for the placebo group. Percentage of patients improved ranged from 80 to 100% for the glucosamine group and from 20 to 40% for the placebo group. No side effects or changes in clinical lab tests were noted.

Drovanti and coauthors, from the Vigevano General Hospital, University of Pavia and Rota Research Laboratories in Italy, randomly divided 80 patients hospitalized for osteoarthritic flare-up into two groups.[1315] Either placebo or 1.5 g/d of glucosamine sulfate was given by mouth for 30 d in a double-blind manner. Osteoarthritis was located in the spine in 68% of subjects from each group. Placebo treatment during hospitalization led to significant reductions in articular pain, joint tenderness, swelling, and restricted movements. However, the decreases in these parameters were significantly greater in the glucosamine group. When measured weekly, the slope of reduction of symptoms ranged from 1.6 to 2.3 times greater in the glucosamine group. Overall, the placebo group realized a 41% decrease in symptoms, with a time to reduce symptoms by 50% of 36 d. The glucosamine group experienced a 73% reduction of overall symptoms, with a time to reduce symptoms by 50% of 20 d. The frequency of symptom-free patients for all symptoms on glucosamine was 8/40 (20%), compared to 0/40 (0%) for the placebo group. Physician evaluation as excellent or good was 29/40 (72%) in the glucosamine group and 17/40 (42%) in the placebo group. The time course of improvements for glucosamine suggested an improvement of cartilage metabolism rather than a direct antiinflammatory or analgesic effect. Electron microscopy of hip or knee cartilage biopsies of two patients in each group was accomplished after the study period. Both placebo subjects exhibited typical osteoarthritic changes of surface fibrillation with cavities, evaluated as severe osteoarthritis. However, both glucosamine-treated patients showed almost smooth cartilage surfaces, with almost no masking of fibrils. Only minor signs of osteoarthrosis were identified. The authors concluded that although few electron microscopy samples were studied, cartilage seemed to be rebuilt after glucosamine treatment for 30 d. This observation makes this particular study unique, because it offered direct visual evidence of clinical and biochemical attributes accorded to glucosamine: repair of cartilage. It is apparent that reversal of osteoarthritis is possible in some cases after chondroprotective treatment with glucosamine. Longer time intervals of treatment and larger numbers of patients with initial and follow-up biopsies will need to be studied before a statement can be made definitively about reversal of osteoarthritis, but the evidence points to this conclusion.

Vajaradul, from the Department of Orthopedic Surgery at Mahidol University in Bangkok, Thailand, studied the effects of intraarticular injections of glucosamine sulfate in 30 patients with knee osteoarthritis.[1316] Placebo injections of saline were given to another 30 patients. Injections were given once weekly for 5 weeks, and evaluations performed 4 weeks after the last injection. Symptom scores of pain, joint tenderness, joint mobility, and joint function were significantly improved from baseline and from placebo effects in the glucosamine-treated group. Thus, long-lasting clinical improvements were seen for intraarticular injections of glucosamine sulfate with excellent safety.

D'Ambrosio and coauthors, from the Hospital "G Stuard" in Parma, Italy, conducted another blind study on the effects of glucosamine sulfate injections followed by oral maintenance.[1317] Thirty patients hospitalized for chronic degenerative osteoarthritic disorders were randomly allocated to placebo or glucosamine groups. A treatment schedule similar to that of Crolle was followed. Pain scores, joint function, and overall symptom scores were all significantly improved after 21 d of treatment with glucosamine sulfate. The placebo of piperazine/chlorbutanol was more effective on reducing pain than restoring mobility, pointing to the nature of glucosamine as an agent that restores metabolic function of cartilage, allowing it to repair or rebuild, and, thus, improving joint function.

Vaz, from St. John Hospital in Oporto, Portugal, conducted a double-blind study in 40 outpatients with unilateral knee osteoarthritis.[1318] The subjects were divided into two groups of equal size. The reference group was given standard therapy — 1.2 g ibuprofen daily — and the treatment group was given 1.5 g/d of glucosamine sulfate for 8 weeks. Measurements of pain showed that ibuprofen decreased pain quicker than glucosamine sulfate, but by the end of the study, the glucosamine group exhibited significantly less pain than the ibuprofen group. Pain scores (from 0 to 3) started at 2.2 and decreased to 0.8 in the glucosamine group and went from 2.3 to 1.2 in the ibuprofen group. Whereas the ibuprofen group showed a rapid decrease in joint pain, followed by a plateau, the glucosamine group showed a steady decrease in pain throughout the study. Overall treatment efficacy, as evaluated by the physician, was rated as good in 8/18 (44%) glucosamine subjects and as good in 3/20 (15%) of ibuprofen subjects. In the glucosamine group, 2/7 patients with swollen knees returned to normal, while 0/4 patients with swollen knees returned to normal in the ibuprofen group.

Tapadinhas and others reported on the results of a large-scale, multicenter trial of oral glucosamine sulfate in Portugal for management of osteoarthritis.[1319] The results from 1208 unselected patients with osteoarthritis seen by 252 doctors was compared to other treatment for osteoarthritis. Patients were entered into the study over a 9-month period in order to reduce possible seasonal variations in osteoarthritis intensity. Regular medical treatments for other concomitant illnesses or diseases were given during the study period. A daily dose of 1.5 g of glucosamine sulfate was used for an average of 50 d. Oxyphenbutazone or acetaminophen was given in addition to glucosamine in 16% of patients. Pain and mobility scores were assessed, along with physician evaluations. Glucosamine was rated as good in 59%, sufficient in 36%, and insufficient in 5% of patients. Overall scores decreased from 8.7 ± 3.4 to 2.5 ± 2.6 after 8 weeks of glucosamine therapy. In 1614 patients given other treatments for osteoarthritis, oral glucosamine sulfate produced the highest percentage of responders (95%), compared to injectable cartilage extracts (Rumalon) (74%), antiinflammatory agents (70%), and other treatments, usually vitamins (71%). A smaller sample of patients (191) given injectable glucosamine sulfates also produced 95% responders. Glucosamine treatments were significantly more effective than any other treatment. Importantly, follow-up of 31 (3%) of original patients 12 weeks after cessation of glucosamine therapy showed that symptom scores increased to 3.2, perhaps indicating that glucosamine treatment should be intermittent or prolonged past 8 weeks. Very few side effects were reported, with heartburn being the chief complaint. However, the tolerance to oral glucosamine was rated significantly better than for any other treatment. The final comments of the authors sum this and others' clinical experiences with oral glucosamine:

> "The results of this investigation, covering 1506 patients reported on by 252 physicians throughout Portugal, therefore, leads us to conclude that ambulatory oral treatment with glucosamine sulfate manages most arthrosis patients to full or partial recovery, whatever the localization of their arthrosis, concomitant illnesses or treatments, though a dose adjustment may be required in obese patients and in those receiving concomitant diuretic treatment. The improvement appears to last for a period of 6 to 12 weeks after the end of treatment, after which time a new course of treatment is indicated to control possible symptomatic recurrence."

Böhmer and colleagues, from Frankfurt, Germany, studied the effects of oral glucosamine sulfate on chondromalacia patellae in young athletes (average age of 19).[1320] Daily doses of 1500 mg for 40 d, followed by 750 mg/d for the next 90 to 100 d were given to 68 athletes. Knee pain was almost completely reduced after 4 weeks of glucosamine sulfate supplementation and was not present at 8 weeks or thereafter. Pain at pressure and medial and lateral pain were completely abolished after 8 weeks of supplementation, whereas pain at displacement took 12 weeks before complete absence was noted. Apical pressure pain was reduced quickly, but was not completely gone until after 12 weeks. Rubbing noise heard in the knee slowly and consistently decreased in frequency, until only 4/68 subjects had noises after 16 weeks. Thus, glucosamine sulfate supplementation was associated with complete recovery from chondromalacia patellae in 52/68 young athletes. After 4 to 5 months, athletes were able to train at preinjury intensities. A follow-up examination 12 months after supplementation stopped found no evidence of recurrence.

F. SAFETY

Oral toxicity of glucosamine or glucosamine sulfate was not reached in animals or dogs, even after long-term (1 year), daily administration.[1308,1309] The human studies with oral glucosamine also found virtually no adverse side effects. Since glucosamine is a naturally occurring component of body tissues, and is absorbed, metabolized, and excreted very rapidly, there is little cause for concern about toxicity of glucosamine, even for long periods of treatment.

G. SUMMARY

Glucosamine salts exhibited the most impressive clinical performances of any nutrient for musculoskeletal conditions. Reproducible human studies, with a large number of patients, showed the ability of oral glucosamine sulfate to reverse symptoms of osteoarthritis in all joints tested, and even showed the potential to reverse cartilage damage. These findings are very exciting and have been replicated. In European countries, glucosamine salts as drugs are standard therapy for osteoarthritis. However, because of the status of glucosamine salts as natural products, their application as drugs in the U.S. may never be possible, given the current patent laws and very high development costs of new drugs. However, glucosamine salts are becoming increasingly available to the public and physicians via nutritional supplement companies. The sources of glucosamine include European pharmaceutical companies and their suppliers. Thus, although food supplements are not regulated as rigorously as pharmaceuticals, they represent an option for application of glucosamine therapy at present.

One consensus of all studies was that glucosamine was very effective for early or less severe osteoarthritis, and less helpful for severe or late osteoarthritis. This observation indicates that when there is insufficient (or none) cartilage on joints, then its repair cannot be affected by glucosamine (or other chondroprotective agents).

Research on the effects of glucosamine on a common injury seen in sports medicine — chondromalacia patellae — showed promising results, indicating that glucosamine may have broad applications for repair of cartilage, and perhaps other connective tissues, given the known mechanisms of action. All connective tissues and cells must synthesize hyaluronan, GAGs, and collagen in order to regenerate, repair, or produce extracellular matrix. Glucosamine offers a single agent that stimulates synthesis of all macromolecular components of cartilage. Thus, application to other degenerative joint diseases is a logical extension of the known properties of glucosamine. Any conditions that involve repair of cartilage and joints is an indication for glucosamine therapy. Such conditions would include osteoarthritis, rheumatoid arthritis, ankylosing spondylitis, invertebral disc conditions, chondromalacia, tendinitis, bursitis, osteochondrosis, postsurgical repair of traumatic injury to joints, traumatic injury to joints, and tenosynovitis. Speculative uses would include repair of other connective tissues, such as tendon or ligament tears and repair, skin wound healing, and fracture repair.

Glucosamine salts appear to be useful in conjunction with other commonly used analgesic and antiinflammatory agents. There is no indication that glucosamine will interfere with the results of NSAIDs, aspirin, or other antiinflammatory or analgesic medications. In fact, there is some preliminary evidence in animals that glucosamine salts may protect cartilage against the long-term effects of catabolism induced by some antiinflammatory agents. If this suggestion remains applicable, then glucosamine salt administration would allow for lower doses of antiinflammatory medications, or longer periods of treatment before side effects become apparent.

There are several commercially available forms of glucosamine salts. Glucosamine sulfate has been the most widely studied, because of its patent protection as a drug in Europe. Other studies and earlier work noticed no difference between glucosamine·HCl, glucosamine iodide, glucosamine sulfate, or *N*-acetylglucosamine. Thus, all of these salts (with the exception of glucosamine iodide, which is contraindicated for persons with thyroid conditions) should be equally effective in clinical settings at identical doses.

Oral administration of glucosamine salts offers several advantages over parenteral administration. Oral administration is less expensive, and can be continued and maintained for long time periods. Oral administration offers excellent pharmacokinetic profiles, similar to injectable routes. Continuous supply of glucosamine to connective tissue cells via oral administration may optimize cartilage repair compared to intermittent supply by weekly injections. Thus, oral administration of glucosamine salts appears to be advantageous for repair of joints and cartilage.

H. GUIDELINES FOR USE

Glucosamine salts are indicated for the conditions listed in Table 8. Daily doses of 1500 mg, divided into two or three doses, have shown clinical efficacy. It is uncertain whether higher doses would lead to improved results; however, higher doses (3 to 6 g/d) appear to be quite safe. A minimum effective dose is also not known and would undoubtably vary among individuals. Glucosamine offers a well-tested and successful means of restoring damaged cartilage via nutritional means.

TABLE 8   Indications for Use of Glucosamine Salts

Degenerative Joint Conditions

Osteoarthritis
Rheumatoid arthritis
Invertebral disc disease
Ankylosing spondylitis
Chondromalacia patellae
Cartilage eburnation
Tendinitis (tendinosis, paratenonitis, epicondylitis, tenosynovitis)
Bursitis

Speculative Uses

Fracture repair
Tendon tears and repair
Ligament tears and repair
Ligament sprains
Skin wound healing (postsurgery)
Carpal tunnel syndrome

Chapter 13

NONESSENTIAL DIETARY COMPONENTS: _____ BIOFLAVONOIDS AND CURCUMIN

I. BIOFLAVONOIDS

A. INTRODUCTION

Bioflavonoids are a ubiquitous class of compounds found in plants.[1321-1327] Table 1 lists the five chemical classes of bioflavonoids and some more common representatives from each category. Over 20 million possible structures exist for bioflavonoids, and over 500 separate structures have been characterized to date. In addition, synthetic (e.g., Cromolyn) and semisynthetic flavonoids have also been produced in an effort to patent the biological activities found for naturally occurring bioflavonoids. Since bioflavonoids are common plant components, bioflavonoids are part of a normal diet. At one time, bioflavonoids were thought to be essential dietary components for preventing capillary permeability, hence the now disregarded synonym of vitamin P. Flavonoids have received renewed interest in the life sciences by virtue of their powerful effects on enzymes and cells. Many of these actions have potential therapeutic applications in regards to healing of injuries or joint diseases.

B. ROLES AND FUNCTIONS

Table 2 lists some of the known functions of bioflavonoids *in vitro* that are pertinent to musculo-skeletal healing.[1321-1327] Because of their common structures, bioflavonoids share properties of enzyme inhibitions, especially for cyclooxygenase, lipoxygenases, phospholipases, and hyaluronidases. In fact, the field of bioflavonoid effects on enzymes becomes confusing quickly since different bioflavonoids often exert completely different activities. Also, it is difficult to extrapolate results from *in vitro* studies on purified enzymes or whole cells to tissues and intact organisms. Nevertheless, it is apparent that bioflavonoids exert potent effects on enzyme activities which have therapeutic potential.

Most bioflavonoids exhibited antioxidant activity of one form or another.[1321-1327] Scavenging of hydroxyl radicals, lipid peroxides, and reactive oxygen species has been repeatedly documented for many bioflavonoids, especially quercetin.[1321-1331] One mechanism is binding of free iron or other heavy metals that catalyze free radical formation. Antioxidant activity has been potent enough to protect collagen and hyaluronan from breakdown by experimental generated free radicals. These findings are of potential importance to degenerative and inflammatory joint conditions.

C. INTAKES AND DIETARY SOURCES

An average intake of bioflavonoids is around 0.5 to 1 g/d from mixed diets.[1322] Since bioflavonoids are found in plants, vegetarians may consume even more bioflavonoids daily, up to several grams. While all plant foods contain bioflavonoids, some are richer sources of bioflavonoids. In general, green tea, berries, onions, citrus fruits, and stone fruits (cherries, plums) have the highest contents of bioflavonoids.[1322] Bee propolis is an extremely rich source of bioflavonoids, but is generally not eaten. Fresh fruits, fresh vegetables, seeds, and whole grains are also rich dietary sources. Animal products have virtually no bioflavonoid content. The amounts of individual bioflavonoids consumed is less clear, since different plants have different occurrences of bioflavonoids classes.

TABLE 1　Major Chemical Classes of Bioflavonoids

Flavans
　Catechins, epicatechins
Flavanones
　Hesperidin, hesperetin, naringin, naringenin
Flavones
　Chrysin, apigenin, luteolin
Flavonols
　Quercetin, rutin, rhamnetin, kaempferol, myricetin
Chalcones
　Hesperidin methyl chalcone, phloretin
Anthocyanidins, proanthocyanidins
　Colored compounds in berries

**TABLE 2　Functions of Bioflavonoids Pertinent
to Musculoskeletal Healing**

Inhibition of enzyme activity
　Cyclooxygenases
　Lipoxygenases
　Prostaglandin synthetases
　Phosphodiesterases
　Hyaluronidases
　Phospholipase A_2
　Aldose reductase
　Histidine decarboxylase
　Catechol-*O*-methyltransferases
　Calcium-dependent ATPase
　Protein kinase C
Complexation of heavy metals
Antioxidant effects (free radical scavenging)

TABLE 3　Biological Effects of Bioflavonoids

Antiinflammatory
Antiulcer preventive
Spare oxidation of ascorbate
Protect against hyaluronate and collagen destruction by free radicals
Antihistamine effects (inhibit release)
Inhibit arachidonic acid release (eicosanoid synthesis)
Possible spasmolytic effects
Antiviral effects
Stabilization of capillary membranes

　　Studies on the absorption of bioflavonoids in humans have found very low uptakes (1% or less) for quercetin, but substantial uptake when glycosylated bioflavonoids (e.g., rutin) were ingested.[1321-1323,1332,1333] Thus, it appears that some bioflavonoids will exhibit biological activity based on chemical structure. This issue is quite important since clinical lack of effect may be due to failure of delivery to target tissues.

D. ANIMAL STUDIES

　　A wealth of animal studies have been performed, mainly in terms of prevention of experimental inflammation.[1321-1327] Occasionally, other compounds (ascorbate, proteases) have been coadministered with bioflavonoids.[1334,1335] Such combinations were reported to be as effective or more so than NSAIDs against histamine-induced wheals, dextran- or carrageenin-induced edema, and capillary permeability after oral administration to rats.[1334,1335]

Czernicki of the Department of Neurology at the Polish Academy of Sciences in Warsaw, Poland investigated the effects of intravenous Trasylol, a synthetic bioflavonoid-like pharmaceutical, and Aescorin, a mixture of the bioflavonoids rutin, hesperidin, escukine, and sparteine, on experimental brain edema in cats.[1336] Trasylol decreased brain edema after experimental surgery, while Aescorin reduced edema after sudden brain compression and decompression. A mechanism of protease inhibition was postulated for Trasylol, and of vascular stabilization for Aescorin.

E. HUMAN STUDIES

The coadministration of ascorbate with 600 mg citrus bioflavonoids in a case study of subpatellar bursitis has been described in the chapter on vitamin C.[703] Citrus bioflavonoids, with or without ascorbate, were found to be more effective than placebo or ascorbate alone for the recovery rate from athletic injuries.[1337] Recovery was twice as rapid in the bioflavonoid groups. Another study administered 1800 mg/d of citrus bioflavonoids or placebo to football players 10 d before practice season.[1338] During the football season, incidence of injuries was equivalent for each group, but the bioflavonoid group exhibited an average of 0.67 d lost playing time postinjury, compared to 2.2 d for the placebo group. Thus, a few studies have shown interesting results for enhancement of healing from athletic injuries. However, studies were small in scale and used subjective methods of measurement. The results do suggest that further testing on the healing effects of bioflavonoids for athletic injuries is feasible.

F. SAFETY

No apparent toxicity from flavonoids after ingestion of foodstuffs has been conclusively demonstrated. However, *in vitro* studies of purified quercetin (and other closely related flavanols) have definitely shown mutagenic action in the Ames bacterial test.[1339] However, other bioflavonoids exhibited antimutagenic activity, and in more appropriate tests for carcinogenicity (long-term animal feeding, induction of bone marrow micronuclei, induction of sister chromatid exchanges), no cancer-causing effects have been found. Thus, it appears that the oral administration of bioflavonoids in general, including quercetin, has no greater risk of causing cancer than consumption of fresh fruits and vegetables.

Bioflavonoids are generally safe and nontoxic when ingested. Due to their relatively poor uptake and extensive metabolism by intestinal microflora, bioflavonoids are considered to be safe with no harm at intakes of at least 1 g/d. Since many humans ingest greater than 1 g/d of bioflavonoids, the upper limit for toxicity has not been found and is probably beyond practical reach.

G. SUMMARY

Bioflavonoids are a common food component consisting of hundreds of different structures. The primary bioflavonoids with commercial availability are mixtures of citrus bioflavonoids, rutin, quercetin, hesperidin, catechins, Gingko biloba extracts, milk thistle seed extracts, and wine proanthocyanidins. These compounds are commonly found in multivitamin/mineral products, vitamin C products, and some antioxidant mixtures. The biopotency of different bioflavonoids is not completely known, but appears to be sufficient for clinical use when daily doses of 1 to 2 g are ingested. Bioflavonoids appear to act as accessory antioxidants, inhibitors of eicosanoid synthesis, and chelators of toxic metals to exert antiinflammatory actions. Thus, bioflavonoids could have activity for enhanced recovery from inflammatory conditions commonly encountered in athletic injuries, such as sprains, strains, bruises, hematomas, and contusions. Another potential application is for degenerative joint conditions, since bioflavonoids are known to partially improve osteolathyrism,[1340] and stabilize collagen and hyaluronan, but clinical studies are lacking. Bioflavonoids appear to render other nutrients more effective as antiinflammatory agents, especially ascorbate and proteases.

**TABLE 4   Clinical Indications for
Bioflavonoid Supplementation**

Acute injuries
    Sprains
    Strains
    Hematomas, bruises, contusions, ecchymoses
Degenerative joint conditions ?

H. GUIDELINES FOR USE

Table 4 lists some clinical indications for bioflavonoid use along with identity of commercially available bioflavonoids. Bioflavonoids are considered applicable to acute traumatic injuries and as adjuncts to ascorbate and proteases uses. Daily doses should range from 1 to 2 g/d for clinical responses to be apparent. Overall, the evidence supporting the use of bioflavonoids is limited, but stands on firm hypothetical grounds.

II. CURCUMIN (TURMERIC)

A. INTRODUCTION

Curcumin [diferuloyl methane; 1,7-bis(4-hydroxy-3-methoxyphenyl)-1,6-heptadiene-3,5-dione; $C_{21}H_{20}O_6$; formula weight 368.37] is the major brilliant yellow-colored compound in *Curcuma longa* and other closely related *Curcuma* species.[1341,1342] Curcumin consists of two molecules of ferulic acid linked by a methane group. Interestingly, the popular NSAID, phenylbutazone, has a similar molecular structure to curcumin. *Curcuma longa*, a member of the family that includes ginger (*Zingiber officinalis*), has enjoyed a long history as a food, seasoning, spice, dye, and herbal medicine, especially in India and Southeast Asia.[1342] Synonyms include Ukon in Japan, Haldi or Haridara in India, and Kurkum in the Middle East (from which curcumin derived its name). Traditionally, the plant is cultivated for its roots, composed of a central bulb and finger-like rhizomes.[1342] Rhizomes are boiled in water for a few hours immediately after harvesting and cleaning, and dried by the sun or mechanical driers for several days or weeks to yield dried turmeric root.[1342]

Turmeric is then powdered and used mostly as a component of curry spice, a staple commodity in India and Southeast Asia. Typically, curry is composed of 10 to 35% turmeric, with coriander, fenugreek, and cumin being other major ingredients.[1342] In addition, turmeric itself can be used as a spice and coloring agent for foods. When turmeric is mixed with lime, the bright yellow color is changed to a deep red color, making the base for a red powder known as kum-kum, regularly used by Indian women to mark their foreheads.[1342] Recently, turmeric oleoresin is being increasingly used as a flavoring for processed foods.[1342] Oleoresins are extracted from bulk powders by acetone or alcohol extraction and are comprised of a mixture of volatile oils, resins, nonvolatile fats, and other compounds which retain the distinctive flavor of a spice. Turmeric oleoresin contains approximately 5% curcuminoids, while turmeric powder contains approximately 1 to 2% curcuminoids by weight.[1341,1342]

B. ROLES AND FUNCTIONS

Turmeric has had a long history of use as a household remedy for topical treatment of sprains and painful inflammatory conditions in Ayurvedic (Indian herbal) medicine.[1342,1343] In addition, turmeric was ingested as a stimulant or carminative, for treating dyspepsia, flatulence, or afflictions of the skin. Indonesian herbal medicines almost always include *Curcuma* species as a component, especially for liver and digestive difficulties. European work on therapeutic use of *Curcuma* species centered around choleretic and liver stimulatory abilities; however, these attributes were later shown to be due to artifactual addition of *p*-dimethyl benzyl alcohol.[1342] Ayurvedic uses led to exploration of turmeric by Indian scientists using Western medical and scientific approaches to find if it possessed active components of any potential commercial value. Thus, attention was focused on antiinflammatory properties of turmeric and its extracts. The major component of turmeric, curcumin, was quickly singled out as the major active ingredient.

The volatile oil of turmeric exhibited inhibition of trypsin and hyaluronidase *in vitro*.[1344] This indicates that inhibition of lysosomal enzymes may be one mechanism of action for antiinflammatory effects of turmeric and curcumin, although applicability of these findings to *in vivo* situations remains to be determined.

C. ANIMAL STUDIES

In 1964, fractions of turmeric were tested for protection against histamine-induced gastric ulceration in rats, but no activity was found.[1345] In 1971, Arora and others from the Department of Pharmacology at the All-India Institute of Medical Sciences in New Delhi, India evaluated the antiinflammatory activity of petroleum ether extracts of turmeric rhizomes in rat models, and compared the results to phenylbutazone (a compound with related structure to curcumin) and hydrocortisone.[1346] At an intraperitoneal dose of 1.0 mg/100 g body weight, extract A (a deep red, viscous oil giving a single spot by TLC) and extract B (an unidentified sterol-like compound) gave similar and significant reductions in granuloma formation after cotton pellet implantation as 0.5 mg/100 g body weight of hydrocortisone acetate. At the same dosages, reductions in formalin-induced arthritis and granuloma pouch inflammatory exudates were identical for turmeric extracts and hydrocortisone. Extract A (10 mg/100 g body weight) given by oral administration inhibited development of adjuvant-induced arthritis as well as an equal oral dose of phenylbutazone. Both turmeric extracts reduced skin histamine and serotonin levels in cotton pellet granuloma rats to 50% of control levels. These results suggested that lipid-soluble components of turmeric possess antiinflammatory activity.

In 1972, Chandra and Gupta from the Department of Pharmacology at Gandhi Medical School in Bhopal, India examined antiinflammatory and antiarthritic effects of volatile (essential) oil from *Curcuma longa* rhizomes.[1347] Volatile oil obtained by fractional steam distillation (80 to 110°C) of dried turmeric rhizomes was emulsified in milk (1:10) and given to rats in daily oral doses of 0.1 ml oil/kg, starting 1 day before injection of Freund's adjuvant to produce arthritis. Compared to cortisone (10 mg/kg/d p.o.), turmeric oil illustrated similar significant preventions in hind paw volume (reduction in swelling) after 3, 10, and 13 days postinjection. This effect was attributed to pituitary–adrenal axis mediation.

Talc-induced tenosynovitis was induced by injection of talc in gum acacia/water vehicle into the left intratarsal joints of pigeons (n = 20 per group) 1 h after oral administration of control (milk), turmeric volatile oil (0.1 ml/kg), or cortisone acetate (10 mg/kg).[1347] Functional joint impairment was measured as the time in minutes to assume a one-footed position. Turmeric oil both delayed occurrence of maximal response to talc injections as well as reduced percent responders (11/20 compared to 20/20 for controls). This effect was attributed to reductions in histamine.

In 1973, Srimal and Dhawan from the Division of Pharmacology of the Central Drug Research Institute in Lucknow, India studied antiinflammatory activities of curcumin in mice, rats, and cats.[1348] Curcumin suspended in 2% gum acacia was administered orally 1 h before other treatments in most experiments. Curcumin pretreatment reduced carrageenin-induced paw edema in both rats and mice at doses equivalent to phenylbutazone and cortisone (Table 5). Curcumin reduced joint edema in rats with formalin-induced arthritis to the same extent as phenylbutazone after the 4th day postinjection. On day 8 postinjection, rats with formalin-induced arthritis exhibited increased serum SGOT (271%) and SGPT (580%) values over controls. However, curcumin (80 mg/kg) and phenylbutazone (20 mg/kg) administered to rats with formalin-induced arthritis exhibited normal levels of SGOT and SGPT.

In the cotton pellet granuloma model, curcumin (21.5% inhibition at 80 mg/kg dose) exhibited the same inhibition of granuloma formation as phenylbutazone (19.0% inhibition at 80 mg/kg dose).[1348] Likewise, in the pouch granuloma model, curcumin significantly reduced granuloma formation, although at three times the dose of phenylbutazone for the same effect. Curcumin (40 mg/kg) was tested for effects on adrenal function. Unlike corticosteroids or NSAIDs (phenylbutazone was tested in this

TABLE 5　Comparative Intraperitoneal Doses of Antiinflammatory Drugs and Curcumin and Turmeric Extracts Exhibiting Activity in Rat Models of Inflammation

Substance	Effective Dose (mg/kg)
Curcumin	20
Water extract of turmeric	10–20
Alcohol extract of turmeric	400
Petroleum ether extract of turmeric	800
Hydrocortisone	25
Indomethacin	4–5
Oxyphenbutazone	100
Sodium salicylate	400

study), curcumin did not change leukocyte counts or the leukocyte differential. Curcumin did not affect adrenal cholesterol or ascorbic acid levels, suggesting that increased adrenal cortex activity is not involved in curcumin's mechanism of action. Thus, curcumin did not have the same mode of action as corticosteroids or NSAIDs. Curcumin did elevate liver ATPase activity like phenylbutazone, but at twice the dose needed for phenylbutazone (40 vs. 20 mg/kg). In rats fed ulcerogenic compounds for 6 d, curcumin administration exhibited a lower ulcerogenic index (0.60) than an equivalent dose of phenylbutazone (1.70). However, curcumin failed to illustrate analgesic or antipyretic actions in standard rat models. In anaesthetized cats, curcumin given intravenously at doses up to 10 mg/kg did not affect blood pressure, respiration, or contraction of the nictating membrane, indicating a lack of autonomic effects for curcumin.

Thus, in this series of experiments, curcumin exhibited antiinflammatory effects in both acute and chronic models of inflammation *in vivo*, with similar potency to phenylbutazone for some models, and one half to one third the potency in other models. Since there was no mortality from curcumin given at oral doses up to 2000 mg/kg (compared to an oral LD_{50} of 418 mg/kg for phenylbutazone),[1348] curcumin can be given in larger doses than phenylbutazone with fewer side effects. However, curcumin did not show the ability to reduce pain or fever, which phenylbutazone significantly reduced.

In 1976, Yegnanarayan and others from the Department of Pharmacology at B.P. Medical College in Poona, India compared the antiinflammatory effects of curcumin and petroleum ether, alcohol, and water extracts of turmeric rhizomes to antiinflammatory drugs in current usage (sodium salicylate, hydrocortisone, oxyphenbutazone, and indomethacin).[1349] All extracts and compounds were given as intraperitoneal injections to rats. Various doses of each substance were administered and ED_{50} doses calculated.

In the carrageenin-induced paw edema model, all turmeric extracts showed antiinflammatory activity, although curcumin and the water extract were most effective.[1349] Potencies of curcumin (ED_{50} = 8.7 mg/kg at 4 h) and water extract (ED_{50} = 4.7 mg/kg) were similar to indomethacin (5 mg/kg). The granuloma pouch method illustrated effective doses of turmeric extracts at doses similar to antiinflammatory drugs. Cotton pellet granuloma formation was likewise significantly inhibited by curcumin, all turmeric extracts, and drugs at comparable doses. As indicated by these results, petroleum ether and water extracts of turmeric exhibited maximum antiinflammatory activities during the prostaglandin-mediated phase of inflammation, while the alcohol extract showed maximum inhibition during the histamine-mediated phases.[1349] Effective doses of each substance are listed in Table 5.

In 1982, Rao and others from the Department of Pharmacology at the All-India Institute of Medical Sciences in New Delhi, India reported on antiinflammatory activities of sodium curcuminate and naturally occurring curcumin analogs (curcuminoids).[1350] Carrageenin-induced paw edema in rats was significantly inhibited by all curcuminoids at oral doses up to 30 mg/kg, although, at higher doses, less inhibition was found, indicating a biphasic antiinflammatory response. This suggests that some doses of curcumin may act as a counter-irritant. The analog 4-hydroxyferuloyl methane exhibited greater

TABLE 6   Comparative Effectiveness of Curcumin and Its Analogs on Carrageenin-Induced Rat Paw Edema

Substance	ED_{50} (p.o. mg/kg)
Phenylbutazone	45, 48, 48
Curcumin	36, 48
Sodium curcuminate	17, 19
Feruloyl, 4-hydroxycinnamoyl methane	9
Bis (4-hydroxycinnamoyl) methane	—[a]
Tetrahydrocurcumin	20
Triethylcurcumin	—[b]
Diacetylcurcumin	—[c]

[a] Doses of 30 mg/kg produced a 35% inhibition of paw edema, but higher doses resulted in no inhibition. Therefore, an ED_{50} was never reached.

[b] Doses of 10 mg/kg produced a 43% inhibition of paw edema, but higher doses resulted in no inhibition or increased edema.

[c] Doses of 3 mg/kg produced a 17% inhibition of paw edema, but higher doses resulted in no inhibition or increased edema.

antiinflammatory activity than curcumin. Antiinflammatory activity of curcuminoids was comparable to or better than phenylbutazone. Table 6 lists the ED_{50} doses for the compounds tested.

Sodium curcuminate exhibited dose-dependent inhibitions of contractions of isolated guinea pig ileum induced by nicotine, acetylcholine, serotonin, and barium chloride.[1350] ED_{50} values ranged from 3.0 μg/ml for nicotine to 17 μg/ml for barium chloride. Also, sodium curcuminate exhibited dose-dependent decreases in isolated rabbit intestine tone and pendular movements. These results suggest that curcumin decreased prostaglandin biosynthesis, similar to known NSAIDs.[1351]

Another series of experiments reported in 1982 by Mukhopadhay and others from the Department of Pharmacology at the All-India Institute of Medical Sciences in New Delhi, India examined curcumin and semisynthetic analogs in an attempt to find more potent antiinflammatory compounds.[1352] Ferulic acid, curcumin, sodium curcuminate, diacetylcurcumin, triethylcurcumin, and tetrahydrocurcumin were compared to phenylbutazone for antiinflammatory activities in rats using the carrageenin-induced paw edema and cotton pellet granuloma formation models of inflammation. All compounds were administered by mouth in aqueous suspensions of 1% gum acacia (except for sodium curcuminate, which was simply dissolved in water).

In the carrageenin-induced paw edema experiments, ferulic acid and diacetylcurcumin showed an increased inflammatory reaction over controls, while curcumin and other analogs showed dose-dependent increases in inhibition of edema followed by lack of inhibition at higher doses, similar to findings of Rao[1350] from naturally occurring curcuminoids.[1352] The ED_{50} values are listed in Table 6. It can be seen that curcumin and sodium curcuminate are more effective than phenylbutazone at equivalent doses by weight. For both curcumin and sodium curcuminate, maximum inhibition of paw edema was 67% at doses of 60 and 30 mg/kg, respectively, whereas this level of inhibition was not reached by phenylbutazone until 70 mg/kg was reached. However, higher doses of curcumin and sodium curcuminate exhibited less inhibition, while phenylbutazone showed further inhibition at higher doses. Curcumin, sodium curcuminate, diacetylcurcumin, and phenylbutazone showed similar effectiveness for reduction of cotton pellet granuloma formation, while triethylcurcumin showed the greatest reductions.[1352] Ferulic acid and tetrahydrocurcumin were ineffective.

When curcumin and sodium curcuminate were administered simultaneously with carrageenin or cotton pellets to assess their irritant activity, the same pattern as oral administration was seen, indicating that both antiinflammatory and local irritant activities compete at higher doses.[1352] In other experiments, intravenous sodium curcuminate did not affect plasma cortisol levels in dogs and did not replace effects of hydrocortisone on carrageenin-induced paw edema in adrenalectomized rats.[1352] Thus, curcumin did not mimic or affect corticosteroid function.

Curcumin and sodium curcuminate were tested in the acetic acid-induced writhing test in mice and showed no analgesic effects, while phenylbutazone showed significant analgesic activity.[1352] Fever induced by subcutaneous injection of dried yeast into rats was not affected by sodium curcuminate. Aggregation of platelets by ADP, epinephrine, or collagen in platelet-rich human plasma was not affected by sodium curcuminate *in vitro* at doses up to 0.1 mM.[1352] These series of studies indicated that the mechanism of action for curcumin is not identical to NSAIDs, i.e., inhibition of prostaglandins may not be a central mechanism for antiinflammatory effects of curcumin.

In 1985, Srivastava and Srimal, from the Division of Pharmacology at the Central Drug Research Institute, Lucknow, India, attempted to further elucidate the mechanism for antiinflammatory effects of curcumin by comparison with ibuprofen, an NSAID with known antiinflammatory activity and known mechanisms.[1353] The effects of oral doses of curcumin on uncoupling of oxidative phosphorylation, stabilization of lysosomal membranes, release of adrenal steroid hormones, and inhibition of prostaglandin biosynthesis (known mechanisms of NSAIDs) were measured in rats. Ibuprofen was 10 times more effective by weight than curcumin at reduction of granuloma formation in the granuloma pouch and sponge pellet models (200 mg/kg of curcumin was equipotent to 20 mg/kg of ibuprofen). Acid phosphatase and cathepsin-D enzyme activities in livers and granuloma tissues of these rats were both reduced by curcumin and ibuprofen. Lysosomal integrity was maintained to a greater degree by curcumin than ibuprofen at doses up to 1 mM. Likewise, inhibition of lysosomal β-glucuronidase activity was inhibited by curcumin at high doses, but not by ibuprofen. Both curcumin and ibuprofen elevated ATPase activity in liver and granuloma tissues, with ibuprofen being 10 times more effective than curcumin.

Administration of curcumin or ibuprofen for 6 d to rats with granuloma pouches normalized elevated adrenal cholesterol levels, but did not affect adrenal ascorbate levels.[1353] However, plasma cortisol was greatly increased by curcumin treatment (29.4 compared to 8.2 nM at 200 mg curcumin per kg) in rats with granuloma pouches. Normal rats showed a plasma cortisol level of 15.7 nM, and ibuprofen-treated, inflamed rats had plasma cortisol levels of 13.8 mM. Both curcumin and ibuprofen treatment reduced PGE_2-like activity in pouch granuloma inflammatory exudates by half. Both curcumin and ibuprofen caused complete inhibition of spontaneous contractions of isolated pregnant rat uterus. All these results suggested that a possible mechanism for antiinflammatory action of curcumin may include the following: (1) stabilization of lysosomal membranes, (2) release of endogenous corticosteroids, (3) uncoupling of oxidative phosphorylation, and (4) weak inhibition of prostaglandin biosynthesis. Thus, curcumin showed some similarities and differences from NSAIDs in the mechanism of antiinflammatory action. Curcumin was less potent by weight than ibuprofen. Nevertheless, curcumin possessed significant antiinflammatory actions, some of which could possibly be explained by antioxidant activity.[1353]

Curcumin was screened for its activity as a prostaglandin biosynthesis inhibitor as reported in 1986 by Wagner and others from the Institute of Biologic Pharmacology at the University of Munich in Munich, Germany.[1354] Addition of curcumin to an *in vitro* system of cyclooxygenase from sheep seminal vesicles followed by HPLC separation of arachidonic acid metabolites led to inhibition of prostaglandin biosynthesis. Other essential oils and phenolic compounds (eugenol, thymol, carvacrol, urushiol, and capsaicin) with biochemical properties (both antiinflammatory and irritant attributes) similar to curcumin also showed inhibition of prostaglandin biosynthesis. This study provided further evidence that curcumin may inhibit prostaglandin synthesis, which is a major mechanism of action for aspirin and NSAIDs.

D. HUMAN STUDIES

1. Rheumatoid Arthritis

The Rheumatology Clinic of the Central Drug Research Institute in Lucknow, India has been assessing the antirheumatic activity of indigenous herbs. Deodhar and others reported on a preliminary,

TABLE 7   Effects of Curcumin (1200 Mg Daily) and Phenylbutazone (300 Mg Daily) on Rheumatoid Arthritis Symptoms

		Mean ± SE	
Measurement	Baseline	Curcumin	Phenylbutazone
Observer assessment[a]	3.8 ± 0.2	3.4 ± 0.1[b]	3.1 ± 0.2[b]
Patient assessment[a]	4.2 ± 0.2	3.9 ± 0.3[b]	3.3 ± 0.2[b]
Time to fatigue (h)	3.8 ± 0.6	3.9 ± 0.5	5.4 ± 0.7[b]
Morning stiffness (min)	132 ± 17	124 ± 17[b]	97 ± 17[b]
Walking time for 25 ft (s)	15.4 ± 1.2	13.8 ± 1.5[b]	12.4 ± 1.0[b]
Joint swelling	16.8 ± 3.3	12.5 ± 2.4[b]	11.2 ± 2.6[b]
Articular index	80 ± 10	76 ± 11	73 ± 10
Grip strength (mm Hg)	68 ± 7	66 ± 6	70 ± 6
Erythrocyte sedimentation rate (mm/h)	40 ± 4	46 ± 3	40 ± 5

Note: Data from Reference 1355.

[a]   5 = poor to 1 = very much better.
[b]   Significantly different ($p <0.05$) compared to baseline value.

short-term, randomized-order, double-blind, crossover study on 18 patients with definite rheumatoid arthritis.[1355] Patients (16 females and 2 males) exhibited articular symptoms an average of 39 months and were not taking corticosteroids or second-line drugs. Patients did not have peptic ulcers, hepatic dysfunction, or renal impairment, and all antiinflammatory medications were halted 4 d before baseline measurements. Clinical effects of curcumin (1200 mg total daily dose) was compared to phenylbutazone (300 mg total daily dose). Both compounds were taken in three equivalent doses per day. The length of treatment periods was not specified, but described as "short-term".

Table 7 lists the results of curcumin and phenylbutazone therapies compared to baseline values. Overall, effects of curcumin treatment were comparable to phenylbutazone treatment. Both therapies demonstrated a moderate but significant reduction in morning stiffness, time to walk 25 feet, joint swelling, and overall observer assessment. Phenylbutazone was superior for reduction of fatigue and subjective patient assessment, consistent with animal studies showing analgesic action. Neither compound affected grip strength, articular index, or erythrocyte sedimentation rates. No side effects were encountered.

These results were limited by the unspecified short duration of study, lack of dose-response data, presence of long-standing joint damage, and the previously known lack of analgesic effect for curcumin.[1348,1352] However, results suggested that curcumin possessed some antiinflammatory activity and lack of adverse effects in symptomatic rheumatoid arthritis. Longer treatment times or higher doses of curcumin deserve further study as antiinflammatory therapy for rheumatoid arthritis.

2. Postsurgery Healing

The Departments of Surgery, Pharmacology, and Clinical Pharmacology of Seth G. S. Medical College in Bombay, India conducted a placebo-controlled, randomized-order, double-blind study on antiinflammatory effects of placebo, curcumin, or phenylbutazone after surgery for inguinal hernia repair and/or hydrocele.[1356] There were 40 male patients (15 to 68 years) operated on and given either placebo (750 mg total daily dose of lactose), curcumin (1200 mg total daily dose), or phenylbutazone (300 mg total daily dose) in three equivalent doses per day for a period of 5 d from the first postsurgical day. All patients were given 500 mg q.i.d. Ampicillin and no other drugs.

Evaluations of spermatic cord edema, spermatic cord tenderness, surgical site pain, and surgical site tenderness were made by calculating total intensity scores (0 to 12 possible points) from grading symptoms on a scale from 0 to 3 (0 = absent; 1 = mild; 2 = moderate; 3 = severe). Table 8 lists the reduction in total intensity score for each treatment group. Curcumin was effective in reducing all four parameters of postsurgical inflammation, while phenylbutazone was effective in all but wound site

Table 8   Reduction in assessment of spermatic cord and wound site pain and tenderness between day 1 and day 6 postsurgery by placebo, curcumin (1200 mg/d), or phenylbutazone (300 mg/d)

Treatment Group	Reduction in Total Intensity Score (TIS)[a]			
	Mean ± SE	% Reduction	d1 TIS	d6 TIS
Placebo (n = 13)	1.0 ± 0.8	62	2.6	1.0
Curcumin (n = 13)	2.4 ± 0.6[b]	84[b]	3.9	0.6
Phenylbutazone (n = 14)	1.6 ± 0.6[c]	86[c]	2.1	0.3

Note: Date from Reference 1356.

[a] Total intensity score (TIS) was assessed from the following scale: 0 = absent; 1 = mild; 2 = moderate; 3 = severe. Initial TIS for the curcumin group was significantly greater than both placebo and phenylbutazone group initial TIS values.
[b] Significant difference ($p < 0.01$) between d6 value and d1 value.
[c] Significant difference ($p < 0.05$) between d6 value and d1 value.

tenderness. Placebo was effective in reducing wound site pain and cord tenderness. Curcumin reduced cord edema and cord tenderness significantly better compared to placebo and phenylbutazone. Phenylbutazone was better at reducing wound site pain than placebo or curcumin. No side effects were observed during the study period.

Thus, curcumin was shown to possess significant antiinflammatory activity following minor surgery in humans. This study was limited by the subjective nature of pain and tenderness assessments. In fact, the authors reported that in an earlier, unpublished study on 60 women with episiotomy pain, there was no significant difference between placebo, curcumin, or phenylbutazone.[1356] Once again, curcumin did not demonstrate analgesic properties. However, estimation of cord edema was less subjective than parameters of pain and tenderness. Since curcumin showed significant reduction of cord edema, some valid antiinflammatory properties of curcumin were found in humans at a daily dose of 1200 mg/d.

E. SUMMARY

Curcumin, the major active principle in turmeric, has exhibited potent antiinflammatory properties in animal models and two human studies. In direct comparisons to NSAIDs, curcumin possessed similar antiinflammatory effects in two human studies. However, curcumin did not exhibit analgesic properties in any setting. Doses of curcumin were four times the weight of NSAIDs, but still within safety and tolerance limits. In many hundreds of years of use as a spice and herbal medicine, there have been no reports of turmeric or curcumin toxicity in humans. Thus, curcumin appears to be safe for human consumption, at least for short time intervals, at relatively high doses of 1 to 2 g daily. In addition, curcumin has exhibited potent antioxidant properties,[1357-1364] antimutagenic or anticarcinogenic properties in animals,[1365-1368] and anti-platelet aggregatory properties,[1369] indicating the potential usefulness and broad application potential of curcumin. Curcumin may represent an alternative to NSAID therapy in those patients known to be sensitive to NSAID side effects. Curcumin deserves further study for specific effects on healing of sports injuries.

Chapter 14

NUTRIENTS APPLIED TO INJURY
REHABILITATION AND SPORTS MEDICINE

The preceding chapters of this book have dealt with individual nutrients and their effects on aspects of musculoskeletal healing. This chapter will attempt to put the findings from previous chapters to practical application. It is exceedingly difficult to beneficially alter a complex and dynamic system by modulation of a single component. When modulation of several components in a rational manner is accomplished, then consistent results are more likely to be attained. This rationale is the basis for the suggestions described in this chapter. Nutritional protocols will be given for acute injuries and chronic conditions. This book represents the first attempt to combine research and clinical evidence on the effects of nutrients on healing with application of logical nutrient combinations on sports injuries. Guidelines for practical clinical application are presented, which may seem controversial to some and helpful to others. In any case, the guidelines presented in this chapter offer a starting point for further research and application of comprehensive nutritional protocols in musculoskeletal healing.

I. GENERAL DIETARY GUIDELINES

A. DIETARY GUIDELINES

Table 1 lists general dietary guidelines incorporated from the chapters discussing total calories, protein, and fats. Making certain that sufficient calories are consumed is critical for proper healing and recovery; however, dietary goals should stress provision of high quality calories rather than merely high quantity. In this way, excess body fat during inactivity, which is not desirable for most athletes, will be easier to avoid. Simply substituting "whole" foods for "junk" foods can greatly improve micronutrient density of the diet. Shifting fat intakes from the usual American consumption of high intakes of potentially oxidized fats to fats known to provide precursors for antiinflammatory eicosanoids is another dietary goal.

B. DIETARY SUPPLEMENTATION
1. Comprehensive Dietary Supplements

In making suggestions and guidelines for nutrient intake, dietary supplementation is frequently involved in order to administer known amounts of nutrients, rather than depend upon variable food contents and intakes. There are two basic types of dietary supplements which concern this chapter: (1) comprehensive dietary supplements that can replace foods; and (2) specific combinations of micronutrients with little or no caloric value. Comprehensive dietary supplements usually consist of protein, carbohydrates, and perhaps fats (either whole foodstuffs or, more frequently, isolated from foodstuffs), along with combinations of vitamins, minerals, and other nutrients. Examples of comprehensive dietary supplements include Ensure®, Sustacal®, Exceed®, Isocal®, Resource®, Nutren®, Replete®, Entrition®, and other similar products that are available in grocery stores in some areas of the country. Pharmacies are another source for comprehensive dietary supplements and may be able to order specific products. Health food stores, gyms, and fitness centers also offer many such products in both liquid and powder forms. Indeed, it is difficult not to find comprehensive dietary supplements, as many designed for weight

TABLE 1   General Dietary Goals During Musculoskeletal Healing

1. Maintain adequate caloric intake (at least 35 kcal/kg/d); more calories may be necessary if injury is severe.
2. Decrease or remove "junk" foods (highly refined or processed foods) from the diet.
3. Replace "junk" foods with "whole" foods (fresh fruits, fresh vegetables, whole grains).
4. Avoid fried foods, greasy foods, or excess use of fat condiments (butter, margarine, gravies, mayonnaise, cream cheese, salad dressings, cheeses); exceptions for high fat foods include use of foods rich in medium-chain triglycerides (coconuts, coconut milk, unhydrogenated coconut oil, palm kernel oil).
5. Substitute fish, poultry, extra lean cuts of red meat, eggs, or nonfat dairy products for fatty red meats (hamburger, hot dogs, many luncheon meats, sausages, bacon, steaks, most pork cuts).
6. Maintain protein intake of 1.0–1.5 g/kg/d (70–100 g protein daily for 70-kg [150-pound] person).

loss may be excellent supplements when combined with meals. For listings of specific pharmaceutical comprehensive dietary supplements used mostly in hospital or home health care settings, the reader is referred to several reviews.[7,168-170] Some of the pharmaceutical companies that offer a variety of comprehensive dietary supplements include Baxter-Travenol, Kendall-McGaw, Mead-Johnson, Ross Laboratories, Sandoz, and other companies.

Comprehensive dietary supplements are excellent sources of protein, carbohydrate, and fat, but many do not contain sufficient amounts of micronutrients (usually vitamins, specific amino acids, specific fats, antioxidant vitamins, proteases, bioflavonoids, or curcumin) to meet the guidelines listed in this chapter. Therefore, comprehensive dietary supplements should be considered equivalent to foodstuffs, and either substituted for undesirable foods (see Table 1) or be added to usual food intakes. Most comprehensive dietary supplements fit the guidelines listed in Table 1. Another advantage of comprehensive dietary supplements is that their nutrient content is clearly listed on the label. Thus, an individual knows exactly which nutrients and how much of each nutrient are ingested. This allows for more accurate determination of nutrient intake when desired.

2. Specific Dietary Supplements

Specific dietary supplements are more commonly known as vitamin pills. The genre has become quite sophisticated, and grocery stores, pharmacies, health food stores, gyms, fitness centers, some physicians' offices, and numerous mail-order companies are sources for finding specific dietary supplements. These products supply purified proteins, amino acid mixtures, single amino acids, specific fats (n3 fatty acids or MCTs), vitamins in almost any conceivable combination, minerals in mixtures or singly, antioxidants alone or in combination, proteases, bioflavonoids and curcumin, and combinations of specific micronutrients. These products usually have little or no caloric value and are designed to provide supplemental amounts of specific dietary components. In other words, one cannot live on pills alone. The advantage of specific dietary supplements is control over dosage of individual nutrients. This allows for safe dosing and prevention of overdosing.

It is not the position of this book to recommend specific products, brands, or companies. The nutrients and nutrient combinations listed in this chapter are definitely available from many sources. Exact matches of products to guidelines may not be immediately found. As long as the critical points of each guideline are followed, exact compliance with the listed numbers is not absolutely necessary. In other words, close enough is good enough.

II. ACUTE INJURIES

In general, acute traumatic injuries comprise the majority of sports injuries. Most are not severe enough to trigger adverse metabolic consequences; however, most are severe enough to limit physical function, training, and competition. The desire to return to full function must be carefully balanced with healing rate to prevent reinjury. Most acute sports injuries will heal without intervention. Is there an advantage to modulating nutrient intake for healing of acute injuries? Research has consistently shown that specific nutrients can accelerate healing rates and shorten recovery to full function for sports injuries (proteases in particular). Other nutrients play supporting roles that are not as conclusive as proteases, but may offer additional benefits to health. From the research findings to date, when acceleration of healing was reported, the healing appeared to be normal and not an artificial situation. Thus, the quicker recovery produced normal tissue function after healing.

In comprehensive protocols, several nutrient combinations keep reappearing. Nutrient combinations with uses for multiple types of injuries include (1) multiple vitamin/minerals, (2) multiple antioxidants, and (3) multiple proteases. Therefore, Tables 2 to 4 list ideal formulas for each type of nutrient combination. For the multiple vitamin/mineral mixture, the different categories of B vitamins, minerals, and fat-soluble vitamins have been considered as separate units. This allows flexibility to reduce overlap between multiple vitamin/mineral products and antioxidant mixtures, which share β-carotene, vitamin E, vitamin C, and selenium.

For each condition, key nutrients which have shown greatest or best-studied benefits are listed first. Optional or more speculative nutrients are listed next. Refer to Tables 2 to 4 for contents of multiple vitamin/mineral mixtures, antioxidant mixtures, or protease mixtures. Whenever possible, overlap of nutrients has been reduced. Some conditions may require different key nutrients during different phases of healing. Thus, some key nutrients may change from inflammatory to repair to remodeling phases of healing. These time periods are indicated in each table describing nutrient protocols for each condition.

A. SPRAINS AND DISLOCATIONS[9-11,18,155-157]

Sprain is a generic term for acute joint trauma after joint movement was forced beyond normal limits. Injury involves joint structures (tendons, ligaments, cartilage, synovium, sheaths) with or without

TABLE 2 Ideal Multiple Vitamin/Mineral Formula for Musculoskeletal Healing

Fat-Soluble Vitamins	**Daily Dose**
Vitamin A (as retinyl palmitate)	5,000 IU (1000 RE or 2.7 mg)
β-carotene	5,000–25,000 IU
Vitamin D (cholecalciferol)	100–400 IU
Vitamin E (d-α-tocopherol)	100–400 IU (67–268 mg)

B Complex Vitamins	
Vitamin B_1 (thiamin)	100 mg
Vitamin B_2 (riboflavin)	50 mg
Vitamin B_3 (niacinamide)	20–100 mg
Vitamin B_6 (pyridoxine)	10–50 mg
Vitamin B_{12} (cyanocobalamin)	0.1 mg
Folic acid	0.4 mg
Pantothenate	100 mg
Biotin	0.1–0.3 mg

Vitamin C (ascorbate)	100–500 mg

Minerals	
Calcium (as citrate, citrate-malate, etc.)	200–500 mg
Magnesium (as oxide, citrate, glycinate, etc.)	200–500 mg
Iron	Not indicated
Zinc (as methionate, citrate, picolinate, etc.)	15 mg
Manganese (as ascorbate, gluconate, etc.)	5–15 mg
Copper (as histidinate, gluconate, etc.)	2–5 mg
Chromium (as polynicotinate or picolinate)	50–250 µg
Selenium (as selenite or selenomethionine)	50–250 µg
Boron (as borate)	3 mg
Iodine	Not indicated
Optional minerals: molybdenum, vanadium, germanium.	

Note: Amounts listed are for total daily supplemental intake. With most products, this means taking more than one unit (tablet, capsule, or powder) daily. In this case, multiple units should be taken in divided doses with meals.

TABLE 3 Ideal Antioxidant Mixture

Key Antioxidants	Daily Dose
β-Carotene	25,000–250,000 IU
Vitamin E (*d*-α-tocopherol or mixed tocopherols) (*d*-α-tocopheryl succinate or acetate)	400–800 IU (400–800 mg)
Vitamin C (ascorbic acid, mineral ascorbates)	1000–5000 mg
Selenium (1:1 ratio from selenite, selenomethionine)	100–300 µg
Cysteine (*N*-acetyl-L-cysteine)	500–2000 mg

Additional Antioxidants	
Bioflavonoids (citrus, catechins, silymarins)	500–2000 mg
Coenzyme Q_{10} (Ubiquinone)	10–200 mg
Taurine	500–4000 mg
L-Methionine	500–2000 mg
Curcumin	100–1000 mg
Rosemary or sage extracts	100–1000 mg
Ferulic acid or gamma oryzanol	100–1000 mg
Garlic	100–1000 mg
Proanthocyanidins	50–500 mg

Note: Amounts listed are for total daily supplemental intake. With most products, this means taking more than one unit (tablet, capsule, or powder) daily. In this case, multiple units should be taken in divided doses with meals. In most cases, more vitamin C is required than can be put into an antioxidant mixture product; therefore, vitamin C can be taken separately, and the amount of vitamin C in an antioxidant mixture does not have to meet the amounts listed.

TABLE 4 Ideal Protease (Proteolytic Enzymes) Mixture

Enzyme	Total Daily Dose (mg)
Pancreatin	1000–4000
Trypsin/chymotrypsin	500–1000
Bromelain	500–2000
Papain	500–1000
±Fungal proteases	500–2000

Note: Since proteases are reported in a wide variety of units that have limited relativity to protease activity, daily doses are given in mg of purified enzyme. Protease products are to be taken on an empty stomach (30 min before meals) four times daily. More frequent dosing is possible, but difficult to achieve in practice. Given the measured activity of protease products, 4 to 10 tablets per dose should be taken to ensure absorption of activity. Protease supplementation should be started as soon after injury as possible (or 6 to 12 h before a known event), and continued for at least 3 d, and up to 1 week.

bleeding. Usually, ligaments are stretched or torn, with varying grades of severity and joint laxity. Pain, tenderness, swelling, ecchymoses, joint instability, and inability to use joint or extremity affected are characteristic signs of sprains. Thus, sprains represent acute inflammation. The nutrient protocol for sprains, dislocations, and other acute joint trauma is listed in Table 5. In general, the most effective nutrients of resolution of acute inflammation are proteases, bioflavonoids, curcumin, and perhaps ascorbates. Other nutrients have hypothetical benefits, but insufficient clinical data to be key nutrients.

Dislocations represent an extreme case of sprain, where disruption of the mechanical structure of the joint occurs, and bone ends are no longer in contact. Fractures of bone surrounding the joint may also be present, and ligaments are usually torn. For dislocations, during the second phase of healing

TABLE 5   Nutrient Protocols for Acute Joint Trauma: Sprains, Strains, Dislocations

PHASE 1: Start as soon as possible after injury, continue for 1 week.

Key Nutrients	Daily Doses
Protease mixture	4–10 units q.i.d. empty stomach
Vitamin C (ascorbate)	4000 mg (1000 mg q.i.d.)
Bioflavonoids (citrus)	2000 mg (500 mg q.i.d.)
Curcumin	2000 mg (500 mg q.i.d.)

Optional Nutrients	
Multiple vitamin/mineral mixture	See Table 2
Antioxidant mixture	See Table 3

PHASE 2: If extensive joint damage has occurred, and healing has not progressed by 1 week postinjury, then the following protocol can be started at 1 week postinjury, and continued until adequate healing has occurred.

Key Nutrients	
Vitamin C (ascorbates)	4000 mg (1000 mg q.i.d.)
Bioflavonoids	2000 mg (500 mg q.i.d.)
Vitamin B_1 (thiamin)	1000 mg (500 mg b.i.d.)
Pantothenate	2000 mg (500 mg q.i.d.)
Multiple vitamin/mineral	See Table 2

Additional Nutrients	
Glucosamine salts	2000 mg (500 mg q.i.d.)
Chondroitin sulfates	2000 mg (500 mg q.i.d.)
Antioxidant mixture	See Table 3

(after 1 week), glucosamine salts and chondroitin sulfates become key nutrients. Nutrient supplementation may have to be extended for dislocations, depending on severity.

B. STRAINS (MUSCLE PULLS)[9-11,18,155-157]

Strains result from sudden overload of musculotendinous units, causing tears or ruptures in muscle fibers and tendon attachments. Strains are an acute inflammatory event and are characterized by pain, muscle spasms, loss of strength, and loss of function. See Table 5 for the nutrient protocol for strains, which are shared with sprains.

C. BRUISES, HEMATOMAS, CONTUSIONS, ECCHYMOSES[9-11,18,155-157]

Bleeding in soft tissues is caused by blunt trauma which crushes tissues and blood vessels beneath the skin. Blood leaking from damaged vessels forms a lump (hematoma) or discolors the skin (ecchymosis). Bruises may accompany other musculoskeletal trauma, such as sprains, strains, or fractures. Table 6 describes the nutrient protocol for bruising and bleeding in soft tissues.

D. LIGAMENT AND TENDON TEARS[9-11,18,155-157]

Some acute traumatic injuries, especially in contact sports, involve mostly the partial or complete tear of ligaments around joints (particularly the knee joint). Sometimes, tendons may detach from bone or joint capsules (an extreme case of a strain). Such injuries have poorer prognosis of complete functional recovery than other acute traumatic injuries, and surgery is often required to repair, reattach, or remove damaged components. Nutrients may assist tendon and ligament healing by reducing inflammation and resulting adhesions, and by providing precursors for matrix biosynthesis. Table 7 lists the nutrient protocol for ligament and tendon tears.

TABLE 6   Nutrient Protocols for Acute Trauma: Bruises, Hematomas, Contusions, Ecchymoses

PHASE 1: Start as soon as possible after injury, continue for 1 week.

Key Nutrients	Daily Dose
Protease mixture	4–10 units q.i.d. empty stomach
Vitamin C (ascorbate)	4000 mg (1000 mg q.i.d.)
Bioflavonoids (citrus)	2000 mg (500 mg q.i.d.)
Antioxidant mixture	See Table 3

Additional Nutrients

Multiple vitamin/mineral mixture	See Table 2

TABLE 7   Nutrient Protocols for Acute Trauma: Ligament and Tendon Tears

PHASE 1: Start as soon as possible after injury, continue for 1 week.

Key Nutrients	Daily Dose
Protease mixture	4–10 units q.i.d. empty stomach
Vitamin C (ascorbate)	4000 mg (1000 mg q.i.d.)
Bioflavonoids (citrus)	2000 mg (500 mg q.i.d.)
Antioxidant mixture	See Table 3
Glucosamine salts	2000 mg (500 mg q.i.d.)
Chondroitin sulfates	2000 mg (500 mg q.i.d.)

Additional Nutrients

Multiple vitamin/mineral mixture	See Table 2
Vitamin B$_1$ (thiamin)	1000 mg (500 mg b.i.d.)
Pantothenate	2000 mg (500 mg q.i.d.)

PHASE 2: After 1 week, repair and remodeling phases may last for long time periods (1–2 years); continued supplementation with glucosamine and chondroitin sulfates is suggested to assist in remodeling.

E.   FRACTURES[9-11,18,155-157]

Fractures are a break in bone continuity caused by excessive forces applied to bones. Fractures range in severity from small cracks to complete breakage of bone (closed compound) with protrusion from skin (open compound). Cracks may be small and localized, or extensive and spiral-shaped (greenstick). Epiphyseal fractures involve crushing, cracking, or breaking the epiphyseal growth plate in young persons. Fractures usually involve bleeding and are an acute inflammatory event. However, the special dietary needs of bones add other nutrients into the key category, especially during callus formation. Also, with more severe fractures, adverse metabolic consequences may arise. For a more extensive description of bone healing, see Chapter 1. Table 8 lists nutrient protocols for fracture healing.

F.   LACERATIONS, ABRASIONS, SURGICAL WOUNDS, SKIN DAMAGE[9-11,18,155-157]

Skin is frequently damaged by athletic activities. Surgery is intentional skin wounding. Healing from both processes is similar and well studied (see Chapter 1). Skin has some unique nutritional needs, including vitamin A (retinols) and zinc, that have been documented as helpful in many conditions of skin healing. Table 9 lists nutrient protocols for healing of skin damage, regardless of cause.

TABLE 8 Nutrient Protocols for Acute Trauma: Bone Fractures

PHASE 1: Administer the following supplements as soon after injury as possible and until soft callus forms (2–3 weeks).

Key Nutrients	Daily Dose
Protease mixture	4–10 units q.i.d. empty stomach
Multiple vitamin/mineral mixture	See Table 2
Vitamin C (ascorbate)	4000 mg (1000 mg q.i.d.)
Bioflavonoids (citrus)	2000 mg (500 mg q.i.d.)
Antioxidant mixture	See Table 3
Glucosamine salts	2000 mg (500 mg q.i.d.)
Chondroitin sulfates	2000 mg (500 mg q.i.d.)

Additional Nutrients (especially if adverse metabolic changes are noticed)

Arginine	10 g (in 3 daily doses)
Ornithine-α-ketoglutarate (OKG)	10 g (5 g b.i.d.)

PHASE 2: Administer during soft and hard callus formation (2–8 weeks postinjury).

Key Nutrients	Daily Dose
Multiple vitamin/mineral mixture	See Table 2
Vitamin C (ascorbate)	4000 mg (1000 mg q.i.d.)
Antioxidant mixture	See Table 3
Glucosamine salts	2000 mg (500 mg q.i.d.)
Chondroitin sulfates	2000 mg (500 mg q.i.d.)

PHASE 3: After callus recedes, remodeling still occurs.

Multiple vitamin/mineral mixture	See Table 2

Note: With severe fractures, increase dietary caloric intake by 1.5 times for 4–6 weeks. Decrease dietary fat and increase dietary carbohydrates and proteins to prevent accumulation of excess body weight during inactivity.

III. CHRONIC INJURIES AND CONDITIONS

Chronic injuries may result from previous acute injuries that did not resolve completely, or from repetitive, overuse scenarios. Chronic inflammation may be apparent for long time periods and is characterized by slow onset and gradual loss of functions. Other factors (age, tissue, blood supply) frequently impact chronic injuries adversely. Nutrient administration has the primary goal of enhancing or stimulating normal repair of injured tissues. Secondly, modulation of chronic inflammatory processes is sought, since chronic conditions may take longer to resolve than acute injuries. Modulation of inflammatory processes can occur by protection of tissues or direct effects on inflammatory cells or mediators. Thus, while there is much overlap with specific nutrients used for acute injuries, other nutrients become key for chronic injuries.

A. DEGENERATIVE JOINT CONDITIONS

"The changes in cartilage occurring with aging and disease are primarily due to changes in nutrition."[1370] This statement was published in 1961 in a pathology textbook. What was apparent to pathologists then has still not become widely practiced at present. Degenerative joint conditions have many forms, but the predominant form is osteoarthritis of articular joints.[45,549,1371-1378] Osteoarthritis has the highest incidence of all diseases, with almost universal occurrence after 50 years of age, although all cases are not severe and some are not noticeable. Over 5 million Americans per year are disabled

TABLE 9 Nutrient Protocols for Acute Trauma: Lacerations, Surgical Wounds, Abrasions, Skin Damage

PHASE 1: Start as soon as possible after injury, continue for 1 week.

Key Nutrients	Daily Dose
Protease mixture	4–10 units q.i.d. empty stomach
Vitamin C (ascorbate)	4,000 mg (1,000 mg q.i.d.)
Bioflavonoids (citrus)	2,000 mg (500 mg q.i.d.)
Antioxidant mixture	See Table 3
Curcumin	2,000 mg (500 mg q.i.d.)
Vitamin A (retinols)	25,000 IU (single dose)
Zinc	50 mg (1 or 2 doses daily)

PHASE 2: Administer the following nutrients starting 1 week after injury until healing or scarring is complete.

Multiple vitamin/mineral mixture	See Table 2
Antioxidant mixture	See Table 3

by osteoarthritis, along with millions more from invertebral disc disease and other degenerative joint conditions. Osteoarthritis has long been thought of as irreversible and progressive to the point of disability and need for joint replacement.[1370-1378] However, there is substantial evidence that osteoarthritis can be reversed.[1379-1381] For example, juvenile chronic arthritis can be halted by long-term, intense physical therapy and drugs. Chronic passive joint mobilization has reversed osteoarthritis in animals. Redistribution of joint loads by surgical techniques, polio, paralysis, and strokes has led to cessation of arthritic progression. The proper types of electrical and mechanical stimulation of chondrocytes are under investigation. Chondroprotective agents described in Chapter 12 were associated with reversal of osteoarthritis in some studies. All told, cartilage has the innate ability to repair itself if given the correct conditions and time. Table 10 lists the nutrients with chondroprotective abilities found in human trials. Their combined usage has not been investigated yet, but each works via different mechanisms of action. The use of chondroprotective nutrients with physical therapy and rational drug therapy augers well for the future of degenerative joint disease treatment.

Other degenerative joint diseases share similar characteristics with osteoarthritis. Invertebral disc disease, chondromalacia patellae, and results of previous joint trauma all have similar mechanisms and therapies to osteoarthritis. Thus, the guidelines in Table 10 are applicable to all forms of degenerative joint conditions.

B. RHEUMATOID ARTHRITIS

Another common musculoskeletal condition is rheumatoid arthritis. Unlike osteoarthritis, there is definite evidence of immune system involvement, cytokine involvement, and severe joint inflammation in rheumatoid arthritis.[424] Nutrient roles in rheumatoid arthritis include modulation of inflammation by eicosanoid precursor supply, effects on immune system cells, chondroprotection for damaged joints, and antiinflammatory effects of nutrients. Table 11 lists the nutrients with these properties.

C. CONNECTIVE TISSUE INFLAMMATIONS (TENDINITIS, BURSITIS, TENOSYNOVITIS, CARPAL TUNNEL SYNDROME)

A large number of conditions commonly seen in sports medicine practices are chronic overuse injuries resulting in limb or joint pain and dysfunction.[9-11,18,155-157] These conditions are inflammatory in nature and chronic. Included are bursitis (inflammation of bursae), tendinitis, paratenonitis, tendinosis, peritendinitis, tenosynovitis, metatarsalgia, fibrositis, fibromyalgia, and other chronic inflammations of

TABLE 10   Nutrient Protocols for Chronic Injuries: Degenerative Joint Conditions (Osteoarthritis, Chondromalacia, Invertebral Disc Disease)

Key Nutrients	Daily Dose
Niacinamide	250 mg every 3–4 h (see Table 5 in Chapter 6)
Antioxidant mixture	See Table 3
Glucosamine salts	2000 mg (500 mg q.i.d.)
Chondroitin sulfates	2000 mg (500 mg q.i.d.)
S-Adenosyl methionine (SAM)	1500 mg (500 mg t.i.d.)
Multiple vitamin/mineral mixture	See Table 2
Additional Nutrients	
Vitamin C (ascorbate)	4000 mg (1000 mg q.i.d.)
Bioflavonoids (citrus)	2000 mg (500 mg q.i.d.)
Pantothenate	2000 mg (500 mg q.i.d.)

Table 11   Nutrient Protocols for Chronic Injuries: Rheumatoid Arthritis

Key Nutrients	Daily Dose
Multiple vitamin/mineral mixture	See Table 2
Pantothenate	2000 mg (500 mg q.i.d.)
Antioxidant mixture	See Table 3
Vitamin C (ascorbate)	4000 mg (1000 mg q.i.d.)
Bioflavonoids (citrus)	2000 mg (500 mg q.i.d.)
Glucosamine salts	2000 mg (500 mg q.i.d.)
Chondroitin sulfates	2000 mg (500 mg q.i.d.)
Flaxseed oil	1–2 TBSP daily
Fish oils (n3 fatty acids)	9 capsules daily (3 units t.i.d.)
GLA oil (evening primrose, borage, or blackcurrant seed)	6 capsules daily (2 t.i.d.)
Additional Nutrients	
Curcumin	1000 mg (500 mg b.i.d.)
Niacinamide	250 mg every 3–4 h (see Table 5 in Chapter 6)
Copper (histidine salt)	10 mg copper daily for 3 months
Histidine	10 g in 2 divided doses

joints structures, tendons, sheaths, etc. These syndromes are all characterized by pain, dysfunction, and inflammation. Nutrient protocols for this heading of symptoms are listed in Table 12.

D. BONE LOSS DISORDERS (OSTEOPENIA, OSTEOPOROSIS, OSTEOMALACIA, ATHLETIC AMENORRHEA)

Bone loss is the imbalance of bone resorption with bone resynthesis. Provision of adequate amounts of each essential mineral, especially magnesium, is paramount for prevention of bone loss or its reversal. Other factors include lack of estrogen, corticosteroid therapy, osteoarthritic processes, overtraining, and insufficient caloric/protein intake. Table 13 lists the nutrient protocol for bone loss disorders.

E. CHRONIC PAIN

Although chronic pain is found in many conditions, sometimes pain is not alleviated by standard analgesics in a few persons. Alternative analgesic methods are then available from nutrients. However, it must be stressed that nutrient analgesics were never completely effective and worked sufficiently well in a subset of all subjects. Nevertheless, nutrient analgesics seemed to be safe alternatives when standard analgesics had to be discontinued due to adverse side effects. Some nutrients appeared to be analgesics by virtue of pain reductions during healing. However, the nutrient effect was not strictly analgesic, but a repair of structures to the point where they no longer exhibited pain.

TABLE 12   Nutrient Protocols for Chronic Injuries: Connective Tissue Inflammations (Bursitis, Tendinitis, Synovitis, Fibrositis, Carpal Tunnel Syndrome)

PHASE 1: Reduction of inflammation may require 2–4 weeks of nutrient administration.

Key Nutrients	Daily Dose
Protease mixture	4–10 units q.i.d. empty stomach (continue for 1–2 weeks only)
Multiple vitamin/mineral mixture	See Table 2
Vitamin B_6	100 mg
Magnesium	500 mg daily in 2 divided doses
Antioxidant mixture	See Table 3
Glucosamine salts	2000 mg (500 mg q.i.d.)
Chondroitin sulfates	2000 mg (500 mg q.i.d.)

Additional Nutrients	
Vitamin C (ascorbate)	4000 mg (1000 mg q.i.d.)
Bioflavonoids (citrus)	2000 mg (500 mg q.i.d.)
Pantothenate	2000 mg (500 mg q.i.d.)
Flaxseed oil	1–2 TBSP daily
Fish oils (n3 fatty acids)	9 capsules daily (3 units t.i.d.)
GLA oil (evening primrose, borage, or black-currant seed)	6 capsules daily (2 t.i.d.)

TABLE 13   Nutrient Protocols for Chronic Injuries: Bone Loss Disorders (Osteopenia, Osteoporosis, Osteomalacia, Athletic Amenorrhea)

Key Nutrients	Daily Dose
Multiple vitamin/mineral mixture	See Table 2
Vitamin K (phylloquinones, menaquinones)	100 µg
Bone meal (microcrystalline hydroxyapatite)	4000 mg daily (1000 mg q.i.d.)

Additional Nutrients	
Silicon	1000 mg daily
Boron (as borate)	6 mg daily
Chondroitin sulfates	1000 mg (500 mg b.i.d.)

TABLE 14   Nutrient Protocols for Chronic Injuries: Chronic Pain

Key Nutrients	Daily Dose
D-Phenylalanine	2000 mg (500 mg q.i.d. on empty stomach)[a]
Vitamin B_6	100 mg
Vitamin B_1 (thiamin)	1000 mg (500 mg b.i.d.)
Pantothenate	1000 mg (500 mg b.i.d.)
Vitamin B_{12} (cyanocobalamin or cobamamide)	1.0 mg daily

Additional Nutrients	
Protease mixture	4–10 units q.i.d. empty stomach
Antioxidant mixture	See Table 3
Multiple vitamin/mineral mixture	See Table 2

[a]   Do not administer D-phenylalanine for more than 3 months.

Chapter **15**

_____ SUMMARY AND CONCLUSIONS

An extensive amount of laboratory research and clinical work has been accumulated on the therapeutic use of individual nutrients, as evidenced in the first 14 chapters. Much of this research has been performed for different specialties, such as surgical nutrition, sports medicine, rheumatology, pain management, orthopedics, and physical therapy. This book has attempted to collate the known effects of nutrients on musculoskeletal healing, in order to determine whether nutrient modulation would have a positive clinical impact on healing of injuries and procedures common to sports medicine and athletic settings.

The human body does not care whether an injury was caused by a careless slip and fall or a 250-pound linebacker. Similarly, the human body does not care if its nutrient intake is from whole foods or pills. The bottom line is that the human body will do its best to heal each injury with the biochemical, physiological, and nutritional components given to it. If the available milieu favors quicker healing, then that is what will occur. At this time, it is apparent that certain nutrients exhibit beneficial effects on healing that have a good chance to be noticed in clinical settings. For acute inflammation, proteases have well-documented effects at reducing inflammation sooner and, at the same time, enhancing the rate of recovery. While not as powerful at reducing pain as common analgesics, proteases do not defeat the body's ability to heal. Chronic injuries took considerable lengths of time to become clinically significant, and represent a failure of the body to balance synthesis and degradation. Supplying key metabolites or nutrients often has allowed the balance of synthesis and degradation to tilt in favor of synthesis, as shown by effects of glucosamine salts on osteoarthritis. Chapter 14 lists the conditions that should show some benefits even in persons with adequate nutrient intake and status (the usual situation). A new slogan for nutrients can be imagined: "Nutrients — they're not just for repleting deficiencies anymore."

However, the impression that taking certain nutrients can return any situation to normal or beyond after an injury is not true. A shotgun approach of supplying all different kinds of nutrients to the body and letting physiological wisdom sort out the actual requirements has been superseded by specific, targeted nutrient administration with doses known to affect a given system or pathway. Much good science has supported this concept.

Nutrients are not advocated in this book as replacements for drugs or other medical care. In fact, most subjects of the numerous research studies conducted on nutrient effects on healing were already receiving drugs and other medical care. Pharmaceutical companies were the primary sponsors of research on proteases. Thus, nutrition can be applied to injury rehabilitation as an adjunct to standard care. Except for the case of vitamin K supplementation interfering with anticoagulant medications (coumarin), there is no consistent evidence to show that nutrient modulation can counteract effects of pharmaceutical agents. Thus, combining drugs and nutrients offers a powerful means to enhance healing through as many avenues as possible. Since the body actually uses nutrients to form new tissues and cells, it makes better empirical sense to modulate nutrient intakes before specific pharmacological approaches are started.

The protocols listed in Chapter 14 have not been rigorously tested in large, multicenter, placebo-controlled, double-blind, crossover studies. To insist on this type of study as proof of effectiveness is a fantasy. Nevertheless, a preponderance of evidence has been accumulated from which, when known and understood, only one obvious conclusion can be drawn — correct manipulation of specific nutrient intakes does indeed improve healing of musculoskeletal conditions. This point was graphically demonstrated to this author. An individual known to this author underwent surgical removal of a malignancy with lymph node removal as well. The individual had no previous health problems and was never hospitalized prior to this incident; therefore, this person was physically active and in excellent nutritional status. Dietary analysis and other laboratory testing showed no obvious nutrient deficiencies. The protocol for skin damage healing was followed, along with additional vitamin A. After removal of bandages the day of surgery (which lasted 5 h), there was no bruising or swelling that was normally expected. Pain medication was greatly reduced from usual amounts in this type of surgery. Two weeks after surgery, radiation therapy was initiated, and the wound site was directly in the radiation field. Supplementation with the guidelines listed for skin damage was maintained throughout radiotherapy and beyond for many months. No side effects from the radiotherapy that were expected were ever observed. After 3 years, the surgical scar is still strong, pliable, and colored, compared to the hard white tissue normally encountered after irradiation of surgical sites. A physician who later examined this person stated that they did not know which side of the body was irradiated if there was no scar. Attending physicians all remarked about the unusual lack of side effects and rapid healing they observed. This is not the only case this author has observed that derived clinical benefit from nutrient manipulation after injury. Thus, this author has seen what can happen when nutrient intake is modified in a rational, safe, and scientific manner to assist healing.

Cost effectiveness is a major issue with health care delivery. The retail cost of the nutritional programs listed in the tables of Chapter 14 can range from $50 to $200 per month, depending upon what specific products are purchased. Many persons are unwilling to pay this additional amount for what they perceive as dubious value. After all, they are going to heal anyway, right? Yes, but how fast and how well? Athletes in particular have a desire or requirement to return to full function as soon as possible. The stresses of athletic competition often mean that even missing certain segments of training will seriously impair chances for success. Thus, extra effort to heal quickly and completely is desirable to many athletes and their coaches, trainers, or physicians.

The doses listed in Chapter 14 are within accepted safety limits found in normal and diseased humans. Thus, there is every reason to expect that the doses are both safe and adequate for athletes. In the case of very large persons, some doses may need to be doubled to achieve expected results. The user of the listed nutrient protocols is encouraged to be flexible and adaptable. Dosage is a major reason why some studies failed to show benefits while others did. Significant intakes must be accomplished to affect status of nutrients in short-term settings.

In conclusion, there is much scientific evidence to indicate that specific nutrients, when used judiciously, can safely accelerate healing of injuries and musculoskeletal conditions common to athletes and the general population. Combinations of specific nutrients may have the potential to significantly impact healing to a greater degree than single agents.

1. Rosse, C. and Clawson, D.K., The musculoskeletal system, in *The Musculoskeletal System in Health and Disease*, Rosse, C. and Clawson, D.K., Eds., Harper & Row, Hagerstown, 1980, 1.

2. Ballinger, W.F., Collins, J.A., Drucker, W.R., Dudrick, S.J., and Zeppa, R., Eds., *Manual of Surgical Nutrition*, W.B. Saunders, Philadelphia, 1975.

3. Fischer, J.E., Ed., *Total Parenteral Nutrition*, 2nd ed., Little, Brown, Boston, 1991.

4. Grant, J.P., *Handbook of Total Parenteral Nutrition*, 2nd ed., W.B. Saunders, Philadelphia, 1992.

5. Jeejeebhoy, K.N., *Total Parenteral Nutrition in the Hospital and at Home*, CRC Press, Boca Raton, FL, 1983.

6. Lee, H.A. and Raman, G.V., Eds., *A Handbook of Parenteral Nutrition*, Chapman and Hall, London, 1990.

7. Rombeau, J.L. and Caldwell, M.D., Eds., *Clinical Nutrition. Enteral and Tube Feeding*, 2nd ed., W.B. Saunders, Philadelphia, 1990.

8. Eby, G.A., Davis, D.R., and Holcomb, W.W., Reduction in duration of common colds by zinc gluconate lozenges in a double-blind study, *Antimicrob. Agents Chemother.*, 25, 20, 1984.

9. Rosse, C. and Clawson, G.K., Eds., *The Musculoskeletal System in Health and Disease*, Harper & Row, Hagerstown, 1980.

10. Poland, J.L., Hobart, D.J., and Payton, O.D., *The Musculoskeletal System*, 2nd. ed., Medical Examination Publishing, Garden City, NY, 1981.

11. Birnbaum, J.S., *The Musculoskeletal Manual*, Academic Press, New York, 1982.

12. Wilson, F.C., Ed., *The Musculoskeletal System. Basic Processes and Disorders*, 2nd ed., Lippincott, Philadelphia, 1983.

13. Nelson, C.L. and Dwyer, A.P., *The Aging Musculoskeletal System*, Collamore Press, Lexington, KY, 1984.

14. Kuhn, K. and Krieg, T., Eds., *Connective Tissue: Biological and Clinical Aspects*, Vol. 10, in *Rheumatology. An Annual Review*, Schattenkirchner, M., Ed., S. Karger, Basel, 1986.

15. Gamble, J.G., *The Musculoskeletal System. Physiological Basics*, Raven Press, New York, 1988.

16. Silver, F.H., *Biological Materials: Structure, Mechanical Properties, and Modeling of Soft Tissues*, New York University Press, New York, 1987.

17. Marieb, E.N., *Human Anatomy and Physiology*, Benjamin/Cummings, Redwood City, CA, 1989.

18. American Academy of Orthopaedic Surgeons, *Athletic Training and Sports Medicine*, 2nd ed., American Academy of Orthopedic Surgeons, Park Ridge, IL, 1991.

19. Hargens, A.R., Ed., *Tissue Nutrition and Viability*, Springer-Verlag, New York, 1986.

20. Urban, J.P.G., Solute transport in articular cartilage and the invertebral disc, in *Connective Tissue Matrix Part 2*, Hukins, D.W.L., Ed., CRC Press, Boca Raton, FL, 1990, 44.

21. McKibbin, B. and Maroudas, A., Nutrition and metabolism, in *Adult Articular Cartilage*, Freeman, M.A.R., Ed., Pitman Medical, Kent, 1979, 461.

22. Gordon, A.M. and Rosse, C., Skeletal muscle, in *The Musculoskeletal System in Health and Disease*, Rosse, C. and Clawson, G.K., Eds., Harper & Row, Hagerstown, MD, 1980, 119.

23. Poland, J.L., Hobart, D.J., and Payton, O.D., Morphology and physiology of muscle, in *The Musculoskeletal System*, 2nd. ed., Medical Examination Publishing, Garden City, NY, 1981, 1.

24. Wilson, F.C., Ed., Basic processes in muscle, in *The Musculoskeletal System. Basic Processes and Disorders*, Part 5, 2nd ed., Lippincott, Philadelphia, 1983, 167.

25. Gamble, J.G., Nerve and muscle, in *The Musculoskeletal System. Physiological Basics*, Raven Press, New York, 1988, 116.

26. Marieb, E.N., Muscles and muscle tissue, in *Human Anatomy and Physiology*, Benjamin/Cummings, Redwood City, CA, 1989, 239.

27. Purslow, P.P. and Duance, V.C., Structure and function of intramuscular connective tissue, in *Connective Tissue Matrix Part 2*, Hukins, D.W.L., Ed., CRC Press, Boca Raton, FL, 1990, 127.

28. Dantzig, J.A. and Goldman, Y.E., Muscle, in *Arthritis Surgery*, Sledge, C.B., Ruddy, S., Harris, E.D., and Kelley, W.N., Eds., W.B. Saunders, Philadelphia, 1994, 94.

29. Rosse, C. and Ross, R., Tissues of the musculoskeletal system, in *The Musculoskeletal System in Health and Disease*, Rosse, C. and Clawson, G.K., Eds., Harper & Row, Hagerstown, MD, 1980, 3.

30. Hukins, D.W.L., Tissue components, in *Connective Tissue Matrix*, Hukins, D.W.L., Ed., Macmillan, London, 1984, 1.

31. Leblond, C.P. and Laurie, G.W., Morphological features of connective tissues, in *Connective Tissue: Biological and Clinical Aspects*, Vol. 10, Kuhn, K. and Krieg, T., Eds., in *Rheumatology. An Annual Review*, Schattenkirchner, M., Ed., S. Karger, Basel, 1986, 1.

32. Marieb, E.N., Tissues: the living fabric, in *Human Anatomy and Physiology*, Benjamin/Cummings, Redwood City, CA, 1989, 100.

33. Sledge, C.B., Biology of the joint, in *Arthritis Surgery*, Sledge, C.B., Ruddy, S., Harris, E.D., and Kelley, W.N., Eds., W.B. Saunders, Philadelphia, 1994, 1.

34. American Academy of Orthopedic Surgeons, The musculoskeletal system, in *Athletic Training and Sports Medicine*, 2nd ed., American Academy of Orthopedic Surgeons, Park Ridge, IL, 1991, 192.

35. Freeman, M.A.R., Ed., *Adult Articular Cartilage*, 2nd ed., Pittman Medical Publishing, Kent, England, 1979.
36. Sokoloff, L., Ed., *The Joints and Synovial Fluid*, Vol. 2, Academic Press, New York 1980.
37. Ghadially, F.N., *Fine Structure of Synovial Joints*, Butterworths, London, 1983.
38. Wilson, F.C., Ed., Basic processes in joints, in *The Musculoskeletal System. Basic Processes and Disorders*, 2nd ed., Lippincott, Philadelphia, 1983, 207.
39. Chrisman, O.D., The biology of aging cartilage, in *The Aging Musculoskeletal System*, Nelson, C.L. and Dwyer, A.P., Eds., Collamore Press, Lexington, KY, 1984, 59.
40. Kuettner, K.E., Schleyerbach, R., and Hascall, V.C., Eds., *Articular Cartilage Biochemistry*, Raven Press, New York, 1985.
41. Silver, F.H., Microscopic and macroscopic structure of tissues, in *Biological Materials: Structure, Mechanical Properties, and Modeling of Soft Tissues*, New York University Press, New York, 1987, 69.
42. Gamble, J.G., Joints, synovium, articular cartilage, in *The Musculoskeletal System. Physiological Basics*, Raven Press, New York, 1988, 100.
43. Mow, V.C., Fithian, D.C., and Kelly, M.A., Fundamentals of articular cartilage and meniscus biomechanics, in *Articular Cartilage and Knee Joint Function*, Ewing, J.W., Ed., Raven Press, New York, 1990, 1.
44. Buckwalter, J.A., Rosenberg, L.C., and Hunziker, E.B., Articular cartilage: composition, structure, response to injury, and methods of facilitating repair, in *Articular Cartilage and Knee Joint Function*, Ewing, J.W., Ed., Raven Press, New York, 1900, 19.
45. Kuettner, K.E., Schleyerbach, R., Peyron, J.G., and Hascall, V.C., Eds., *Articular Cartilage and Osteoarthritis*, Raven Press, New York, 1991.
46. Hall, B. and Newman, S., Eds., *Cartilage: Molecular Aspects*, CRC Press, Boca Raton, FL, 1991.
47. Hardingham, T.E. and Caterson, B., Biochemistry of articular cartilage and joint disease, in *Osteoarthritis: Current Research and Prospects for Pharmacological Intervention*, Russell, R.G.G. and Dieppe, P.A., Eds., IBC Technical Services, London, 1991, 51.
48. Bayliss, M.T., Responses in human articular cartilage in relation to age, in *Osteoarthritis: Current Research and Prospects for Pharmacological Intervention*, Russell, R.G.G. and Dieppe, P.A., Eds., IBC Technical Services, London, 1991, 115.
49. Woessner, J.F. and Howell, D.S., Eds., *Joint Cartilage Degradation. Basic and Clinical Aspects*, Marcel Dekker, New York, 1993.
50. Horton, W.A., Morphology of connective tissue: cartilage, in *Connective Tissue and Its Heritable Disorders. Molecular, Genetic, and Medical Aspects*, Royce, P.M. and Steinmann, B., Eds., Wiley-Liss, New York, 1993, 73.
51. Poole, A.R., Cartilage in health and disease, in *Arthritis and Allied Conditions. A Textbook of Rheumatology*, Vol. 1, McCarty, D.J. and Koopman, W.J., Eds., Lea & Febiger, Philadelphia, 1993, 293.
52. Wilson, F.C., Ed., Basic processes in bones, in *The Musculoskeletal System. Basic Processes and Disorders*, 2nd ed., Lippincott, Philadelphia, 1983, 87.
53. Veis, A., Bones and teeth, in *Extracellular Matrix Biochemistry*, Piez, K.A. and Reddi, A.H., Elsevier, New York, 1984, 329.
54. Gamble, J.G., Bone morphology and histology, in *The Musculoskeletal System. Physiological Basics*, Raven Press, New York, 1988, 81.
55. Marieb, E.N., Bones and bone tissue, in *Human Anatomy and Physiology*, Benjamin/Cummings, Redwood City, CA, 1989, 152.
56. Simmons, D.J., Ed., *Nutrition and Bone Development*, Oxford University Press, New York, 1990.
57. Coe, F.L. and Favus, M.J., Eds., *Disorders of Bone and Mineral Metabolism*, Raven Press, New York, 1992.
58. Rosse, C. and Simkin, P.A., Joints, in *The Musculoskeletal System in Health and Disease*, Rosse, C. and Clawson, G.K., Eds., Harper & Row, Hagerstown, MD, 1980, 77.
59. Ewing, J.W., Ed., *Articular Cartilage and Knee Joint Function. Basic Science and Arthroscopy*, Raven Press, New York, 1990.
60. Norkin, C.C. and Levangie, P.K., Eds., *Joint Structure & Function. A Comprehensive Analysis*, 2nd ed., F.A. Davis, Philadelphia, 1992.
61. Mankin, H.J. and Radin, E.L., Structure and function of joints, in *Arthritis and Allied Conditions. A Textbook of Rheumatology*, Vol. 1, McCarty, D.J. and Koopman, W.J., Eds., Lea & Febiger, Philadelphia, 1993, 181.
62. McCarty, D.J., The physiology of the normal synovium, in *The Joints and Synovial Fluid*, Vol. 2, Sokoloff, L., Ed., Academic Press, New York, 1980, 294.
63. Henderson, B. and Edwards, J.C.W., *The Synovial Lining in Health and Disease*, Chapman and Hill, London, 1987.
64. Simkin, P.A., Synovial physiology, in *Arthritis and Allied Conditions. A Textbook of Rheumatology*, Vol. 1, McCarty, D.J. and Koopman, W.J., Eds., Lea & Febiger, Philadelphia, 1993, 199.
65. Bandara, G. and Evans, C.H., Intercellular regulation by synoviocytes, in *Biological Regulation of the Chondrocytes*, Adolphe, M., Ed., CRC Press, Boca Raton, FL, 1992, 205.
66. DeHaven, K.E., The role of the meniscus, in *Articular Cartilage and Knee Joint Function. Basic Science and Arthroscopy*, Ewing, J.W., Ed., Raven Press, New York, 1990, 103.
67. Muir, I.H.M., The chemistry of the ground substance of joint cartilage, in *The Joints and Synovial Fluid*, Vol. 2, Sokoloff, L., Ed., Academic Press, New York, 1980, 28.
68. Varma, R.S. and Varma, R., Eds., *Glycosaminoglycans and Proteoglycans in Physiological and Pathological Processes of Body Systems*, S. Karger, Basel, 1982.
69. Heinegard, D. and Paulsson, M., Structure and metabolism of proteoglycans, in *Extracellular Matrix Biochemistry*, Piez, K.A. and Reddi, A.H., Elsevier, New York, 1984, 277.
70. Bayliss, M.T., Proteoglycans: structure and molecular organizations in cartilage, in *Connective Tissue Matrix*, Hukins, D.W.L., Ed., Macmillan, London, 1984, 55.

71. Rosenberg, L.C. and Buckwalter, J.A., Cartilage proteoglycans, in *Articular Cartilage Biochemistry*, Kuettner, K.E., Schleyerbach, R., and Hascall, V.C., Eds., Raven Press, New York, 1985, 39.

72. Lohmander, L.S. and Kimura, J.H., Biosynthesis of cartilage proteoglycan, in *Articular Cartilage Biochemistry*, Kuettner, K.E., Schleyerbach, R., and Hascall, V.C., Eds., Raven Press, New York, 1985, 93.

73. Hardingham, T.E., Structure and biosynthesis of proteoglycans, in *Connective Tissue: Biological and Clinical Aspects*, Vol. 10, Kuhn, K. and Krieg, T., Eds., in *Rheumatology. An Annual Review*, Schattenkirchner, M., Ed., S. Karger, Basel, 1986, 143.

74. Silbert, J.E., Advances in the biochemistry of proteoglycans, in *Connective Tissue Disease. Molecular Pathology of the Extracellular Matrix*, Uitto, J. and Perejda, A.J., Eds., Marcel Dekker, New York, 1987, 83.

75. Wight, T.N. and Mecham, R.P., Eds., *Biology of the Proteoglycans*, Academic Press, Orlando, 1987.

76. Gamble, J.G., Structural components, in *The Musculoskeletal System. Physiological Basics*, Raven Press, New York, 1988, 57.

77. Kuettner, K.E., Schleyerbach, R., Peyron, J.G., and Hascall, V.C., Part I: Structural components of cartilage: proteoglycans, in *Articular Cartilage and Osteoarthritis*, Kuettner, K.E., Schleyerbach, R., Peyron, J.G., and Hascall, V.C., Eds., Raven Press, New York, 1991, 1.

78. Weitzhandler, M. and Bernfield, M.R., Proteoglycan conjugates, in *Wound Healing. Biochemical & Clinical Aspects*, Cohen, I.K., Diegelmann, R.F., and Lindblad, W.J., Eds., W.B. Saunders, Philadelphia, 1992, 195.

79. Handley, C.J. and Ng, C.K., Proteoglycan, hyaluronan, and noncollagenous matrix protein metabolism by chondrocytes, in *Biological Regulation of the Chondrocytes*, Adolphe, M., Ed., CRC Press, Boca Raton, FL, 1992, 85.

80. Neame, P.J., Extracellular matrix of cartilage: proteoglycans, in *Joint Cartilage Degradation. Basic and Clinical Aspects*, Woessner, J.F. and Howell, D.S., Eds., Marcel Dekker, New York, 1993, 109.

81. Rosenberg, L., Structure and function of proteoglycans, in *Arthritis and Allied Conditions. A Textbook of Rheumatology*, Vol. 1, McCarty, D.J. and Koopman, W.J., Eds., Lea & Febiger, Philadelphia, 1993, 229.

82. Heinegard, D. and Oldberg, A., Glycosylated matrix proteins, in *Connective Tissue and Its Heritable Disorders. Molecular, Genetic, and Medical Aspects*, Royce, P.M. and Steinmann, B., Eds., Wiley-Liss, New York, 1993, 189.

83. Trelstad, R.L. and Kemp, P.D., Matrix glycoproteins and proteoglycans, in *Arthritis Surgery*, Sledge, C.B., Ruddy, S., Harris, E.D., and Kelley, W.N., Eds., W.B. Saunders, Philadelphia, 1994, 48.

84. Brimacombe, J.S. and Webber, J.M., *Mucopolysaccharides. Chemical Structure, Distribution and Isolation*, Elsevier, Amsterdam, 1964.

85. Quintarelli, G., Ed., *The Chemical Physiology of Mucopolysaccharides*, Little, Brown, Boston, 1968.

86. Varma, R. and Varma, R.S., Eds., *Mucopolysaccharides — Glycosaminoglycans — of Body Fluids in Health and Disease*, Walter de Gruyter, Berlin, 1983.

87. Hardingham, T.E., Fosang, A.J., and Dudhia, J., Aggrecan, the chondroitin sulfate/keratan sulfate proteoglycan from cartilage, in *Articular Cartilage and Osteoarthritis*, Kuettner, K.E., Schleyerbach, R., Peyron, J.G., and Hascall, V.C., Eds., Raven Press, New York, 1991, 5.

88. Karzel, K. and Domenjoz, R., Effects of hexosamine derivatives and uronic acid derivatives on glycosaminoglycan metabolism of fibroblast cultures, *Pharmacology*, 5, 337, 1971.

89. Piez, K., Molecular and aggregate structures of the collagens, in *Extracellular Matrix Biochemistry*, Piez, K.A. and Reddi, A.H., Eds., Elsevier, New York, 1984, 1.

90. Miller, E.J., Chemistry of the collagens and their distribution, in *Extracellular Matrix Biochemistry*, Piez, K.A. and Reddi, A.H., Eds., Elsevier, New York, 1984, 41.

91. Kivirikko, K.I. and Myllylä, R., Biosynthesis of the collagens, in *Extracellular Matrix Biochemistry*, Piez, K.A. and Reddi, A.H., Eds., Elsevier, New York, 1984, 83.

92. Klein, L.K. and Rajan, J.C., The biology of aging human collagen, in *The Aging Musculoskeletal System*, Nelson, C.L. and Dwyer, A.P., Eds., Collamore Press, Lexington, KY, 1984, 37.

93. Tinker, D. and Rucker, R.B., Role of selected nutrients in synthesis, accumulation, and chemical modification of connective tissue proteins, *Physiol. Rev.*, 65(3), 607, 1985.

94. Berg, R.A. and Kerr, J.S., Nutritional aspects of collagen metabolism, *Annu. Rev. Nutr.*, 12, 369, 1992.

95. Burgeson, R.E. and Morris, N.P., The collagen family of proteins, in *Connective Tissue Disease. Molecular Pathology of the Extracellular Matrix*, Uitto, J. and Perejda, A.J., Eds., Marcel Dekker, New York, 1987, 3.

96. Nimni, M.E. and Olsen, B.R., Eds., *Collagen*, Vol. 1–4, CRC Press, Boca Raton, FL, 1988, 1989.

97. Kuettner, K.E., Schleyerbach, R., Peyron, J.G., and Hascall, V.C., Part III: Structural components of cartilage: collagens, in *Articular Cartilage and Osteoarthritis*, Kuettner, K.E., Schleyerbach, R., Peyron, J.G., and Hascall, V.C., Eds., Raven Press, New York, 1991, 115.

98. Van der Rest, M. and Garrone, R., Collagen family of proteins, *FASEB J.*, 5, 2814, 1991.

99. Petit, B., Freyria, A.M., van der Rest, M., and Herbage, D., Cartilage collagens, in *Biological Regulation of the Chondrocytes*, Adolphe, M., Ed., CRC Press, Boca Raton, FL, 1992, 33.

100. Kucharz, E.J., *The Collagens: Biochemistry and Pathophysiology*, Springer-Verlag, Berlin, 1992.

101. Kielty, C.M., Hopkinson, I., and Grant, M.E., Collagen: the collagen family: structure, assembly, and organization in the extracellular matrix, in *Connective Tissue and Its Heritable Disorders. Molecular, Genetic, and Medical Aspects*, Royce, P.M. and Steinmann, B., Eds., Wiley-Liss, New York, 1993, 103.

102. Mayne, R. and Brewton, R.G., Extracellular matrix of cartilage: collagen, in *Joint Cartilage Degradation. Basic and Clinical Aspects*, Woessner, J.F. and Howell, D.S., Eds., Marcel Dekker, New York, 1993, 81.

103. Williams, C.J., Vandenburg, P., and Prockop, D.J., Collagen and elastin, in *Arthritis Surgery*, Sledge, C.B., Ruddy, S., Harris, E.D., and Kelley, W.N., Eds., W.B. Saunders, Philadelphia, 1994, 35.

104. Gosline, J.M. and Rosenbloom, J., Elastin, in *Extracellular Matrix Biochemistry*, Piez, K.A. and Reddi, A.H., Eds., Elsevier, New York, 1984, 191.

105. Robert, L. and Hornebeck, W., Eds., *Elastin and Elastases*, Vols. 1 & 2, CRC Press, Boca Raton, FL, 1989.

106. Winlove, C.P. and Parker, K.H., Physicochemical properties of vascular elastin, in *Connective Tissue Matrix Part 2*, Hukins, D.W.L., Ed., CRC Press, Boca Raton, FL, 1990, 167.

107. Rosenbloom, J., Elastin, in *Connective Tissue and Its Heritable Disorders. Molecular, Genetic, and Medical Aspects*, Royce, P.M. and Steinmann, B., Eds., Wiley-Liss, New York, 1993, 167.

108. Davidson, J.M., Giro, G., and Quaglino, D., Elastin repair, in *Wound Healing. Biochemical & Clinical Aspects*, Cohen, I.K., Diegelmann, R.F., and Lindblad, W.J., Eds., W.B. Saunders, Philadelphia, 1992, 223.

109. Hunt, T.K. and Van Winkle, W., Normal repair, in *Fundamentals of Wound Management*, Hunt, T.K. and Dunphy, J.E., Eds., Appleton-Century-Crofts, New York, 1979, 2.

110. Ross, R., Inflammation, cell proliferation, and connective tissue formation in wound repair, in *Wound Healing and Wound Infection. Theory and Surgical Practice*, Hunt, T.K., Ed., Appleton-Century-Crofts, New York, 1980, 1.

111. Peacock, E.E., *Wound Repair*, 3rd ed., W.B. Saunders, Philadelphia, 1984.

112. Irvin, T.T., The healing wound, in *Wound Healing for Surgeons*, Bucknall, T.E. and Ellis, H., Eds., Balliere Tindall, London, 1984, 3.

113. Hunt, T.K., Knighton, D.R., Thakral, K.K., Andrews, W., and Michaeli, D., Cellular control of repair, in *Soft and Hard Tissue Repair. Biological and Clinical Aspects*, Hunt, T.K., Heppenstall, R.B., Pines, E., and Rovee, D., Eds., Praeger Scientific, New York, 1984, 3.

114. Grotendorst, G.R. and Martin, G.R., Cell movements in wound-healing and fibrosis, in *Connective Tissue: Biological and Clinical Aspects*, Vol. 10, Kuhn, K. and Krieg, T., Eds., in *Rheumatology. An Annual Review*, Schattenkirchner, M., Ed., S. Karger, Basel, 1986, 385.

115. Gamble, J.G., Subcellular organelles and cells, in *The Musculoskeletal System. Physiological Basics*, Raven Press, New York, 1988, 16.

116. American Academy of Orthopedic Surgeons, Physiology of tissue repair, in *Athletic Training and Sports Medicine*, 2nd ed., American Academy of Orthopedic Surgeons, Park Ridge, 1991, 96.

117. Cohen, I.K., Diegelmann, R.F., and Lindblad, W.J., Biological processes involved in wound healing, in *Wound Healing. Biochemical & Clinical Aspects*, Cohen, I.K., Diegelmann, R.F., and Lindblad, W.J., Eds., W.B. Saunders, Philadelphia, 1992, 20.

118. Mainardi, C.L., Fibroblast function and fibrosis, in *Arthritis Surgery*, Sledge, C.B., Ruddy, S., Harris, E.D., and Kelley, W.N., Eds., W.B. Saunders, Philadelphia, 1994, 123.

119. Annefeld, M., The chondrocyte — the living element of articular cartilage, in *Articular Cartilage and Osteoarthrosis*, Fassbender, H.G., Annefeld, M., Wilhelmi, G., and Maier, R., Eds., Hans Huber Publishers, Bern, 1983, 30.

120. Kuettner, K.E., Schleyerbach, R., Peyron, J.G., and Hascall, V.C., Part V: Chondrocyte metabolism, in *Articular Cartilage and Osteoarthritis*, Kuettner, K.E., Schleyerbach, R., Peyron, J.G., and Hascall, V.C., Eds., Raven Press, New York, 1991, 235.

121. Adolphe, M., Ed., *Biological Regulation of the Chondrocytes*, CRC Press, Boca Raton, FL, 1992.

122. Leibovich, S.J. and Ross, R., The role of the macrophage in wound repair: a study with hydrocortisone and antimacrophage serum, *Am. J. Pathol.*, 78, 71, 1975.

123. Diegelmann, R.F., Cohen, I.K., and Kaplan, A.M., The role of macrophages in wound repair: a review, *Plast. Reconstr. Surg.*, 68, 107, 1981.

124. Leibovich, S.J., Mesenchymal cell proliferation in wound repair: the role of macrophages, in *Soft and Hard Tissue Repair. Biological and Clinical Aspects*, Hunt, T.K., Heppenstall, R.B., Pines, E., and Rovee, D., Eds., Praeger Scientific, New York, 1984, 329.

125. Pike, M.C. and Snyderman, R., Structure and function of monocytes and macrophages, in *Arthritis and Allied Conditions. A Textbook of Rheumatology*, Vol. 1, McCarty, D.J. and Koopman, W.J., Eds., Lea & Febiger, Philadelphia, 1993, 347.

126. McGhee, J.R., Lymphoid function and antibody synthesis, in *Biology of Wound Healing*, Menaker, L., Ed., Harper & Row, Hagerstown, MD, 1975, 97.

127. Suzuki, N., Kansas, G.S., and Engleman, E.G., Lymphocytes: structure and function, in *Arthritis and Allied Conditions. A Textbook of Rheumatology*, Vol. 1, McCarty, D.J. and Koopman, W.J., Eds., Lea & Febiger, Philadelphia, 1993, 377.

128. Cronstein, B.N. and Weissmann, G., Neutrophil structure and function, in *Arthritis and Allied Conditions. A Textbook of Rheumatology*, Vol. 1, McCarty, D.J. and Koopman, W.J., Eds., Lea & Febiger, Philadelphia, 1993, 389.

129. Pepys, J. and Edwards, A.M., *The Mast Cell. Its Role in Health and Disease*, University Park Press, Baltimore, 1979.

130. Gruber, B.L. and Kaplan, A.P., Mast cells and rheumatic diseases, 1, in *Arthritis and Allied Conditions. A Textbook of Rheumatology*, Vol. 1, McCarty, D.J. and Koopman, W.J., Eds., Lea & Febiger, Philadelphia, 1993, 417.

131. Moreno, H., Platelet function, in *Biology of Wound Healing*, Menaker, L., Ed., Harper & Row, Hagerstown, MD, 1975, 6.

132. Michaeli, D., Hunt, T.K., and Knighton, D.R., The role of platelets in wound healing: demonstration of angiogenic activity, in *Soft and Hard Tissue Repair. Biological and Clinical Aspects*, Hunt, T.K., Heppenstall, R.B., Pines, E., and Rovee, D., Eds., Praeger Scientific, New York, 1984, 380.

133. Saleh, M. and LoBuglio, A., Platelets in rheumatic diseases, in *Arthritis and Allied Conditions. A Textbook of Rheumatology*, Vol. 1, McCarty, D.J. and Koopman, W.J., Eds., Lea & Febiger, Philadelphia, 1993, 437.

134. Wright, N. and Aluison, M., *The Biology of Epithelial Cell Populations*, Vol. 1, Clarendon Press, Oxford, 1984.

135. Simionescu, N. and Simionescu, M., Eds., *Endothelial Cell Biology in Health and Disease*, Plenum Press, New York, 1988.

136. Ryan, U.S., Ed., *Endothelial Cells*, Vols. 1, 2, & 3, CRC Press, Boca Raton, FL, 1988.

137. Fox, R.I. and Kang, H., Structure and function of synoviocytes, in *Arthritis and Allied Conditions. A Textbook of Rheumatology*, Vol. 1, McCarty, D.J. and Koopman, W.J., Eds., Lea & Febiger, Philadelphia, 1993, 263.

138. Cerra, F.B., Nutrient modulation of inflammatory and immune function, *Am. J. Surg.*, 161, 230, 1991.

139. Cerra, F.B., Role of nutrition in the management of malnutrition and immune dysfunction in trauma, *J. Am.Coll. Nutr.*, 11(5), 512, 1992.

140. Boucek, R.J., Factors affecting wound healing, *Otolaryngol. Clin. N. Am.*, 17(2), 243, 1984.

141. Jacobs, D.O., Black, P.R., and Wilmore, D.W., Hormone-substrate interactions, in *Clinical Nutrition. Enteral and Tube Feeding*, 2nd ed., Rombeau, J.L. and Caldwell, M.D., Eds., W.B. Saunders, Philadelphia, 1990, 34.

142. Dahn, M.S., Neuro-humoral regulation in starvation and injury, in *Nutrition and Metabolism in the Surgical Patient*, Kirkpatrick, J.R., Ed., Futura Publishing, Mount Kisco, NY, 1983, 89.

143. Menaker, L., Ed., *Biology of Wound Healing*, Harper & Row, Hagerstown, MD, 1975.

144. Hunt, T.K. and Dunphy, J.E., Eds., *Fundamentals of Wound Management*, Appleton-Century-Crofts, New York, 1979.

145. Hunt, T.K., Ed., *Wound Healing and Wound Infection. Theory and Surgical Practice*, Appleton-Century-Crofts, New York, 1980.

146. Irvin, T.T., *Wound Healing. Principles and Practice*, Chapman and Hall, London, 1981.

147. Bucknall, T.E. and Ellis, H., Eds., *Wound Healing for Surgeons*, Balliere Tindall, London, 1984.

148. Hunt, T.K., Heppenstall, R.B., Pines, E., and Rovee, D., Eds., *Soft and Hard Tissue Repair. Biological and Clinical Aspects*, Praeger Scientific, New York, 1984.

149. Davis, J.C. and Hunt, T.K., *Problem Wounds. The Role of Oxygen.*, Elsevier, New York, 1988.

150. Glauert, A.M., Ed., *The Control of Tissue Damage*, Elsevier, Amsterdam, 1988.

151. Janssen, H., Rooman, R., and Robertson, J.I.S., *Wound Healing*, Wrightson Biomedical Publishing, Petersfield, England, 1991.

152. Cohen, I.K., Diegelmann, R.F., and Lindblad, W.J., Eds., *Wound Healing. Biochemical & Clinical Aspects*, W.B. Saunders, Philadelphia, 1992.

153. Gallin, J.I., Goldstein, I.M., and Snyderman, R., Eds., *Inflammation. Basic Principles and Clinical Correlates*, 2nd ed., Raven Press, New York, 1992.

154. Norris, C.M., Healing, in *Sports Injuries. Diagnosis and Management for Physiotherapists*, Butterworth-Heinemann, Oxford, 1993, 21.

155. Torg, J.S., Welsh, R.P., and Shephard, R.J., Eds., *Current Therapy in Sports Medicine — 2*, B.C. Decker, Toronto, 1990.

156. Grana, W.A. and Kalenak, A., Eds., *Clinical Sports Medicine*, W.B. Saunders, Philadelphia, 1991.

157. Norris, C.M., *Sports Injuries. Diagnosis and Management for Physiotherapists*, Butterworth-Heinemann, Oxford, 1993.

158. Wright, P.H. and Brashear, H.R., The local response to trauma, in *The Musculoskeletal System. Basic Processes and Disorders*, 2nd ed., Wilson, F.C., Ed., Lippincott, Philadelphia, 1983, 261.

159. Wornom, I.L. and Buchman, S.R., Bone and cartilaginous tissue, 2, in *Wound Healing. Biochemical & Clinical Aspects*, Cohen, I.K., Diegelmann, R.F., and Lindblad, W.J., Eds., W.B. Saunders, Philadelphia, 1992, 344.

160. Williams, J.M., Uebelhart, D., Ongichi, D.R., Kuettner, K.E., and Thonar, E.J.A., Animal models of articular cartilage repair, in *Articular Cartilage and Osteoarthritis*, Kuettner, K.E., Schleyerbach, R., Peyron, J.G., and Hascall, V.C., Eds., Raven Press, New York, 1991, 511.

161. Buckwalter, J.A. and Mow, V.C., Cartilage repair in osteoarthritis, , in *Osteoarthritis. Diagnosis and Medical/Surgical Management*, 2nd ed., Moskowitz, R.W., Howell, D.S., Goldberg, V.M., and Mankin, H.J., Eds., W.B. Saunders, Philadelphia, 1992, 71.

162. Amadio, P.C., Tendon and ligament, in *Wound Healing. Biochemical & Clinical Aspects*, Cohen, I.K., Diegelmann, R.F., and Lindblad, W.J., Eds., W.B. Saunders, Philadelphia, 1992, 356.

163. Levenson, S.M. and Demetriou, A.A., Metabolic factors, 5, in *Wound Healing. Biochemical & Clinical Aspects*, Cohen, I.K., Diegelmann, R.F., and Lindblad, W.J., Eds., W.B. Saunders, Philadelphia, 1992, 248.

164. Levenson, S.M. and Siefter, E., Dysnutrition, wound healing and resistance to infection, *Clin. Plast. Surg.*, 4(3), 375, 1977.

165. Gadisseux, P., Ward, J.D., Young, H.F., and Becker, D.P., Nutrition and the neurosurgical patient, *J. Neurosurg.*, 60, 219, 1984.

166. Souba, W.W. and Wilmore, D.W., Diet and nutrition in the care of the patient with surgery, trauma, and sepsis, in *Modern Nutrition in Health and Disease*, 7th ed., Shils, M.E. and Young, V.R., Eds., Lea & Febiger, Philadelphia, 1988.

167. Ruberg, R.L., Role of nutrition in wound healing, *Surg. Clin. N. Am.*, 64(4), 705, 1984.

168. Anonymous, Standards for Nutrition Support: Hospitalized Patients, ASPEN Publishing, Washington, D.C., 1984.

169. Brooks, D., Ed., *Suggested Guidelines for Nutrition Management of the Critically Ill Patient*, American Dietetic Association, Chicago, 1984.

170. Alpers, D.H., Clouse, R.E., and Stenson, W.F., Eds., *Manual of Nutritional Therapeutics*, 2nd ed., Little, Brown, Boston, 1988.

171. Hill, G.L., *Disorders of Nutrition and Metabolism in Clinical Surgery*, Churchill Livingstone, Edinburgh, 1992.

172. Kreitzman, S.N., Nutrition in wound healing, in *Nutrition in Oral Health and Disease*, Pollack, R.L. and Kravitz, E., Eds., Lea & Febiger, Philadelphia, 1985, 131.

173. Willcutts, H.D., Nutritional assessment of 1000 surgical patients in an affluent suburban community hospital, *JPEN*, 1, 25A, 1977.

174. Bishop, C.W., Bowen, P.E., and Ritchey, S.J., Norms for nutritional assessment of American adults by upper arm anthropometry, *Am. J. Clin. Nutr.*, 34, 2530, 1981.

175. Lohman, T.G., Roche, A.F., and Martorell, R., Eds., *Anthropometric Standardization Reference Manual*, abridged Ed., Human Kinetics Books, Champaign, IL, 1991.

176. Niinikoski, J., Kivisaari, J., and Vijanto, J., Local hyperalimentation of experimental granulation tissue, *Acta Chir. Scand.*, 143, 201, 1977.

177. Viljanto, J. and Raekallio, J., Local hyperalimentation of open wounds, *Br. J. Surg.*, 63, 427, 1973.

178. Hill, G.L., Effects of nutritional therapy, in *Disorders of Nutrition and Metabolism in Clinical Surgery*, Churchill Livingstone, Edinburgh, 1992, 85.

179. Vogel, R.I. and Alvares, O.F., Nutrition and periodontal disease, in *Nutrition in Oral Health and Disease*, Pollack, R.L. and Kravitz, E., Eds., Lea & Febiger, Philadelphia, 1985, 136.

180. Haw, M.P., Bell, S.J., and Blackburn, G.L., Potential of parenteral and enteral nutrition in inflammation and immune dysfunction: a new challenge for dietitians, *J. Am. Diet. Assoc.*, 91, 701, 1991.

181. Haydock, H.A. and Hill, G.L., Improved wound healing response in surgical patients receiving intravenous nutrition, *Br. J. Surg.*, 74, 320, 1987.

182. Ringsdorf, W.M. and Cheraskin, E., Periodontal pathosis in man. IV. Effect of protein versus placebo supplementation upon gingivitis, *J. Dent. Med.*, 18, 92, 1963.

183. Ringsdorf, W.M. and Cheraskin, E., Periodontal pathosis in man. V. Effect of protein versus placebo supplementation upon sulcus depth, *Parodontologie*, 18, 83, 1963.

184. Cheraskin, E. and Ringsdorf, W.M., Periodontal pathosis in man. VIII. Effect of protein versus placebo supplementation upon clinical tooth mobility, *Periodontics*, 2, 69, 1964.

185. Cheraskin, E. and Ringsdorf, W.M., Periodontal pathosis in man. IX. Effect of combined versus animal protein supplementation upon gingival state, *J. Dent. Med.*, 19, 82, 1964.

186. Cheraskin, E. and Ringsdorf, W.M., Periodontal pathosis in man. X. Effect of combined versus animal protein supplementation upon sulcus depth, *J. Oral Ther. Pharmacol.*, 1, 497, 1965.

187. Cheraskin, E., Ringsdorf, W.M., Setyaadmadja, A.T.S.H., and Ray, D.W., An ecologic analysis of tooth mobility: effect of prophylaxis and protein supplementation, *J. Periodontol.*, 38, 227, 1967.

188. Cheraskin, E., Ringsdorf, W.M., Setyaadmadja, A.T.S.H., and Barrett, R.A., An ecologic analysis of gingival state: effect of prophylaxis and protein supplementation, *J. Periodontol.*, 39, 316, 1968.

189. Tkatch, L., Rapin, C.H., Rizzoli, R., Slosman, D., Nydegger, V., Vasey, H., and Bonjour, J.P., Benefits of oral protein supplementation in elderly patients with fracture of the proximal femur, *J. Am. Coll. Nutr.*, 11(5), 519, 1992.

190. Dudrick, P.S. and Souba, W.W., Amino acids in surgical nutrition. Principles and practice, *Surg. Clin. N. Am.*, 71(3), 459, 1991.

191. Short, S.H., Surveys of dietary intake and nutrition knowledge of athletes and their coaches, 6, in *Nutrition in Exercise and Sport*, 2nd ed., Wolinksy, I. and Hickson, J.F., Eds., CRC Press, Boca Raton, FL, 1994, 367.

192. Smith, R.J., Glutamine metabolism and its physiological importance, *JPEN*, 14(4) Suppl., 40S, 1990.

193. Visek, W., Arginine needs, physiological state and usual diets — a reevaluation, *J. Nutr.*, 116, 36, 1986.

194. Barbul, A., Arginine biochemistry, physiology and therapeutic implications, *JPEN* 19, 227, 1986.

195. Barbul, A., Arginine and immune function, *Nutrition*, 6, 53, 1990.

196. Kirk, S.J. and Barbul, A., Role of arginine in trauma, sepsis, and immunity, *JPEN*, 14(Suppl.), 226S, 1990.

197. Barbul, A., Rettura, G., Levenson, S.M., and Seifter, E., Arginine: a thymotropic and wound healing promoting agent, *Surg. Forum*, 28, 101, 1977.

198. Seifter, E., Rettura, G., Barbul, A., and Levenson, S.M., Arginine: an essential amino acid for injured rats, *Surgery*, 84, 224, 1978.

199. Barbul, A., Rettura, G., Levenson, S.M., and Seifter, E., Wound healing and thymotropic effects of arginine: a pituitary mechanism of action, *Am. J. Clin. Nutr.*, 37, 786, 1983.

200. Chuyn, J.H. and Griminger, P., Improvement of nitrogen retention by arginine and glycine supplementation and its relation to collagen synthesis in traumatized mature and aged rats, *J. Nutr.*, 144, 1687, 1984.

201. Barbul, A., Fishel, R.S., Shimazu, S., Wasserkrug, H.L., Yoshimura, N.N., Tao, R.C., and Efron, G., Intravenous hyperalimentation with high arginine levels improved wound healing and immune function, *J. Surg. Res.*, 38, 328, 1985.

202. Natsvlishvili, N.A., Samonina, G.E., and Ashmarin, I.P., The antiulcer action of antidepressants. II. The effect of the antidepressants inkazan, azafen, and OF-743 in combination with arginine on ethanol-evoked damage to the gastric mucosa in rats, *Biol. Nauki.*, (7), 52, 1991.

203. Sitren, H.S. and Fisher, H., Nitrogen retention in rats fed on diets enriched with arginine and glycine, *Br. J. Nutr.*, 37, 195, 1977.

204. Leon, P., Redmond, H.P., Shou, J., Kelly, C.J., Schluter, M.D., Stein, T.P., and Daly, J.M., Arginine supplementation improves fibrinogen and hepatic protein synthesis after surgical trauma, *Surg. Forum*, 42, 5, 1991.

205. Barbul, A., Rettura, G., Levenson, S.M., and Siefter, E., Thymotropic effects of arginine, ornithine, and growth hormone, *Fed. Proc.,* 37, 264, 1978.

206. Rettura, G., Barbul, A., Levenson, S.M., and Seifter, E., Citrulline does not share the thymotropic properties of arginine and ornithine, *Fed. Proc.,* 38, 289, 1979.

207. Rettura, G., Padawer, J., Barbul, A., Levenson, S.M., and Seifter, E., Supplemental arginine increases thymic cellularity in normal and murine sarcoma virus-inoculated mice and increases the resistance to murine sarcoma virus tumor, *JPEN,* 3, 409, 1979.

208. Barbul, A., Wasserkrug, H.L., Sisto, D.A., Seifter, E., Rettura, G., Levenson, S.M., and Efron, G., Thymic and immune stimulatory actions of arginine, *JPEN,* 4, 446, 1980.

209. Barbul, A., Wasserkrug, H.L., Seifter, E., Rettura, G., Levenson, S.M., and Efron, G., Immunostimulatory effects of arginine in normal and injured rats, *J. Surg. Res.,* 29, 228, 1980.

210. Barbul, A., Sisto, D.A., Wasserkrug, H.L., Yoshimura, N.N., and Efron, G., Metabolic and immune effects of arginine in post-injury hyperalimentation, *J. Trauma,* 21, 970, 1981.

211. Saito, H., Trocki, O., Wang, S.L., Gonce, S.J., Joffe, S.N., and Alexander, J.W., Metabolic and immune effects of dietary arginine supplementation after burn, *Arch. Surg.,* 122, 784, 1987.

212. Madden, H.P., Breslin, R.J., Wasserkrug, H.L., Efron, G., and Barbul, A., Stimulation of T cell immunity by arginine enhances survival in peritonitis, *J. Surg. Res.,* 44(6), 658, 1988.

213. Reynolds, J.V., Zhang, S.M., Thom, A.K., Ziegler, M.M., Naji, A., and Daly, J.M., Arginine as an immunomodulator, *Surg. Forum,* 38, 415, 1987.

214. Reynolds, J.V., Thom, A.K., Zhang, S.M., Ziegler, M.M., Naji, A., and Daly, J.M., Arginine, protein malnutrition, and cancer, *J. Surg. Res.,* 45(6), 513, 1988.

215. Reynolds, J.V., Daly, J.M., Zhang, S., Evantash, E., Shou, J., Sigal, R., and Ziegler, M.M., Immunomodulatory mechanisms of arginine, *Surgery,* 104, 142, 1988.

216. Hinds, A., Nutrients as modulators of immune function, *Can. Med. Assoc. J.,* 145, 35, 1991.

217. Kirk, S.J., Regan, M.C., Wasserkrug, H.L., Sodeyama, M., and Barbul, A., Arginine enhances T-cell responses in athymic nude mice, *JPEN,* 16(5), 429, 1992.

218. Anonymous, Does supplemental arginine alter immune function following major surgery?, *Nutr. Rev.,* 51(2), 54, 1993.

219. Elsair, J., Poey, J., and Issad, H., Effect of arginine chlorohydrate on nitrogen balance during the first three days following routine surgery in man, *Biomed. Press.,* 29, 312, 1978.

220. Barbul, A., Wasserkrug, H.L., Yoshimura, N., Tao, R., and Efron, G., High arginine levels in intravenous hyperalimentation abrogate post-traumatic immune suppression, *J. Surg. Res.,* 36, 624, 1984.

221. Daly, J.M., Reynolds, J., Thom, A., Kinsley, L., Dietrick-Gallagher, M., Shou, J., and Ruggieri, B., Immune and metabolic effects of arginine in the surgical patient, *Ann. Surg.,* 208(4), 512, 1988.

222. Barbul, A., Lazarou, S.A., Efron, D.T., Wasserkrug, H.L., and Efron, G., Arginine enhances wound healing and lymphocyte immune responses in humans, *Surgery,* 108, 331, 1990.

223. Cerra, F.B., Lehmann, S., Konstantinides, N., Dzik, J., Fish, J., Konstantinides, F., LiCari, J.J., and Holman, R.T., Improvement in immune function in ICU patients by enteral nutrition supplemented with arginine, RNA, and menhaden oil is independent of nitrogen balance, *Nutrition,* 7, 193, 1991.

224. Barbul, A., Sisto, D.A., Wasserkrug, H.L., and Efron, G., Arginine stimulates lymphocyte immune responses in healthy humans, *Surgery,* 90, 244, 1981.

225. Hibbs, J.B., Taintor, R.R., and Vavrin, Z., Functional changes in human lymphocytes and monocytes after *in vitro* incubation with arginine, *Nutr. Res.,* 7, 719, 1987.

226. Sigal, R.K., Shou, J., and Daly, J.M., Parenteral arginine infusion in humans: nutrient substrate or pharmacologic agent?, *JPEN,* 16(5), 423, 1992.

227. Knopf, R.F., Conn, J.W., Falans, S.S., Floyd, J.C., Guntsche, E.M., and Rull, J.A., Plasma growth hormone responses to intravenous administration of amino acids, *Clin. Endocrinol.,* 25, 1140, 1965.

228. Rabinowitz, D., Merimee, T.J., Burgess, J.A., and Riggs, L., Growth hormone and insulin release after arginine: indifference to hyperglycemia and epinephrine, *J. Clin. Endocrinol.,* 26, 1170, 1966.

229. Merimee, T.J., Rabinowitz, D., Riggs, L., Burgess, J.A., Rimoin, D.L., and McKusick, V.A., Plasma growth hormone after arginine infusion. Clinical experiences, *N. Engl. J. Med.,* 276, 434, 1967.

230. Rakoff, J.S., Siler, T.M., Sinha, Y.N., and Yen, S.S.C., Prolactin and growth hormone release in response to sequential stimulation by arginine and synthetic TRF, *J. Clin. Endocrinol.,* 37, 641, 1973.

231. Bratusch-Marrain, P. and Waldhausl, W., The influence of amino acids and somatostatin on prolactin and growth hormone release in man, *Acta Endocrinol.,* 90, 403, 1979.

232. Mathieni, G., Growth hormone secretion by arginine stimulus: the effect of both low doses and oral arginine, *Boll. Soc. Ital. Sper. Biol.,* 56, 2254, 1980.

233. Besset, L., Increase in sleep related growth hormone and prolactin secretion after chronic arginine aspartate administration, *Acta Endocrinol.,* 99, 18, 1982.

234. Elsair, C., Effets de l'arginine, administrie par voie orale, *C. R. Soc. Biol.,* 179, 608, 1985.

235. Saggese, G., Cesaretti, G., and Ghirri, P., Use of arginine hydrochloride in non-endocrine growth disorders, *Minerva Pediatr.,* 42, 449, 1990.

236. Pittari, A.M., Becherucci, P., LaCauza, F., and Seminara, S., Therapy with arginine chlorohydrate in children with short constitutional stature, *Minerva Pediatr.,* 45, 61, 1993.

237. Herranz-Jordan, B., Moreno-Romero, F., Cardesa-Garcia, J.J., Santos-Hurtado, I., Aparicio-Palomino, A., and Requena-Guerrero, F., Controlled clinical assay in Clonidine, arginine aspartate, alpha-ketoglutarate of ornithine and ciproheptadine as growth stimulants in children with short stature, *An. Esp. Pediatr.*, 38, 509, 1993.

238. Isidori, A., Lo Monaco, A., and Cappa, M., A study of growth hormone release in man after oral administration of amino acids, *Curr. Med. Res. Opinion*, 7, 475, 1981.

239. Prudden, J.F., Nishihara, G., and Ocampo, L., Studies on growth hormone. III. The effect on wound tensile strength of marked postoperative anabolism induced with growth hormone, *Surg. Gynecol. Obstet.*, 107, 481, 1958.

240. Shernan, S.K., Demling, R.H., Lalonde, C., Lowe, D.K., Eriksson, E., and Wilmore, D.W., Growth hormone enhances reepithelialization of human split-thickness skin graft donor sites, *Surg. Forum*, 40, 37, 1989.

241. Steenfos, H., Spencer, E.M., and Hunt, T.K., Insulin-like growth factor I has a major role in wound healing, *Surg. Forum*, 40, 68, 1989.

242. Billiar, T.R. and Simmons, R., The therapeutic use of L-arginine to increase nitric oxide production, *Nutrition*, 8, 371, 1992.

243. Agostini, A., Marasini, B., Biondi, M.L., Bassani, C., and Cazzaniga, A., L-arginine therapy in Raynaud's phenomenon?, *Int. J. Clin. Lab. Res.*, 21, 202, 1991.

244. Das, U.N., L-Arginine, nitric oxide and collagen vascular diseases: a potential relationship?, *Nutrition*, 8, 371, 1992.

245. Harima, A., Shimizu, H., and Takagi, H., Analgesic effect of L-arginine in patients with persistent pain, *Eur. Neuropsychopharmacol.*, 1(4), 529, 1991.

246. Takagi, H., Physiological and pharmacological actions of a neuroactive dipeptide, kyotorphin, and its precursor, L-arginine, and clinical application, *Nippon Yakurigaku Z.*, 96(3), 85, 1990.

247. Elam, R.P., Morphological changes in adult males from resistance exercise and amino acid supplementation, *J. Sports Med.*, 28, 35, 1988.

248. Bucci, L.R., Nutritional ergogenic aids, in *Nutrition in Exercise and Sport*, 2nd ed., Wolinsky, I. and Hickson, J.F., Eds., CRC Press, Boca Raton, FL, 1994, 295.

249. Bucci, L.R., Micronutrient supplementation and ergogenesis — metabolic intermediates, in *Nutrients as Ergogenic Aids for Sports and Exercise*, CRC Press, Boca Raton, FL, 1993, 41.

250. Liljenquist, J.E., Lacy, W.W., Chaisson, J.L., and Rabinowitz, D., Regulation of alanine and BCAA metabolism in intact man, in *Clinical Nutrition Update: Amino Acids*, Greene, H.L., Holliday, M.A., and Munro, H.N., Eds., AMA, Chicago, 1979, 22.

251. Walser, M. and Williamson, J.R., Eds., *Metabolism and Clinical Implications of Branched Chain Amino Acids and Ketoacids*, Elsevier, New York, 1981.

252. Blackburn, G.L., Grant, J.P., and Young, V.R., Eds., *Amino Acids. Metabolism and Medical Applications*, John Wright/PSG, Boston, 1983.

253. Harper, A.E., Miller, R.H., and Block, K.P., Branched-chain amino acid metabolism, *Annu. Rev. Nutr.*, 4, 409, 1984.

254. Freund, H., Hoover, H.C., Atamian, A., and Fischer, J.E., Infusion of the BCAAs in postoperative patients. Anticatabolic properties, *Ann. Surg.*, 190(1), 18, 1979.

255. Cerra, F.B., Upson, D., Angelico, R., Wiles, C., Lyons, J., Faulkenbach, L., and Paysinger, J., Branched chains support postoperative protein synthesis, *Surgery*, 92, 192, 1982.

256. Desai, S.P., Bistrian, B.R., Moldawer, L.L., Miller, M.M., and Blackburn, G.L., Plasma amino acid concentrations during branched-chain amino acid infusions in stressed patients, *J. Trauma*, 22, 747, 1982.

257. Kern, K.A., Bower, R.H., Atamian, S., Matarese, L.E., Ghory, M.J., and Fischer, J.E., The effect of a new branched chain-enriched amino acid solution on postoperative catabolism, *Surgery*, 92, 780, 1982.

258. Schmitz, J., Dölp, R., Grünert, A., and Ahnefeld, F., The effect of solutions of varying branched chain concentration on the plasma amino acid pattern and metabolism in intensive care patients, *Clin. Nutr.*, 1, 147, 1982.

259. Cerra, F.B., Mazuski, J., Teasley, K., Nuwer, N., Lysne, J., Shronts, E., and Konstantinides, F., Nitrogen retention in critically ill patients is proportional to the BCAA load, *Crit. Care Med.*, 11(10), 775, 1983.

260. Nuwer, N., Cerra, F.B., Shronts, E.P., Lysne, J., Teasley, K.M., and Konstantinides, F.N., Does modified amino acid total parenteral nutrition alter immune response in high level surgical stress?, *JPEN*, 7, 521, 1983.

261. Cerra, F.B., Mazuski, J., Chute, E., Nuwer, N., Teasley, K., Lysne, J., Shronts, E.P., and Konstantinides, F.N., Branched chain metabolic support. A prospective, randomized, double-blind trial in surgical stress, *Ann. Surg.*, 199, 286, 1984.

262. Echenique, M.M., Bistrian, B.R., Moldawer, L.L., Palombop, J.D., Mille, M.M., and Blackburn, G.L., Improvement in amino acid use in the critically ill patient with parenteral formulas enriched with BCAAs, *Surg. Gynecol. Obstet.*, 159, 233, 1984.

263. Desai, S.P., Bistrian, B.R., Moldawer, L.L., and Blackburn, G.L., Whole-body nitrogen and tyrosine metabolism in surgical patients receiving branched-chain amino acid solutions, *Arch. Surg.*, 120, 1345, 1985.

264. Iapichino, G., Radrizzani, D., Bonetti, G., Colombo, A., Damia, G., Della Torre, P., Ferro, A., Leoni, L., Ronzoni, G., and Scherini, A., Parenteral nutrition of injured patients: effect of manipulation of amino acid infusion (increasing branched chain while decreasing aromatic and sulphurated amino acids), *Clin. Nutr.*, 4, 121, 1985.

265. Bower, R.H., Muggia-Sullan, M., Vallgren, S., and Fischer, J., Branched chain amino-acid enriched solutions in the septic patient: a randomized, prospective trial, *Ann. Surg.*, 203, 13, 1986.

266. Brennan, M., Cerra, F., Daly, J., Fischer, J., Moldawer, L., Smith, R., Vinnars, E., Wannemacher, R., and Young, V.R., Report of a research workshop: BCAAs in stress and injury, *JPEN*, 10, 446, 1986.

267. Takala, J. and Klossner, J., Branched chain amino acid enriched parenteral nutrition in surgical intensive care patients, *Clin. Nutr.*, 5, 167, 1986.

268. Vander Woude, P., Morgan, R.E., Kosta, J.M., Davis, A.T., Scholten, D.J., and Dean, R.E., Addition of BCAAs to parenteral nutrition of stressed critically ill patients, *Crit. Care Med.,* 14(8), 685, 1986.

269. Bonau, R., Ang, S., Jeevanandam, M., and Daly, J., High-BCAA solutions. Relationship of composition to efficacy, *JPEN,* 8, 622, 1987.

270. Cerra, F., Hirsch, J., Mullen, K., Blackburn, G., and Luther, W., The effect of stress level, amino acid formula, and nitrogen dose on nitrogen retention in traumatic and septic stress, *Ann. Surg.,* 205, 282, 1987.

271. Desai, S.P., Bistrian, B.R., Palombo, J.D., Moldawer, L.L., and Blackburn, G.L., Branched-chain amino acid administration in surgical patients. Effects on amino acid and fuel substrate profiles, *Arch. Surg.,* 122, 760, 1987.

272. Hammarqvist, F., Wernerman, J., von der Decken, A., and Vinnars, E., The effects of branched chain amino-acids upon postoperative muscle protein synthesis and nitrogen balance, *Clin. Nutr.,* 7, 171, 1988.

273. Mattox, T.W. and Teasley-Strausburg, K.M., Brief communication: clinical experience with high branched-chain parenteral nutrition, *J. Am. Coll. Nutr.,* 11, 25, 1993.

274. Kvamme, E., Ed., *Glutamine and Glutamate in Mammals,* Vols. 1 & 2, CRC Press, Boca Raton, FL, 1988.

275. Häussinger, D. and Sies, H., Eds., *Glutamine Metabolism in Mammalian Tissues,* Springer-Verlag, Berlin, 1984.

276. Bender, D.A., *Amino Acid Metabolism,* 2nd ed., John Wiley & Sons, Chichester, 1985.

277. Lacey, J.M. and Wilmore, D.W., Is glutamine a conditionally essential amino acid?, *Nutr. Rev.,* 48(8), 297, 1990.

278. Lehtinen, P., Takala, I., and Kulonen, E., Dependence of collagen synthesis by embryonic chick tendon cells on the extracellular concentrations of glutamine, *Connect. Tissue Res.,* 6, 155, 1978.

279. Handley, C.J., Speight, G., Leyden, K.M., and Lowther, D.A., Extracellular matrix metabolism by chondrocytes. VII. Evidence that L-glutamine is an essential amino acid for chondrocytes and other connective tissue cells, *Biochim. Biophys. Acta,* 627, 324, 1980.

279a. Shive, W., Snider, R.N., DuBilier, B., Rude, J.C., Clark, G.E., and Ravel, J.O., Glutamine in treatment of peptic ulcer, *Tex. State J. Med.,* 53, 840, 1957.

280. Wernerman, J., Hammarkvist, F., Ali, M.R., and Vinnars, E., Glutamine and ornithine-α-ketoglutarate but not BCAAs reduce the loss of muscle glutamine after surgical trauma, *Metabolism,* 38 (Suppl.1), 63, 1989.

281. Vinnars, E., Hammarqvist, F., von der Decken, A., and Wernerman, J., Role of glutamine and its analogs in posttraumatic muscle protein and amino acid metabolism, *JPEN,* 14 (Suppl.), 125S, 1990.

282. Ziegler, T.R., Benfell, K., Smith, R.J., Young, L.S., Brown, E., Ferrari-Baliviera, E., Lowe, D.K., and Wilmore, D.W., Safety and metabolic effects of L-glutamine administration in humans, *JPEN,* 14 (Suppl.), 137S, 1990.

283. Mobrahan, S., Glutamine: a conditionally essential nutrient or another nutritional puzzle, *Nutr. Rev.,* 50, 331, 1993.

284. Hammarqvist, F., Wernerman, J., Ali, R., von der Decken, A., and Vinnars, E., Addition of glutamine to total parenteral nutrition after elective abdominal surgery spares free glutamine in muscle, counteracts the fall in muscle protein synthesis, and improves nitrogen balance, *Ann. Surg.,* 209, 455, 1989.

285. Karner, J., Roth, E., Ollenschläger, G., Fürst, P., Simmel, A., and Karner, J., Glutamine-containing dipeptides as infusion substrates in the septic state, *Surgery,* 106, 893, 1989.

286. Kapadia, C.R., Colpoys, M.R., Jiang, Z.M., Johnson, D.J., Smith, R.J., and Wilmore, D.W., Maintenance of skeletal muscle intracellular glutamine during standard surgical trauma, *JPEN,* 9, 583, 1985.

287. Kasai, K., Kobayashi, M., and Shimoda, S., Stimulatory effect of glycine on human growth hormone secretion, *Metabolism,* 27, 201, 1978.

288. Kasai, K., Suzuki, H., Nakamura, T., Shiina, H., and Shimoda, S., Glycine stimulates growth hormone in man, *Acta Endocrinol.,* 93, 283, 1980.

289. Braverman, E. R. and Pfeiffer, C. C., Glycine, in *The Healing Nutrients Within. Facts, Findings and New Research on Amino Acids,* Keats Publishing, New Canaan, CT, 1986, 237.

290. Fitzpatrick, D.W. and Fisher, H., Carnosine, histidine, and wound healing, *Surgery,* 91, 56, 1982.

291. Vizioli, M.R. and Almeida, O.P., Effects of carnosine on the development of rat sponge-induced granulation. I. General morphology and glycosaminoglycans histophotometry, *Cell. Mol. Biol.,* 23, 267, 1978.

292. Perelman, M.I., Kornilova, Z.K., Paukov, V.S., Boikov, A.K., and Priimak, A.A., The effect of carnosine on the healing of a lung wound, *Biull. Eksp. Biol. Med.,* 108(9), 352, 1989.

293. Guliaeva, N.V., Dupin, A.M., Levshina, I.P., Obidin, A.B., and Boldyrev, A.A., Carnosine prevents the activation of free-radical lipid oxidation during stress, *Biull. Eksp. Biol. Med.,* 107, 144, 1989.

294. Formaziuk, V.E. and Sergienko, V.I., The use of carnosine in medical practice. Priorities: past and future, *Biokhimiia,* 57, 1404, 1992.

295. Arakawa, T., Satoh, H., Nakamura, A., Nebiki, H., Fukuda, T., Sakuma, H., Nakamura, H., Ishikawa, M., Seiki, M., and Kobayashi, K., Effects of zinc L-carnosine on gastric mucosal and cell damage caused by ethanol in rats. Correlation with endogenous prostaglandin E2, *Dig. Dis. Sci.,* 35, 559, 1990.

296. Seiki, M., Ueki, S., Tanaka, Y., Soeda, M., Hori, Y., Aita, H., Yoneta, T., Morita, H., Tagashira, E., and Okabe, S., Studies on anti-ulcer effects of a new compound, zinc L-carnosine (Z-103), *Folia Pharmacol. Jpn.,* 95, 257, 1990.

297. Yoshikawa, T., Naito, Y., Tanigawa, T., Yoneta, T., Yasuda, M., Ueda, S., Oyamada, H., and Kondo, M., Effect of zinc-carnosine chelate compound (Z-103), a novel antioxidant, on acute gastric mucosal injury induced by ischemia-reperfusion in rats, *Free Radical Res. Commun.,* 14, 289, 1991.

298. Cho, C.H., Luk, C.T., and Ogle, C.W., The membrane-stabilizing action of zinc carnosine (Z-103) in stress-induced gastric ulceration in rats, *Life Sci.,* 49(23), PL189, 1991.

299. Tanigawa, T., Yoshikawa, T., Naito, Y., Yoneta, T., Ueda, S., Oyamada, H., Takemura, T., Morita, Y., Tainaka, K., and Yoshida, N., Antioxidative action of zinc-carnosine compound (Z-103), *Adv. Exp. Med. Biol.*, 264, 223, 1990.

300. Yoshikawa, T., Naito, Y., Tanigawa, T., Yoneta, T., and Kondo, M., The antioxidant properties of a novel zinc-carnosine chelate compound, N-(3-aminopropionyl)-L-histidinato zinc, *Biochim. Biophys. Acta*, 1115, 15, 1991.

301. DSouza, R.S. and Dhume, V.G., Gastric cytoprotection, *Indian J. Physiol. Pharmacol.*, 35, 88, 1991.

302. Gerber, D.A., Decreased concentration of free histidine in serum in rheumatoid arthritis, an isolated amino acid abnormality not associated with generalized hypoaminoacidemia, *J. Rheumatol.*, 2, 384, 1975.

303. Gerber, D.A., Treatment of rheumatoid arthritis with histidine, *Clin. Res.*, 17, 352, 1969.

304. Pinals, R.S., Harris, E.D., Burnett, J.B., and Gerber, D.A., Treatment of rheumatoid arthritis with L-histidine: a randomized, placebo-controlled, double-blind trial, *J. Rheumatol.*, 4, 414, 1977.

305. Halliwell, B. and Gutteridge, J.M.C., *Free Radicals in Biology and Medicine*, 2nd ed., Clarendon Press, Oxford, 1989.

306. Simic, M.G., Taylor, K.A., Ward, J.F., and von Sonntag, C., Eds., *Oxygen Radicals in Biology and Medicine*, Plenum Press, New York, 1987.

307. Bors, W., Saran, M., and Tait, D., *Oxygen Radicals in Chemistry and Biology*, Walter de Gruyter, Berlin, 1984.

308. Localio, S.A., Morgan, M.E., and Hinton, J.W., The biological chemistry of wound healing. I. The effect of dl-methionine on the healing of wounds in protein depleted animals, *Surg. Gynecol. Obstet.*, 86, 582, 1948.

309. Perez-Tamayo, R. and Ihnen, M., The effect of methionine in experimental wound healing; a morphologic study, *Am. J. Path.*, 29, 233, 1953.

310. Williamson, M.B. and Fromm, H.J., The incorporation of sulphur amino acids into proteins of regenerating wound tissue, *J. Biol. Chem.*, 212, 705, 1955.

311. Udupa, K.N., Woessner, J.F., and Dunphy, J.E., The effect of methionine on the production of mucopolysaccharides and collagen in healing wounds of protein-depleted animals, *Surg. Gynecol. Obstet.*, 102, 639, 1956.

312. Edwards, L.C. and Dunphy, J.E., Methionine in wound healing during protein starvation, in *The Healing of Wounds*, Williamson, M.B., Ed., McGraw-Hill, London, 1957, 1.

313. Caldwell, F.T., Rosenberg, I.K., Rosenberg, B.F., and Mishra, O.P., Effect of single amino-acid supplementation upon the tensile strength of wounds in protein-depleted rats, *Surg. Gynecol. Obstet.*, 119, 823, 1964.

314. Stramentinoli, G., Pezzoli, C., and Catto, E., Azione antiflogistica e analgesica della *S*-adenosil-L-metionina (SAMe) in prove sperimentali su animali da laboratorio, *Min. Med.*, 66, 4434, 1975.

315. Gualano, M., Stramentinoli, G., Rossoni, G., and Berti, F., Antiinflammatory activity of S-adenosyl-L-methionine: interference with the eicosanoid system, *Pharmacol. Res. Commun.*, 15, 683, 1983.

316. Polli, E., Cortellaro, M., Parrini, L., Tessari, L., and Cherie-Ligniere, G., Aspetti farmacologici e clinici della solfo-adenosil-etionina (SAMe) nella artropatia degenerativa primaria (osteoartrosi), *Min. Med.*, 66, 4443, 1975.

317. Ballabio, C. and Caruso, I., Le traitement medical de la Coxarthrose, *J. Med. Strasbourg*, 9, 313, 1978.

318. Ceccato, S., Cucinotta, D., Carapezzi, C., and Passeri, M., Indagine Clinica aperta e comparativa sull'impiego della SAMe e del Ketoprofen nella osteoartrosi, *Progresso Med.*, 35, 177, 1979.

319. Ceccato, S., Cucinotta, D., Carapezzi, C., Ferretti, G., and Passeri, M., Studio clinico in doppio cieco sull'effetto terapeutico della SAMe e dell'ibuprofen nella patologia degenerative osteoarticolare, *G. Clin. Med.*, 61, 148, 1980.

320. Marcolongo, R., Girodano, N., Colombo, B., Cherie-Lingerie, G., Todesco, S., Mazzi, A., Mattara, L., Leardini, G., Passeri, M., and Cucinotta, D., Double-blind multicentre study of the activity of S-adenosylmethionine in hip and knee osteoarthritis, *Curr. Ther. Res.*, 37, 82, 1985.

321. diPadova, C., S-adenosylmethionine in the treatment of osteoarthritis. Review of the clinical studies, *Am. J. Med.*, 83(5A), 60, 1987.

322. Müller-Fassbender, H., Double-blind clinical trial of S-adenosylmethionine versus ibuprofen in the treatment of osteoarthritis, *Am. J. Med.*, 83(5A), 81, 1987.

323. Vetter, G., Double-blind comparative clinical trial with S-adenosylmethionine and indomethacin in the treatment of osteoarthritis, *Am. J. Med.*, 83(5A), 78, 1987.

324. Maccagno, A., Di Giorgio, E.E., Caston, O.L., and Sagasta, C.L., Double-blind controlled clinical trial of oral S-adenosylmethionine versus piroxicam in knee osteoarthritis, *Am. J. Med.*, 83(5A), 72, 1987.

325. Caruso, I.K. and Pietrogrande, V., Italian double-blind multi-centre study comparing S-adenosylmethionine, naproxen and placebo in the treatment of degenerative joint disease, *Am. J. Med.*, 83(5A), 66, 1987.

326. Stramentinoli, G., Gualano, M., and Galli-Kienle, M., intestinal absorption of S-adenosyl-L-methionine, *J. Pharmacol. Exp. Ther.*, 209, 323, 1979.

327. Salim, A.S., Role of sulfhydryl-containing agents in the management of venous (varicose) ulceration. A new approach, *Clin. Exp. Dermatol.*, 17, 427, 1992.

328. Salim, A.S., Sulphydryl-containing agents stimulate the healing of duodenal ulceration in man, *Pharmacology*, 45, 170, 1992.

329. Jacob, S.W. and Herschler, R., Introductory remarks: dimethyl sulfoxide after twenty years, *Ann. N.Y. Acad. Sci.*, 411, xiii, 1983.

330. Cynober, L., Ornithine α-ketoglutarate in nutritional support, *Nutrition*, 7(5), 1, 1991.

331. Bessman, S.P., Blood ammonia, *Adv. Clin. Chem.*, 2, 135, 1958.

332. Mutch, B.J.C. and Banister, E.W., Ammonia metabolism in exercise and fatigue: a review, *Med. Sci. Sports Exer.*, 15, 41, 1983.

333. Banister, E.W., Rajendra, W., and Mutch, B.J.C., Ammonia as an indicator of exercise stress: implications of recent findings to sports medicine, *Sports Med.*, 2, 34, 1985.

334. Donnadieu, M., Combourieu, M., and Schimpff, R.M., Comparison de différentes épreuves de stimulation utilisées pour l'étude de la fonction somatotrope chez l'infant, *Pathol. Biol.,* 19, 293, 1971.

335. Gourmalen, M., Donnadieu, M., Schimpff, R.M., Lestradet, H., and Girard, F., Effect of ornithine monochloride on plasma HGH levels, *Ann. Endocrinol.,* 33, 526, 1972.

336. Evian-Brion, D., Donnadieu, M., Roger. M., and Job, J.C., Simultaneous study of somatotrophic and corticotrophic pituitary secretions during ornithine infusion test, *Clin. Endocrinol.,* 17, 119, 1982.

337. Bucci, L.R., Hickson, J.F., Pivarnik, J.M., Wolinsky, I., McMahon, J.C., and Turner, S.D., Ornithine ingestion and growth hormone release in bodybuilders, *Nutr. Res.,* 10, 329, 1990.

338. Fogelholm, G.M., Näveri, H.K., Kiilavuori, K.T.K., and Härkönen, M.H.A., Low-dose amino acid supplementation: no effects on serum growth hormone and insulin in male weightlifters, *Int. J. Sport Nutr.,* 3, 290, 1993.

339. Fricker, P.A., Beasley, S.K., and Copeland, I.W., Physiological growth hormone response of throwers to amino acids, eating and exercise, *Aust. J. Sci. Med. Sport,* 20, 21, 1988.

340. Lambert, M.I., Hefer, J.A., Millar, R.P., and Macfarlane, P.W., Failure of commercial oral amino acid supplements to increase serum growth hormone concentrations in male bodybuilders, *Int. J. Sport Nutr.,* 3, 298, 1993.

341. Bucci, L.R., Hickson, J.F., Wolinsky, I., and Pivarnik, J.M., Ornithine supplementation and insulin release in bodybuilders, *Int. J. Sport Nutr.,* 2, 287, 1992.

342. Cynober, L., Coudray-Lucas, C., de Bandt, J.P., Guéchot, J., Aussel, C., Salvucci, M., and Giboudeau, J., Action of ornithine α–ketoglutarate, ornithine hydrochloride, and calcium α-ketoglutarate on plasma amino acid and hormonal patterns in healthy subjects, *J. Am. Coll. Nutr.,* 9, 2, 1990.

343. Grillo, M.A., Metabolism and function of polyamines, *Int. J. Biochem.,* 17, 943, 1985.

344. Oratz, M., Rothschild, M.A., Schrieber, S.S., Burks, A., Mongelli, J., and Matarese, B., The role of the urea cycle and polyamines in albumin synthesis, *Hepatology,* 3, 567, 1983.

345. Silk, D.B.A. and Payne-James, J.J., Novel substrates and nutritional support: possible role of ornithine α-ketoglutarate, *Proc. Nutr. Soc.,* 49, 381, 1990.

346. Cynober, L., Vaubourdelle, M., Dore, A., and Gibodeau, J., Kinetics and metabolic effects of orally administered ornithine α-ketoglutarate in healthy subjects fed with a standardized regimen, *Am. J. Clin. Nutr.,* 39, 514, 1984.

347. Cynober, L., Saizy, R., Dinh, F.N., Lioret, N., and Gibodeau, J., Effect of enterally administered ornithine alpha-ketoglutarate on plasma and urinary amino acid levels after burn injury, *J. Trauma,* 24, 590, 1984.

348. Vaubourdelle, M., Cynober, L., Lioret, N., Coudray-Lucas, C., Aussel, C., Saizy, R., and Gibodeau, J., Influence of enterally administered ornithine α-ketoglutarate on hormonal patterns in burn patients, *Burns,* 13, 349, 1987.

349. Eriksson, L.S., Reihner, E., and Wahren, J., Infusion of ornithine α–ketoglutarate in healthy subjects: effects on protein metabolism, *Clin. Nutr.,* 4, 73, 1985.

350. Molimard, R., Charpentier, C., and Lemonnier, F., Modifications de l'amino acidemie des cirrhotiques sous l'influence de sels d'ornithine, *Ann. Nutr. Metab.,* 26, 25, 1982.

351. Gay, G., Villaume, C., Beaufrand, M.J., Felber, J.P., and Debry, G., Effects of ornithine alphaketoglutarate on blood insulin, glucagon and amino acids in alcoholic cirrhosis, *Biomedicine,* 30, 173, 1979.

352. Krassowski, J., Rousselle, J., Maeder, E., and Felber, J.P., The effect of ornithine-α-ketoglutarate on insulin and glucagon secretion in normal subjects, *Acta Endocrinol.,* 98, 252, 1981.

353. Elalouf, M., Mizrahi, R., Leclère, J., and Harteman, P., Test d'exploration de las fonction somatotrope par l'ornithine chez l'adulte, *Rev. Fr. Endocrinol. Clin.,* 21, 357, 1980.

354. Lecointre, C.L. and Dailly, R., Stimulation de l'hormone de croissance par l'ornithine en pathologie pediatrique: etude de la response insulinique, *Ouest Med.,* 34, 1197, 1981.

355. Bouchon, Y. and Merle, M., Etude de la cicatisation chez 10 patients atteints d'artérite au stade 4 et traités par l'alpha-cétoglutarate d'Ornithine, *Gaz. Med. Fr.,* 88, 1062, 1981.

356. Bouchon, Y. and Merle, M., A controlled clinical study with double-blind test on forty-two cases, comparing ornithine alpha-cetoglutarate to a placebo for the prevention of local complications in plastic surgery, *Ann. Chir. Plast. Esthet.,* 29, 385, 1984.

357. Bouchon, Y., Michon, J., Chanson, L., and Merle, M., Incidence de l'oxoglutarate d'ornithine sur la duree et la qualite de la cicatrisation au cours des grands decollements de la chirurgie reparatrice et plastique, *Ann. Chir. Plast. Esthet.,* 34, 447, 1989.

358. Pradoura, J.P., Carcassone, Y., and Spitalier, J.M., Incidence de l'oxoglutarate d'ornithine (Cetornan) sur la reparation cutanee des malades de carcinologie cervico-faciales operes, *Cah. ORL,* 25, 61, 1990.

359. Wernerman, J., Hammarqvist, F., von der Decken, A., and Vinnars, E., Ornithine-alpha-ketoglutarate improves skeletal muscle protein synthesis as assessed by ribosome analysis and nitrogen use after surgery, *Ann. Surg.,* 206, 674, 1987.

360. Leander, U., Fürst, P., Vesterberg, K., and Vinnars, E., Nitrogen sparing effect of Ornicetil® in the immediate postoperative state: clinical biochemistry and nitrogen balance, *Clin. Nutr.,* 4, 43, 1985.

361. Hammarqvist, F., Wernerman, J., Ali, R., and Vinnars, E., Effects of an amino acid solution enriched with either BCAAs or ornithine-α-ketoglutarate on the postoperative intracellular amino acid concentration of skeletal muscle, *Br. J. Surg.,* 77, 214, 1990.

362. Vesterberg, K., Vinnars, E., Leander, U., and Fürst, P., Nitrogen sparing effect of Ornicetil® in the immediate postoperative state. II. Plasma and muscle amino acids, *Clin. Nutr.,* 6, 213, 1987.

363. Demarcq, J.M., Delbar, M., Trochu, G., and Crignon, J.J., Effets de l'alpha cetoglutarate d'ornithine sur l'etat nutritionnel des malades de reanimation, *Cah. Anesthesiol.,* 32, 3, 1984.

364. Mertes, N., Möllman, M., Pfisterer, M., Fyrst, P., Puchstein, C., Nolte, G., and Winde, G., Nitrogen sparing effect of Ornicetil-supplemented TPN in hypercatabolic septic or polytraumatized patients, in *Advances in Ammonia Metabolism and Hepatic Encephalopathy,* Soeters, P.B., Wilson, J.H.P., Meijer, A.J., and Holm, E., Eds., Elsevier, Amsterdam, 1988, 141.

365. Nicolas, F. and Rodineau, P., Essai controle croise de l'α-cetoglutarate d'ornithine en alimentation enterale, *Ouest Med.,* 35, 711, 1982.

366. Cynober, L., Blonde, F., Lioret, N., Coudray-Lucas, C., Saizy, R., and Gibodeau, J., Arterio-venous differences in amino acids, glucose, lactate and fatty acids in burn patients; effect of ornithine alpha-ketoglutarate, *Clin. Nutr.,* 5, 221, 1986.

367. Cynober, L., Lioret, N., Coudray-Lucas, C., Aussel, C., Ziegler, F., Baudin, B., Saizy, R., and Gibodeau, J., Action of ornithine alpha-ketoglutarate on protein metabolism in burn patients, *Nutrition,* 3, 187, 1987.

368. Pasquali, J.L., Urlacher, A., and Storck, D., La stimulation lymphocytaire *in vitro* par le pokeweed mitogene chex les sujects normaux et les sujets denutris: influence de sels d'ornithine, *Pathol. Biol.,* 31, 191, 1983.

369. Peacock, E.E., Effect of dietary proline and hydroxyproline on tensile strength of healing wounds, *Proc. Soc. Exp. Biol. Med.,* 105, 380, 1960.

370. Nurmikko, T., Pertovaara, A., and Pontinen, P.J., Attenuation of tourniquet-induced pain in man by D-phenylalanine, a putative inhibitor of enkephalin degradation, *Acupuncture Electrother. Res.,* 12, 185, 1987.

371. Kitade, T., Odahara, Y., Shinohara, S., Ikeuchi, T., Sakai, T., Morikawa, K., Minamikawa, M., Toyota, S., Kawachi, A., and Hyodo, M., Studies on the enhanced effect of acupuncture analgesia and acupuncture anesthesia by D-phenylalanine (first report) — effect on pain threshold and inhibition by naloxone, *Acupuncture Electrother. Res.,* 13, 87, 1988.

372. Kitade, T., Odahara, Y., Shinohara, S., Ikeuchi, T., Sakai, T., Morikawa, K., Minamikawa, M., Toyota, S., Kawachi, A., and Hyodo, M., Studies on the enhanced effect of acupuncture analgesia and acupuncture anesthesia by D-phenylalanine (2nd report) — schedule of administration and clinical effects in low back pain and tooth extraction, *Acupuncture Electrother. Res.,* 15, 121, 1990.

373. Balagot, R.C., Ehrenpreis, S., Kubota, K., Greenberg, J., Analgesia in mice and humans by D-phenylalanine: relation to inhibition of enkephalin degradation and enkephalin levels, *Adv. Pain Res. Ther.,* 5, 289, 1983.

374. Budd, K., Use of D-phenylalanine, an enkephalinase inhibitor, in the treatment of intractable pain, *Adv. Pain Res. Ther.,* 5, 305, 1983.

375. Hyodo, M., Kitade, T. and Hosoka, E., Study on the enhanced analgesic effect induced by phenylalanine during acupuncture analgesia in humans, *Adv. Pain Res. Ther.,* 5, 577, 1983.

376. Walsh, N.E., Ramamurthy, S., Schoenfeld, L., and Hoffman, J., Analgesic effectiveness of D-phenylalanine in chronic pain patients, *Arch. Phys. Med. Rehabil.,* 67, 436, 1986.

377. Walsh, N.E., Letter, *Pain,* 25, 409, 1986.

378. Wurtman, R.J. and Fernstrom, J.D., Effects of the diet on brain neurotransmitters, *Nutr. Rev.,* 32, 193, 1974.

379. Haze, J.J., Toward an understanding of the rationale for the use of dietary supplementation for chronic pain management: the serotonin model, *Cranio,* 9, 339, 1991.

380. Seltzer, S., Stoch, R., Marcus, R., and Jackson, E., Alteration of human pain thresholds by nutritional manipulation and L-tryptophan supplementation, *Pain,* 13, 385, 1982.

381. King, R.B., Pain and tryptophan, *J. Neurosurg.,* 53, 44, 1980.

382. Seltzer, S., Dewart, D., Pollack, R.L., and Jackson, E., The effects of dietary tryptophan on chronic maxillofacial pain and experimental pain tolerance, *J. Psychiatr. Res.,* 17, 181, 1982/83.

383. Shpeen, S.E., Morse, D.R., and Furst, M.L., The effect of tryptophan on postoperative endodontic pain, *Oral Surg. Oral Med. Oral Pathol.,* 58, 446, 1984.

384. Stockstill, J.W., McCall, W.D., Gross, A.J., and Piniewski, B., The effect of L-tryptophan supplementation and dietary instruction on chronic myofascial pain, *J. Am. Dent. Assoc.,* 118, 457, 1989.

385. Ceccherelli, F., Diani, M.M., Altafina, L., Varotto, E., Stefecius, A., Casale, R., Costola, A., and Giron, G.P., Postoperative pain treated by intravenous L-tryptophan: a double-blind study versus placebo in cholecystectomized patients, *Pain,* 47, 163, 1991.

386. Broadhurst, A.D., Tryptophan and rheumatic diseases, *Br. Med. J.,* Aug 13, 456, 1977.

387. Russell, I.J., Michalek, J.E., Vipraio, G.A., Fletcher, E.M., and Wall, K., Serum amino acids in fibrosis/fibromyalgia syndrome, *J. Rheumatol.,* 16 (Suppl. 19), 158, 1989.

388. Yunus, M.B., Dailey, J.W., Aldag, J.C., Masi, A.T., and Jobe, P.C., Plasma tryptophan and other amino acids in primary fibromyalgia: a controlled study, *J. Rheumatol.,* 18, 90, 1992.

389. Moldofsky, H. and Warsh, J.J., Plasma tryptophan and musculoskeletal pain in non-articular rheumatism ("fibrositis syndrome"), *Pain,* 5, 65, 1978.

390. Puttini, P.S. and Caruso, I., Primary fibromyalgia syndrome and 5-hydroxy-L-tryptophan: a 90-day open study, *J. Int. Med. Res.,* 20, 182, 1992.

391. Segura, R. and Ventura, J.L., Effect of L-tryptophan supplementation on exercise performance, *Int. J. Sports Med.,* 9, 301, 1988.

392. Muller, E.E., Brambilla, F., Cavagnini, F., Peracchi, M., and Panerai, A., Slight effect of L-tryptophan on growth hormone release in normal human subjects, *J. Clin. Endocrinol. Metab.,* 39, 1, 1974.

393. Woolf, P.D. and Lee, L., Effect of the serotonin precursor, tryptophan, on pituitary hormone secretion, *J. Clin. Endocrinol. Metab.,* 45, 123, 1977.

394. Fraser, W.M., Tucker, H.S., Grubb, S.R., Wigand, J.P., and Blackard, W.G., Effect of L-tryptophan on growth hormone and prolactin release in normal volunteers and patients with secretory pituitary tumors, *Horm. Metab. Res.*, 11, 149, 1979.

395. Glass, A.R., Schaaf, M., and Dimond, R.C., Absent growth hormone response to L-tryptophan in acromegaly, *J. Clin. Endocrinol. Metab.*, 48, 664, 1979.

396. Koulu, M. and Lammintausta, R., Effect of methionine on L-tryptophan and apomorphine-stimulated growth hormone secretion in man, *J. Clin. Endocrinol. Metab.*, 49, 70, 1979.

397. Hartmann, E., L-tryptophan: a rational hypnotic with clinical potential, *Am. J. Psychiatr.*, 134, 366, 1977.

398. Slutsker, L., Eosinophilia-Myalgia Syndrome associated with exposure to tryptophan from a single manufacturer, *J. Am. Med. Assoc.*, 264(2), 213, 1990.

399. Belongia, R., An investigation of the cause of the Eosinophilia-Myalgia Syndrome associated with tryptophan use, *N. Engl. J. Med.*, 323(6), 357, 1990.

400. Jaffe, R., Eosinophilia Myalgia Syndrome secondary to contaminated tryptophan — clinical experience, *J. Nutr. Med.*, 2, 195, 1991.

401. Aldhous, P., Yellow light on L-tryptophan, *Nature*, 353, 490, 1991.

402. Civitelli, R., Villareal, D.T., Agnusdei, D., Nardi, P., Avioli, L.V., and Gennari, C., Dietary L-lysine and calcium metabolism in humans, *Nutrition*, 8, 400, 1992.

403. Dupont, J., Lipids, in *Present Knowledge in Nutrition*, 6th ed., Brown, M.L., Ed., International Life Sciences Foundation, Washington, D.C., 1990, 56.

404. Linscheer, W.G. and Vergroesen, A.J., Lipids, in *Modern Nutrition in Health and Disease*, 7th ed., Shils, M.E. and Young, V.R., Eds., Lea & Febiger, Philadelphia, 1988, 72.

405. Chow, C.K., Ed., *Fatty Acids in Foods and Their Health Implications*, Marcel Dekker, New York, 1992.

406. Simopoulos, A.P., Kifer, R.R., Martin, R.E., and Barlow, S.M., Eds., *Health Effects of ω3 Polyunsaturated Fatty Acids in Seafoods*, Vol. 66, World Review of Nutrition and Dietetics, S. Karger, Basel, 1991.

407. Horrobin, D.F., Ed., *Omega-6 Essential Fatty Acids. Pathophysiology and Roles in Clinical Medicine*, Wiley-Liss, New York, 1990.

408. Willis, A.L., Ed., *CRC Handbook of Eicosanoids: Prostaglandins and Related Lipids*, Vols. 1–3, CRC Press, Boca Raton, FL, 1987.

409. Rudin, D.O. and Felix, C., *The Omega-3 Phenomenon. The Nutrition Breakthrough of the '80s*, Rawson Associates, New York, 1987.

410. Horrobin, D.F., Ed., *Clinical Uses of Essential Fatty Acids*, Eden Press, Montreal, 1982.

411. Chapkin, R.S., Reappraisal of the essential fatty acids, in *Fatty Acids in Foods and Their Health Implications*, Chow, C.K., Ed., Marcel Dekker, New York, 1992, 429.

412. Horrobin, D.F. and Manku, M.S., Clinical biochemistry of essential fatty acids, in *Omega-6 Essential Fatty Acids. Pathophysiology and Roles in Clinical Medicine*, Horrobin, D.F., Ed., Wiley-Liss, New York, 1990, 21.

413. Anderson, G.J. and Connor, W.E., On the demonstration of ω-3 essential-fatty acid deficiency in humans, *Am. J. Clin. Nutr.*, 49, 585, 1989.

414. Bjerve, K.S., ω3 Fatty acid deficiency in man: implications for the requirement of alpha-linolenic acid and long-chain ω3 fatty acids, in *Health Effects of ω3 Polyunsaturated Fatty Acids in Seafoods*, Vol. 66, World Review of Nutrition and Dietetics, Simopoulos, A.P., Kifer, R.R., Martin, R.E., and Barlow, S.M., Eds., S. Karger, Basel, 1991, 133.

415. Horrobin, D.F., Essential fatty acids: a review, in *Clinical Uses of Essential Fatty Acids*, Horrobin, D.F., Ed., Eden Press, Montreal, 1982, 3.

416. Hwang, D., Dietary fatty acids and eicosanoids, in *Fatty Acids in Foods and Their Health Implications*, Chow, C.K., Ed., Marcel Dekker, New York, 1992, 545.

417. Sinclair, H.M., History of essential fatty acids, in *Omega-6 Essential Fatty Acids. Pathophysiology and Roles in Clinical Medicine*, Horrobin, D.F., Ed., Wiley-Liss, New York, 1990, 1.

418. Bruckner, G., Biological effects of polyunsaturated fatty acids, in *Fatty Acids in Foods and Their Health Implications*, Chow, C.K., Ed., Marcel Dekker, New York, 1992, 631.

419. Endres, S., Meydani, S.N., and Dinarello, C.A., Effects of ω3 fatty acid supplements on *ex vivo* synthesis of cytokines in human volunteers. Comparison with oral aspirin and ibuprofen, in *Health Effects of ω3 Polyunsaturated Fatty Acids in Seafoods*, Vol. 66, World Review of Nutrition and Dietetics, Simopoulos, A.P., Kifer, R.R., Martin, R.E., and Barlow, S.M., Eds., S. Karger, Basel, 1991, 401.

420. Endres, S., Ghorbani, R., Kelley, V.E., Georgilis, K., Lonnemann, G., van der Meer, J.W.M., Cannon, J.G., Rogers, T.S., Klempner, M.S., Weber, P.C., Schaefer, E.J., Wolff, S.M., and Dinarello, C.A., The effect of dietary supplementation with ω3 polyunsaturated fatty acids on the synthesis of interleukin-1 and tumor necrosis factor by mononuclear cells, *N. Engl. J. Med.*, 320, 265, 1989.

421. Sperling, R.I., Effects of dietary fish oil on leukocyte leukotriene and PAF generation and on neutrophil chemotaxis, in *Health Effects of ω3 Polyunsaturated Fatty Acids in Seafoods*, Vol. 66, World Review of Nutrition and Dietetics, Simopoulos, A.P., Kifer, R.R., Martin, R.E., and Barlow, S.M., Eds., S. Karger, Basel, 1991, 391.

422. Sperling, R.I., Robin, J.L., Kylander, K.A., Lee, T.H., Lewis, R.A., and Austen, K.F., The effects of n-3 polyunsaturated fatty acids on the generation of platelet-activating factor-acether by human monocytes, *J. Immunol.*, 139, 4186, 1987.

423. Ringer, T.V., Hughes, G.S., Spillers, C.R., Watts, K.C., Francom, S.F., and DeLoof, M.J., Fish oil blunts the pain response to cold pressor testing in normal males, *J. Am. Coll. Nutr.*, 8, 435, 1989.

424. McCarty, D.J. and Koopman, W.J., Eds., *Arthritis and Allied Conditions. A Textbook of Rheumatology*, Vol. 1, Lea & Febiger, Philadelphia, 1993.

425. Kremer, J.M., Bigaouette, J., Michalek, A.V., Timchalk, M.A., Lininger, L., Rynes, R.I., Huyck, C., Zieminski, J., and Bartholomew, L.E., Effects of manipulation of dietary fatty acids on clinical manifestations of rheumatoid arthritis, *Lancet*, 1, 184, 1985.

426. Kremer, J.M., Jubiz, W., Michalek, A., Rynes, R.I., Bartholomew, L.E., Bigaouette, J., Timchalk, M., Beeler, D., and Lininger, L., Fish-oil fatty acid supplementation in active rheumatoid arthritis. A double-blinded, controlled, crossover study, *Ann. Intern. Med.,* 106(4), 497, 1987.

427. Sperling, R.I., Weinblatt, M., Robin, J.L., Ravalese, J., Hoover, R.L., House, F., Coblyn, J.S., Fraser, P.A., Spur, B.W., and Robinson, D.R., Effects of dietary supplementation with marine fish oil on leukocyte lipid mediator generation and function in rheumatoid arthritis, *Arthritis Rheum.,* 30(9), 988, 1987.

428. Magaro, M., Altomonte, L., Zoli, A., Mirone, L., De Sole, P., Di Mario, G., Lippa, S., and Oradei, A., Influence of diet with different lipid composition on neutrophil chemiluminescence and disease activity in patients with rheumatoid arthritis, *Ann. Rheum. Dis.,* 47(10), 793, 1988.

429. Tulleken, J.E. and van Rijswijk, M.H., Fish oil in the treatment of patients with rheumatoid arthritis, *Ned. Tijdschr. Geneeskd.,* 132(41), 1875, 1988.

430. Cleland, L.G., French, J.K., Betts, W.H., Murphy, G.A., and Elliott, M.J., Clinical and biochemical effects of dietary fish oil supplements in rheumatoid arthritis, *J. Rheumatol.,* 15(10), 1471, 1988.

431. Belch, J.J., Ansell, D., Madhok, R., O'Dowd, A., and Sturrock, R.D., Effects of altering dietary essential fatty acids on requirements for non-steroidal antiinflammatory drugs in patients with rheumatoid arthritis: a double blind placebo controlled study, *Ann. Rheum. Dis.,* 47(2), 96, 1988.

432. Tulleken, J.E., Limburg, P.C., and van Rijswijk, M.H., N-3 polyunsaturated acids, interleukin-1 and tumor necrosis factor. Letter, *N. Engl. J. Med.,* 321, 55, 1989.

433. van der Tempel, H., Tulleken, J.E., Limburg, P.C., Muskiet, F.A.J., and van Rijswik, M.H., Effects of fish oil supplementation in rheumatoid arthritis, *Ann. Rheum. Dis.,* 49, 76, 1990.

434. Kremer, J.M., Lawrence, D.A., Jubiz, W., DiGiacomo, R., Rynes, R., Bartholomew, L.E., and Sherman, M., Dietary fish oil and olive oil supplementation in patients with rheumatoid arthritis: clinical and immunological effects, *Arthritis Rheum.,* 33, 810, 1990.

435. Kremer, J.M. and Robinson, D.R., Studies of dietary supplementation with ω3 fatty acids in patients with rheumatoid arthritis, in *Health Effects of ω3 Polyunsaturated Fatty Acids in Seafoods*, Vol. 66, World Review of Nutrition and Dietetics, Simopoulos, A.P., Kifer, R.R., Martin, R.E., and Barlow, S.M., Eds., S. Karger, Basel, 1991, 367.

436. Boissonneault, G.A. and Hayek, M.G., Dietary fat, immunity, and inflammatory disease, in *Fatty Acids in Foods and Their Health Implications*, Chow, C.K., Ed., Marcel Dekker, New York, 1992, 707.

437. Carmichael, H.A., Use of nutritional precursors or prostaglandin E1 in the management of rheumatoid arthritis and chronic coxsackie infection, in *Clinical Uses of Essential Fatty Acids*, Horrobin, D.F., Ed., Eden Press, Montreal, 1982, 139.

438. Hansen, T.M., Lerche, A., Kassis, V., Lorenzen, I., and Søndergaard, J., Treatment of rheumatoid arthritis with prostaglandin E$_1$ precursors *cis*-linoleic acid and γ-linolenic acid, Scand. J. Rheum., 12, 85, 1983.

439. Werbach, M.R., *Nutritional Influences on Illness. A Sourcebook of Clinical Research*, 2nd ed., Third Line Press, Tarzana, CA, 1993.

440. Diboune, M., Ferard, G., Ingenbleek, Y., Tulasne, P.A., Calon, B., Hasselman, M., Suader, P., Spielmann, D., and Metais, P., Composition of phospholipid fatty acids in red blood cell membranes of patients in intensive care units: effects of different intakes of soybean oil, medium-chain triglycerides, and black-currant seed oil, *JPEN,* 16(2), 136, 1992.

441. Gottschlich, M.M., Jenkins, M., Warden, G.D., Baumer, T., Havens, P., Snook, J.T., and Alexander, J.W., Differential effects of three enteral dietary regimens on selected outcome variables in burn patients, *JPEN,* 14, 225, 1990.

442. Bach, A.S. and Babayan, V.K., Medium-chain triglycerides — an update, *Am. J. Clin. Nutr.,* 36, 950, 1982.

443. Babayan, V.K., Medium chain triglycerides and structured lipids, *Nutr. Support Serv.,* 6, 26, 1986.

444. Seaton, T.B., Welle, S.L., Warenko, M.K., and Campbell, R.G., Thermic effect of medium-chain and long-chain triglycerides in man, *Am. J. Clin. Nutr.,* 44, 630, 1976.

445. Hill, J.O., Peters, J.C., Yang, D., Sharp, T., Kaler, M., Abumrad, N.N., and Greene, H.L., Thermogenesis in human overfeeding with medium-chain triglycerides, *Metabolism,* 38, 641, 1989.

446. Johnson, R.C., Young, S.K., Cotter, R., Lin., L., and Rowe, W.B., Medium-chain triglyceride lipid emulsion: metabolism and tissue distribution, *Am. J. Clin. Nutr.,* 52, 502, 1990.

447. Baba, N., Bracco, E.F., and Hashim, S.A., Enhanced thermogenesis and diminished deposition of fat in response to overfeeding with diet containing medium chain triglyceride, *Am. J. Clin. Nutr.,* 35, 678, 1982.

448. Geliebter, A., Torbay, N., Bracco, E.F., Hashim, S.A., and van Itallie, T.B., Overfeeding with medium-chain triglyceride diet results in diminished deposition of body fat, *Am. J. Clin. Nutr.,* 37, 1, 1983.

449. Scalfi, L., Coltorti, A., and Contaldo, F., Postprandial thermogenesis in lean and obese subjects after meals supplemented with medium-chain and long-chain triglyceride, *Am. J. Clin. Nutr.,* 53, 1130, 1991.

450. Dias, V., Effects of feeding and energy balance in adult humans, *Metabolism,* 39, 887, 1990.

451. Blackburn, G.L., Kater, G., Mascoli, E.A., Kowalchuk, M., Babayan, V.K., and Bistrian, B.R., A reevaluation of coconut oil's effect on serum cholesterol and atherogenesis, *J. Philipp. Med. Assoc.,* 65, 144, 1989.

452. Lenaz, G., Ed., *Coenzyme Q. Biochemistry, Bioenergetics and Clinical Applications of Ubiquinone*, John Wiley & Sons, Chichester, 1985.

453. Lenaz, G., Fato, R., Castelluccio, C., Batino, M., Cavazzoni, M., Rauchova, H., and Castelli, G.P., Coenzyme Q saturation kinetics of mitochondrial enzymes: theory, experimental aspects and biomedical implications, in *Biomedical and Clinical Aspects of Coenzyme Q*, Vol. 6, Folkers, K., Yamagami, T., and Littarru, G.P., Eds., Elsevier/North-Holland, Amsterdam, 1991, 11.

454. Littarru, G.P., Nakamura, R., Ho, L., Folkers, K., and Kuzell, W.C., Deficiency of coenzyme Q_{10} in gingival tissue from patients with periodontal disease, *Proc. Natl. Acad. Sci.,* 68, 2232, 1971.

455. Nakamura, R., Littarru, G.P., Folkers, K., and Wilkinson, E.G., Deficiency of coenzyme Q in gingiva of patients with periodontal disease, *Int. J. Vit. Nutr. Res.,* 43, 84, 1973.

456. Hansen, I.L., Iwamoto, Y., Kishi, K., Folkers, K., and Thompson, L.E., Bioenergetics in clinical medicine. IX. Gingival and leucocytic deficiencies of coenzyme Q_{10} in patients with periodontal disease, *Res. Commun. Chem. Pathol. Pharmacol.,* 14, 729, 1976.

457. Iwamoto, Y., Nakamura, R., Folkers, K., and Morrison, R.F., Study of periodontal disease and coenzyme Q, *Res. Commun. Chem. Pathol. Pharmacol.,* 11, 265, 1975.

458. Shizukuishi, S., Hanioka, T., Tsunemitsu, A., Fukunaga, Y., Kishi, T., and Sato, N., Clinical effect of coenzyme Q_{10} on periodontal disease; evaluation of oxygen utilization in gingiva by tissue reflectance spectrophotometry, in *Biomedical and Clinical Aspects of Coenzyme Q*, Vol. 5, Folkers, K. and Yamamura, Y., Eds., Elsevier, Amsterdam, 1986, 359.

459. Tsunemitsu, A. and Matsumura, T., Effects of coenzyme Q administration on hypercitricemia of patients with periodontal disease, *J. Dent. Res.,* 46, 1382, 1967.

460. Wilkinson, E.G., Arnold, R.M., Folkers, K., Hansen, I., Kishi, H., Bioenergetics in clinical medicine. II. Adjunctive treatment with coenzyme Q in periodontal therapy, *Res. Commun. Pathol. Pharmacol.,* 12, 111, 1975.

461. Iwamoto, Y., Watanabe, T., Okamoto, H., Ohta, N., and Folkers, K., in *Biomedical and Clinical Aspects of Coenzyme Q*, Vol. 3, Folkers, K. and Yamamura, Y., Eds., Elsevier, Amsterdam, 1981, 109.

462. Matsumura, T., Saji, S., Nakamura, R., and Folkers, K., Evidence for enhanced treatment of periodontal disease by therapy with coenzyme Q, *Int. J. Vit. Nutr. Res.,* 43, 537, 1973.

463. Lenaz, G., Barnabei, O., Rabbi, A., and Battino, M., Eds., *Highlights in Ubiquinone Research,* Taylor & Francis, London, 1990.

464. Folkers, K. and Yamamura, Y., Eds., *Biomedical and Clinical Aspects of Coenzyme Q,* Elsevier/North-Holland, Amsterdam, 1977.

465. Yamamura, Y., Folkers, K., and Ito, Y., Eds., *Biomedical and Clinical Aspects of Coenzyme Q,* Vol. 2, Elsevier/ North-Holland, Amsterdam, 1980.

466. Folkers, K. and Yamamura, Y., Eds., *Biomedical and Clinical Aspects of Coenzyme Q,* Vol. 3, Elsevier/North-Holland, Amsterdam, 1981.

467. Folkers, K. and Yamamura, Y., Eds., *Biomedical and Clinical Aspects of Coenzyme Q,* Vol. 4, Elsevier/North-Holland Amsterdam, 1984.

468. Folkers, K. and Yamamura, Y., Eds., *Biomedical and Clinical Aspects of Coenzyme Q,* Vol. 5, Elsevier/North-Holland Amsterdam, 1986.

469. Folkers, K., Yamagami, T., and Littarru, G.P., *Biomedical and Clinical Aspects of Coenzyme Q,* Vol. 6, Elsevier/North-Holland, Amsterdam, 1991.

470. Tatum, V. and Chow, C.K., Effects of processing and storage on fatty acids in edible oils, in *Fatty Acids in Foods and Their Health Implications*, Chow, C.K., Ed., Marcel Dekker, New York, 1992, 337.

471. Chow, C.K., Biological effects of oxidized fatty acids, in *Fatty Acids in Foods and Their Health Implications*, Chow, C.K., Ed., Marcel Dekker, New York, 1992, 689.

472. Kinsella, J.E., α-Linolenic acid: functions and effects of linolenic acid metabolism and eicosanoid-mediated reactions, *Adv. Food Nutr. Res.,* 35, 1, 1991.

473. Nordøy, A., Is there a rational use for n-3 fatty acids (fish oils) in clinical medicine?, *Drugs,* 42, 331, 1991.

474. Simopoulos, A.P., Omega-3 fatty acids in health and disease and in growth and development, *Am. J. Clin. Nutr.,* 54, 438, 1991.

475. Fernandes, G. and Venkatraman, J.T., Role of omega-3 fatty acids in health and disease, *Nutr. Res.,* 13 (Suppl. 1), S19, 1993.

476. Moore, T., *Vitamin A,* Elsevier, Amsterdam, 1957, 535.

477. Olson, J.A., Vitamin A, in *Handbook of Vitamins. Second Edition, Revised and Expanded*, 2nd ed., Machlin, L.J., Ed., Marcel Dekker, New York, 1991, 1.

478. Olson, J.A., Vitamin A, in *Present Knowledge in Nutrition*, 6th ed., Brown, M.L., Ed., International Life Sciences Foundation, Washington, D.C., 1990, 96.

479. Olson, J.A., Vitamin A, retinoids, and carotenoids, in *Modern Nutrition in Health and Disease*, 7th ed., Shils, M.E. and Young, V.R., Eds., Lea & Febiger, Philadelphia, 1988, 292.

480. Bender, D.A., Vitamin A: retinol and β-carotene, in *Nutritional Biochemistry of the Vitamins*, Cambridge University Press, Cambridge, 1992, 19.

481. Combs, G.F., Vitamin A, in *The Vitamins. Fundamental Aspects in Nutrition and Health*, Academic Press, San Diego, 1992, 119.

482. Krinsky, N.I. and Denke, S.M., The interaction of oxygen and oxyradicals with carotenoids, *J. Natl. Cancer Inst.,* 69, 205, 1982.

483. Burton, G.W. and Ingold, K.U., β-Carotene, an unusual type of lipid anti-oxidant, *Science,* 224, 569, 1984.

484. Freiman, M., Seifter, E., Connerton, C., and Levenson, S.M., Vitamin A deficiency and surgical stress, *Surg. Forum,* 21, 81, 1970.

485. Pollack, S.V., Wound healing: a review. III. Nutritional factor affecting wound healing, *J. Dermatol. Surg. Oncol.,* 5, 615, 1979.

486. Hunt, T.K., Ehrlich, H.P., Garcia, J.A., and Dunphy, J.E., Effect of vitamin A on reversing the inhibitory effect of cortisone on healing of open wounds in animals and man, *Ann. Surg.,* 170, 633, 1969.

487. Hunt, T.K., Vitamin A and wound healing, *J. Am. Acad. Dermatol.,* 15, 817, 1986.

488. Bendich, A. and Langseth, L., Safety of vitamin A, *Am. J. Clin. Nutr.,* 49, 358, 1989.

489. Gerber, L.E. and Erdmann, J.W., Effect of dietary retinyl acetate, β-carotene and retinoic acid on wound healing in rats, *J. Nutr.,* 112, 1555, 1982.

490. Chernov, M.S., Hale, H.W., and Wood, M., Prevention of stress ulcers, *Am. J. Surg.,* 122, 674, 1971.

491. Chernov, M.S., Cook, F.B., Wood, M., and Hale, H.W., Stress ulcer: a preventable disease, *J. Trauma,* 12, 831, 1972.

492. Rai, K. and Courtemanche, A.D., Vitamin A assay in burned patients, *J. Trauma,* 15, 419, 1975.

493. Patty, I., Benedek, S., Deak, G., Javor, T., Kenez, P., Nagy, L., Simon, L., Tarnok, F., and Mozsik, G., Controlled trial of vitamin A therapy in gastric ulcer, *Lancet,* 2, 876, 1982.

494. Honkanen, V., Konttinen, Y.T., and Mussalo-Rauhamaa, H., Vitamins A and E, retinol binding protein and zinc in rheumatoid arthritis, *Clin. Exp. Rheumatol.,* 7(5), 465, 1989.

495. Cohen, B.E., Gill, G., Cullen, P.R., and Morris, P.J., Reversal of postoperative immunosuppression in man by vitamin A, *Surg. Gynecol. Obstet.,* 149, 658, 1979.

496. Bendich, A., The safety of beta carotene, *Nutr. Cancer,* 11, 207, 1988.

497. Collins, E.D. and Norman, A.W., Vitamin D, in *Handbook of Vitamins. Second Edition, Revised and Expanded,* 2nd ed., Machlin, L.J., Ed., Marcel Dekker, New York, 1991, 59.

498. Norman, A.W., Vitamin D, in *Present Knowledge in Nutrition,* 6th ed., Brown, M.L., Ed., International Life Sciences Foundation, Washington, D.C., 1990, 108.

499. DeLuca, H.F., Vitamin D and its metabolites, in *Modern Nutrition in Health and Disease,* 7th ed., Shils, M.E. and Young, V.R., Eds., Lea & Febiger, Philadelphia, 1988, 313.

500. Bender, D.A., Vitamin D, in *Nutritional Biochemistry of the Vitamins,* Cambridge University Press, Cambridge, 1992, 51.

501. Combs, G.F., Vitamin D, in *The Vitamins. Fundamental Aspects in Nutrition and Health,* Academic Press, San Diego, 1992, 151.

502. Norman, A.W., Ed., *Vitamin D. Molecular Biology and Clinical Nutrition,* Marcel Dekker, New York, 1980.

503. Norman, A.W., Boullion, R., and Thomasset, M., Eds., *Vitamin D. Gene Regulation, Structure-Function Analysis and Clinical Application,* Walter de Gruyter, Berlin, 1991.

504. Chen, T.C., Tian, X., and Holick, M.F., 1α25-Dihydroxyvitamin D: a novel agent for wound healing, in *Vitamin D. Gene Regulation, Structure-Function Analysis and Clinical Application,* Norman, A.W., Boullion, R., and Thomasset, M., Eds., Walter de Gruyter, Berlin, 1991, 435.

505. Farrell, P.M., Vitamin E, 5, in *Modern Nutrition in Health and Disease,* 7th ed., Shils, M.E. and Young, V.R., Eds., Lea & Febiger, Philadelphia, 1988, 340.

506. Machlin, L.J., Vitamin E, in *Handbook of Vitamins. Second Edition, Revised and Expanded,* 2nd ed., Machlin, L.J., Ed., Marcel Dekker, New York, 1991, 99.

507. Bieri, J.G., Vitamin E, 3, in *Present Knowledge in Nutrition,* 6th ed., Brown, M.L., Ed., International Life Sciences Foundation, Washington, D.C., 1990, 117.

508. Bender, D.A., Vitamin E, in *Nutritional Biochemistry of the Vitamins,* Cambridge University Press, Cambridge, 1992, 87.

509. Combs, G.F., Vitamin E, in *The Vitamins. Fundamental Aspects in Nutrition and Health,* Academic Press, San Diego, 1992, 151.

510. Diplock, A.T., Machlin, L.J., Packer, L., and Pryor, W.A., *Vitamin E. Biochemistry and Health Implications,* Vol. 570, *Annals of the New York Academy of Sciences,* New York Academy of Sciences, New York, 1989.

511. Lubin, B. and Machlin, L.J., *Vitamin E: Biochemical, Hematological, and Clinical Aspects,* Vol. 393, *Annals of the New York Academy of Sciences,* New York Academy of Sciences, New York, 1982.

512. Kagan, V.E., Spirichev, V.B., Serbinova, E.A., Witt, E., Erin, A.N., and Packer, L., The significance of vitamin E and free radicals in physical exercise, in *Nutrition in Exercise and Sport,* 2nd ed., Wolinksy, I. and Hickson, J.F., Eds., CRC Press, Boca Raton, FL, 1994, 185.

513. Stuyvesant, V.W. and Jolley, W.B., Antiinflammatory activity of d-α-tocopherol (vitamin E) and linoleic acid, *Nature,* 216, 586, 1967.

514. Kamimura, M., Antiinflammatory effect of vitamin E, *J. Vitaminol.,* 18, 204, 1972.

515. Chan, A.C. and Hamelin, S.S., The effects of vitamin E and corn oil on prostacyclin and thromboxane B_2 synthesis in rats, *Ann. N. Y. Acad. Sci.,* 393, 201, 1982.

516. Khettab, N., Amory, M.C., Briand, G., Bousquet, B., Combre, A., Forlot, P., and Barey, M., Photoprotective effect of vitamins A and E on polyamine and oxygenated free radical metabolism in hairless mouse epidermis, *Biochimie,* 70, 1709, 1988.

517. Hirschelmann, R. and Bekemeier, H., Antiphlogistic effect by antioxidant therapy with vitamin C and E?, *Z. Klin. Med.,* 44, 83, 1988.

518. Brandt, K., Elmadfa, I., Sobirey, M., and Schlotzer, E., Effect of various combinations of DL-α-tocopherol and acetylsalicylic acid on adjuvant arthritis in rats, *Z. Rheumatol.,* 47, 381, 1988.

519. Kheir-Eldin, A.A., Hamdy, M.A., Motawi, T.K., Shaheen, A.A., and Abd El Gawad, H.M., Biochemical changes in arthritic rats under the influence of vitamin E, *Agents Actions,* 36, 300, 1992.

520. Yoshikawa, T., Tanaka, H., and Kondo, M., Effect of vitamin E on adjuvant arthritis in rats, *Biochem. Med.,* 29(2), 227, 1983.

521. Pletsityi, K.D., Nikushkin, E.V., Askerov, M.A., and Ponomarev, L.G., Inhibition of the development of adjuvant arthritis in rats as affected by vitamin E, *Biull. Eksp. Biol. Med.,* 103(1), 43, 1987.

522. Schwartz, E.R., The modulation of osteoarthritic development by vitamins C and E, *Int. J. Vit. Nutr. Res.*, 26 (Suppl.), 141, 1984.

523. Ehrlich, H.P., Tarver, H., and Hunt, T.K., Inhibitory effects of vitamin E on collagen synthesis and wound repair, *Ann. Surg.*, 175, 235, 1972.

524. Peters, C.R., Shaw, T., and Raju, D.R., The influence of vitamin E on capsule formation and contracture around silicone implants, *Ann. Plast. Surg.*, 5, 347, 1980.

525. Caffee, H.H., Vitamin E and capsule contracture, *Ann. Plast. Surg.*, 19, 512, 1987.

526. Kagoma, P., Burger, S.N., Seifter, E., Levenson, S.M., and Demetriou, A.A., The effect of vitamin E on experimentally induced peritoneal adhesions in mice, *Arch. Surg.*, 120, 949, 1985.

527. Hayden, R.E., Yeung, C.S.T., Paniello, R.C., Bello, S.L., and Dawson, S.M., The effect of glutathione and vitamins A, C and E on acute skin flap survival, *Laryngoscope*, 97, 1176, 1987.

528. Taren, D.L, Chvapil, M., and Weber, C.W., Increasing the breaking strength of wounds exposed to pre-operative irradiation using vitamin E supplementation, *Int. J. Vit. Nutr. Res.*, 57, 133, 1987.

529. Iwasa, K., Ikata, T., and Fukuzawa, K., Protective effect of vitamin E on spinal cord injury by compression and concurrent lipid peroxidation, *Free Radical Biol. Med.*, 6, 599, 1989.

530. Anderson, D.K., Saunders, R.D., Demediuk, P., Dugan, L.L., Braughler, M., Hall, E.D., Means, E.D., and Horrocks, L.A., Lipid hydrolysis and peroxidation in injured spinal cord: partial protection with methylprednisolone or vitamin E and selenium, *Cent. Nerv. Sys. Trauma*, 2, 257, 1985.

531. Chen, Z., Meng, X., Feng, J., Wang, S., and Dong, Y., Dynamic changes of lipid peroxides and vitamin E contents in plasma, eschar, liver mitochondria and microsomes after burn injury, *J. Med. Coll. PLA*, 3, 244, 1988.

532. Meng, X., Chen, Z., Wang, S., Dong, Y., and Feng, J., Mechanism of erythrocyte damage after burn injury in rats: interrelationship between lipid peroxides, α-tocopherol, and degree of hydrogen peroxide-induced hemolysis, *J. Med. Coll. PLA*, 3, 250, 1988.

533. Bekiarova, G.I., Markova, M.P., and Kagan, V.E., α-Tocopherol protection of erythrocytes from hemolysis induced by thermal injury, *Biull. Eksp. Biol. Med.*, 107, 413, 1989.

534. Bekiarova, G., Kozarev, I., and Yankova, T., Dependence between the free-radical peroxidation, the activity of the superoxide dismutase glucose-6-phosphate dehydrogenase and erythrocytes hemolysis after thermal trauma and α-tocopherol treatment, *Acta Physiol. Pharmacol. Bulg.*, 15, 68, 1989.

535. Kuroiwa, K., Nelson, J.L., Boyce, S.T., Alexander, J.W., Ogle, C.K., and Inoue, S., Metabolic and immune effect of vitamin E supplementation after burn, *JPEN*, 15, 22, 1991.

536. Fitzgerald, G.A. and Brash, A.R., Endogenous prostacyclin and thromboxane biosynthesis during chronic vitamin E therapy in man, *Ann. N. Y. Acad. Sci.*, 393, 209, 1982.

537. Baehner, R.L., Boxer, L.A., Ingraham, L.M., Butterick, C., and Haak, R.A., The influence of vitamin E on human polymorphonuclear cell metabolism and function, *Ann. N. Y. Acad. Sci.*, 393, 237, 1982.

538. Baker, J.L., The effectiveness of alpha-tocopherol (vitamin E) in reducing the incidence of spherical contracture around breast implants, *Plast. Reconstr. Surg.*, 68, 696, 1981.

539. Lovas, R.M., Erfahrungen mit Vitamin-E-Langzeitapplikation in der ästhetisch-plastichen Chirurgie, in *Vitamin E in der Rehabilitation und ärztlichen Praxis*, Böhlau, V., Ed., Notamed, Melsungen, 1984, 154.

540. Sukolinskii, V.N. and Morozkina, T.S., Prevention of postoperative complications in patients with stomach cancer using an antioxidant complex, *Vopr. Onkol.*, 35, 12142, 1989.

541. Ramasastry, S.S., Angel, M.F., Narayanan, K., Basford, R.A., and Futrell, J.W., Biochemical evidence of lipoperoxidation in venous stasis ulcer. Beneficial role of vitamin E as antioxidant, *Ann. N.Y. Acad. Sci.*, 570, 506, 1989.

542. Mézes, M. and Bartosiewicz, G., Investigations on vitamin E and lipid peroxide status in rheumatic diseases, *Clin. Rheumatol.*, 2, 259, 1983.

543. Mézes, M., Par, A., Bartosiewicz, G., and Nemeth, J., Vitamin E content and lipid peroxidation of blood in some chronic inflammatory diseases, *Acta Physiol. Hung.*, 69(1), 133, 1987.

544. Killeen, R., Response to vitamin E, *South. Med. J.*, 69, 1372, 1976.

545. Rubyk, B.I., Fil'chagin, N.M., and Sabadyshin, R.A., Change in lipid peroxidation in patients with primary osteoarthrosis deformans, *Ter. Arkh.*, 60, 110, 1988.

546. Kienholz, E.W., Vitamin E, selenium, and knee problems, *Lancet*, 1, 531, 1975.

547. Machtey, I. and Ouaknine, L., Tocopherol in osteoarthritis: a controlled pilot study, *J. Am. Ger. Soc.*, 26, 328, 1978.

548. Blankenhorn, G., Clinical effectiveness of Spondyvit (vitamin E) in activated arthroses. A multicenter placebo-controlled double blind study, *Z. Orthop. Ihre Grenzgeb.*, 125, 340, 1986.

549. Swaak, A.J.G. and Koster, J.F., Eds., *Free Radicals and Arthritic Diseases*, Eurage, Rijswijk, 1986.

550. Fujii, T., The clinical effects of vitamin E on purpuras due to vascular defects, *J. Vitaminol.*, 18, 125, 1972.

551. Fiala, B., Lindner, E., and Cermakova, M., On the relationship of the level of vitamin E in blood serum to periodontal diseases, *Cas. Stomat.*, 69, 264, 1969.

552. Goldbach, H., The effect of vitamin E treatment of the periodontal patient, *Bl. Zahnheilk.*, 26, 171, 1965.

553. Goodson, M., Vitamin E therapy and periodontal disease, in *Diet, Nutrition and Periodontal Disease*, Hazen, S., Ed., American Society for Preventive Dentistry, Chicago, 1975, 53.

554. Khmelevski, I., Effect of vitamins A, E and K on the indices of the glutathione antiperoxidase system in gingival tissues in periodontitis, *Vopr. Pitan.*, (4), 54, 1985.

555. Slade, E., Bartuska, D., Rose, L., and Cohen, D., Vitamin E and periodontal disease, *J. Periodontol.*, 47, 352, 1976.

556. Cathcart, R.F., Leg cramps and vitamin E, *JAMA*, 219, 216, 1972.

557. Ayres, S. and Mihan, R., Nocturnal leg cramps (systremna): a progress report on response to vitamin E, *South. Med. J.*, 67, 1308, 1974.

558. Lotzof, L., Vitamin E controls muscle cramps, *Med. J. Aust.*, June 11, 904, 1977.

559. Yuan, C., Mei, Z., FengJu, Q., Hua, K., Wenan, W., Tingzhi, H., and Weiming, Z., Burns and damage by lipid peroxidation, *J. Med. Coll. PLA*, 3, 55, 1988.

560. Bendich, A. and Machlin, L.J., Safety of oral intake of vitamin E, *Am. J. Clin. Nutr.*, 48, 612, 1988.

561. Salkald, R.M., Safety and tolerance of high-dose vitamin E administration in man, *Fed. Regist.*, 44, 16172, 1979.

562. Olson, R.E., Vitamin K, 4, in *Modern Nutrition in Health and Disease*, 7th ed., Shils, M.E. and Young, V.R., Eds., Lea & Febiger, Philadelphia, 1988, 328.

563. Suttie, J.W., Vitamin K, 4, in *Present Knowledge in Nutrition*, 6th ed., Brown, M.L., Ed., International Life Sciences Foundation, Washington, D.C., 1990, 122.

564. Suttie, J.W., Vitamin K, in *Handbook of Vitamins. Second Edition, Revised and Expanded*, 2nd ed., Machlin, L.J., Ed., Marcel Dekker, New York, 1991, 145.

565. Bender, D.A., Vitamin K, in *Nutritional Biochemistry of the Vitamins*, Cambridge University Press, Cambridge, 1992, 106.

566. Combs, G.F., Vitamin K, in *The Vitamins. Fundamental Aspects in Nutrition and Health*, Academic Press, San Diego, 1992, 205.

567. Bouckaert, J.H. and Said, A.H., Fracture healing by vitamin K, *Nature*, 185, 849, 1960.

568. Hart, J.P., Shearer, M.J., Klenerman, L., Shearer, M.J., and Catterall, A., Electrochemical detection of depressed circulating levels of vitamin K in osteoporosis, *J. Clin. Endocrinol. Metab.*, 60, 1268, 1985.

569. Werlen, D., Robert, D., Leclerq, M., Guelpa, G., and Pfister, C.E., Modifications in the urinary excretion of gamma-carboxyglutamic acid induced by vitamin K, *Schweiz. Med. Wochenschr.*, 118(6), 203, 1988.

570. Jie, K.S., Gijsbers, B.L., Knapen, M.H., Hamulyak, K., Frank, H.L., and Vermeer, C., Effects of vitamin K and oral anticoagulants on urinary calcium excretion, *Br. J. Haematol.*, 83, 100, 1993.

571. Shils, M.E. and Young, V.R., Eds., *Modern Nutrition in Health and Disease*, 7th ed., Lea & Febiger, Philadelphia, 1988.

572. Marks, J., *The Vitamins. Their Role in Medical Practice*, MTP Press Unlimited, Lancaster, 1985.

573. Brown, M.L., Ed., *Present Knowledge in Nutrition*, 6th ed., International Life Sciences Foundation, Washington, D.C., 1990.

574. Machlin, L.J., Ed., *Handbook of Vitamins. Second Edition, Revised and Expanded*, 2nd ed., Marcel Dekker, New York, 1991.

575. Combs, G.F., *The Vitamins. Fundamental Aspects in Nutrition and Health*, Academic Press, San Diego, 1992.

576. Bender, D.A., *Nutritional Biochemistry of the Vitamins*, Cambridge University Press, Cambridge, 1992.

577. Anonymous, Vitamin B6 deficiency affects lung elastin crosslinking, *Nutr. Rev.*, 44(1), 24, 1986.

578. Bird, T.A. and Levene, C.I., Lysyl oxidase: evidence that pyridoxal phosphate is a cofactor, *Biochem. Biophys. Res. Commun.*, 108(3), 1172, 1982.

579. Bird, T.A. and Levene, C.I., The effect of a vitamin B-6 antagonist, 4-deoxypyridoxine, on the crosslinking of collagen in the developing chick embryo, *Biochem. J.*, 210, 633, 1983.

580. Greenberg, L.D., Misconi, L.Y., and Wang, A.C., Desmosine and isodesmosine levels of aortic elastin in control and pyridoxine-deficient monkeys, *Res. Commun. Chem. Path. Pharmacol.*, 2(6), 869, 1971.

581. Kang, A.H. and Trelstad, R.L., A collagen defect in homocystinuria, *J. Clin. Invest.*, 52, 2571, 1973.

582. Murray, J.C., Fraser, D.R., and Levene, C.I., The effect of pyridoxine deficiency on lysyl oxidase activity in the chick, *Exp. Mol. Pathol.*, 28, 301, 1978.

583. Prasad, R., Lakshmi, A.V., and Bamji, M.S., Impaired collagen maturity in vitamins B2 and B6 deficiency — probable molecular basis of skin lesions, *Biochem. Med.*, 30, 333, 1983.

584. Rucker, R.B. and O'Dell, B.L., Inhibition of elastin cross-linking by iproniazid and its counteraction by pyridoxal phosphate, *Biochim. Biophys. Acta*, 222, 527, 1970.

585. Starcher, B.C., The effect of pyridoxine deficiency on aortic elastin biosynthesis, *Proc. Soc. Exp. Biol. Med.*, 132, 379, 1969.

586. Brattström, L.E., Hultberg, B.L., and Hardebo, J.E., Folic acid responsive postmenopausal homocysteinemia, *Metabolism*, 34, 1073, 1985.

587. Hautvast, J.G.A.J. and Barnes, M.J., Collagen metabolism in folic acid deficiency, *Br. J. Nutr.*, 32, 457, 1974.

588. Alvarez, O.M. and Gilbreath, R.L., Thiamine influence on collagen production in rat wound healing, *Fed. Proc.*, 38, 707, 1979.

589. Alvarez, O.M. and Gilbreath, R.L., Effect of dietary thiamine on intermolecular collagen crosslinking during wound repair: a mechanical and biochemical assessment, *J. Trauma*, 22(1), 20, 1982.

590. Alvarez, O.M. and Gilbreath, R., Thiamin influence on collagen during the granulation of skin wounds, *J. Surg. Res.*, 32, 24, 1982.

591. Ostrovskii, A. and Nikitin, V.S., Morphological characteristics of cellular elements in the focus of post-traumatic inflammation in thiamin deficiency, *Vopr. Pitan.*, (5), 57, 1987.

592. Nelson, M.N., *Proc. Soc. Exptl. Biol. Med.*, 73, 31, 1950.

593. Aprahamian, M., Humbert, W., Dentinger, A., Stock-Damgé, C., and Grenier, J.F., Efficiency of pantothenic acid on wound healing: effect of an increase of iron and copper content of the tissues?, *Eur. Surg. Res.*, 15 (Suppl.), 61, 1983.

594. Aprahamian, M., Dentinger, A., Stock-Damge, C., Kouassi, J.C., and Grenier, J.F., Effects of supplemental pantothenic acid on wound healing: experimental study in rabbit, *Am. J. Clin. Nutr.*, 41, 578, 1985.

595. Fidanza, A., Bruno, C., Morganti, P., and Oddone, G., Osservazioni al microscopio elettronico a scansione del pelo di ratto in carenza di acido pantotenico, *Bull. Soc. Ital. Biol. Sper.*, 55, 559, 1979.

596. Grenier, J.F., Aprahamian, M., Genot, C., and Dentinger, A., Pantothenic acid (vitamin B_5) efficiency on wound healing, *Acta Vitaminol. Enzymol.*, 4(1–2), 81, 1982.

597. Carmel, R., Cobalamin and osteoblast-specific proteins, *N. Engl. J. Med.*, 319, 70, 1988.

598. Benke, P.J., Fleshood, H.L., and Pitot, H.C., Osteoporotic bone disease in the pyridoxine-deficient rat, *Biochem. Med.*, 6, 526, 1972.

599. Baker, H., Frank, O., and Hutner, S.H., B-Complex vitamin analyses and their clinical value, *J. Appl. Nutr.*, 41, 3, 1989.

600. Bucci, L.R., A functional analytical technique for monitoring nutrient status and repletion, *Am. Clin. Lab.*, 12, 8, 1993.

601. Shive, W., Pinkerton, F., Humphreys, J., Johnson, M.M., Hamilton, W.G., and Matthews, K.S., Development of a chemically defined serum- and protein-free medium for growth of human peripheral lymphocytes, *Proc. Natl. Acad. Sci. U.S.A.*, 83, 9, 1986.

602. Lacroix, B., Didier, E., and Grenier, J.F., Role of pantothenic acid and ascorbic acid in wound healing processes: *in vitro* study on fibroblasts, *Int. J. Vit. Nutr. Res.*, 58, 407, 1988.

603. LaCroix, B., Didier, E., and Grenier, J.F., Effects of pantothenic acid on fibroblastic cell cultures, *Res. Exp. Med.*, 188, 391, 1988.

604. Levenson, S.M., Green, R.W., Taylor, F.H.L., Robinson, P., Paige, R.W., Johnson, R.E., and Lund, C.C., Ascorbic acid, riboflavin, thiamine and nicotinic acid in relation to severe injury, hemorrhage, and infection in the human, *Ann. Surg.*, 124, 840, 1946.

605. Lund, C.C., Levenson, S.M., Green, R.W., Paige, R.W., Robinson, P.E., Adams, M.A., Macdonald, A.H., Taylor, F.H.L., and Johnson, R.E., Ascorbic acid, thiamine, riboflavin and nicotinic acid in relation to acute burns in man, *Arch. Surg.*, 55, 557, 1947.

606. Andreae, W.A., Schenker, V., and Browne, J.S.L., Riboflavin metabolism after trauma and during convalescence in man, *Fed. Proc.*, 5, 3, 1946.

607. Kurashige, S., Akuzawa, Y., Fujii, N., Kishi, S., Takeshita, M., and Miyamoto, Y., Effect of vitamin B complex on the immunodeficiency produced by surgery of gastric cancer patients, *Jpn. J. Exp. Med.*, 58, 197, 1988.

608. Miehlke, K., Liebelt, J., and Bonke, D., Vitamine der B-gruppe. Additive Effekte bei der medikamentösen Therapie rheumatischer Erkrankungen, *Therapiewoche*, 35, 3313, 1985.

609. Bonke, D., Influence of vitamin B_1, B_6, and B_{12} on the control of fine motoric movements, *Bibl. Nutr. Dieta*, 38, 104, 1986.

610. Kuhlwein, A., Meyer, H.J., and Koehler, C.O., Reduced need for Diclofenac with concomitant B-vitamin therapy: results of a double-blind clinical study with reduced Diclofenac-dosage (75 mg Diclofenac vs. 75 mg Diclofenac plus B-vitamins daily) in patients with acute lumbago, *Klin. Wochenschr.*, 68, 107, 1990.

611. Brüggemann, G., Koehler, C.O., and Koch, E.M.W., The therapy of acute lumbago with Diclofenac and B-vitamins — results of a double-blind clinical study, *Klin. Wochenschr.*, 68, 119, 1990.

612. Lettko, M. and Bartoszyk, G.D., Reduced need for Diclofenac with concomitant administration of pyridoxine and other B vitamins. Clinical and experimental studies, *Ann. N.Y. Acad. Sci.*, 585, 510, 1990.

613. Bartoszyk, G.D. and Wild, A., Antinociceptive effects of pyridoxine, thiamine, and cyanocobalamin in rats, *Ann. N.Y. Acad. Sci.*, 585, 473, 1990.

614. Jurna, I., Carlson, K.H., Bonke, D., Fu, Q.G., and Zimmermann, M., Suppression of thalamic and spinal nociceptive response by pyridoxine, thiamine, and cyanocobalamin, *Ann. N.Y. Acad. Sci.*, 585, 492, 1990.

615. Becker, K.W., Kienecker, E.W., Dick, P., and Bonke, D., Enhancement of regeneration of the saphenous nerve after treatment with vitamins B_1, B_6, and B_{12} after cold lesion in the rabbit, *Ann. N.Y. Acad. Sci.*, 585, 477, 1990.

616. Boissier, J.R., Action de la thiamine sur les potentiels des nerfs moteurs de la queue de rat provoqués par stimulations electriques et mécaniques, *Therapie*, 21, 159, 1966.

617. De Castro, J., Synaptanalgésie a base de fortes doses de thiamine, *Med. Hyg. (Geneve)*, 23, 1012, 1965.

618. Lenot, G., Note sur l'aneurine, anesthésique général, *Ann. Anesthesiol. Fr.*, 7 (Suppl). 1, 173, 1966.

619. Mazzoni, P. and Valenti, F., Un nuovo anestetico generale per via endovenosa — la tiamina, *Acta Anaesthesiol. Padova*, 15, 185, 1964.

620. Quirin, H., Pain and vitamin B_1 therapy, *Bibl. Nutr. Dieta*, 38, 110, 1986.

621. Herzog, B. and McCall, J.O., Thiamin hydrochloride as an adjunct in surgical periodontal treatment, *J. Periodontol.*, 24, 116, 1953.

622. Kaufman, W., *The Common Form of Joint Dysfunction: Its Incidence and Treatment*, E.L. Hildreth, Brattleboro, VT, 1949.

623. Kaufman, W., Niacinamide therapy for joint mobility, *Conn. Med. J.*, 17, 584, 1953.

624. Kaufman, W., The use of vitamin therapy to reverse certain concomitants of aging, *J. Am. Ger. Soc.*, 3, 927, 1955.

625. Kaufman, W., Niacinamide: a most neglected vitamin, *J. Int. Acad. Prev. Med.*, 8, 5, 1983.

626. Hoffer, A., Treatment of arthritis by nicotinic acid and nicotinamide, *Can. Med. Assoc. J.*, 81, 235, 1959.

627. Hadler, N.M., Nerve entrapment syndromes, in *Arthritis and Allied Conditions. A Textbook of Rheumatology*, Vol. 2, McCarty, D.J. and Koopman, W.J., Eds., Lea & Febiger, Philadelphia, 1993, 1619.

628. Ellis, J.M., Kishi, T., Azuma, J., and Folkers, K., Therapy of the carpal tunnel syndrome with vitamin B-6, *IRCS Med. Sci.*, 4, 193, 1976.

629. Ellis, J.M., Kishi, T., Azuma. J., and Folkers, K., Vitamin B-6 deficiency in patients with a clinical syndrome including the carpal tunnel defect: biochemical and clinical response to therapy with pyridoxine, *Res. Commun. Chem. Pathol. Pharmacol.*, 13, 743, 1976.

630. Ellis, J.M., Azuma, J., Watanabe, T., and Folkers, K., Survey and new data on treatment with pyridoxine of patients having a clinical syndrome including the carpal tunnel and other defects, *Res. Commun. Chem. Pathol. Pharmacol.*, 17, 165, 1977.

631. Folkers, K., Saji, S., Kaji, M., and Ellis, J.M., Biochemical evidence for a deficiency of vitamin B-6 in the carpal tunnel syndrome, *Acta Pharm. Suec.*, 14 (Suppl.), 38, 1977.

632. Folkers, K., Ellis, J., Watanabe, T., Saji, S., and Kaji, M., Biochemical evidence for a deficiency of vitamin B-6 in the carpal tunnel syndrome based on a cross-over clinical study, *Proc. Natl. Acad. Sci. U.S.A.*, 75, 3410, 1978.

633. Ellis, J., Folkers, K., Watanabe, T., Kaji, M., Saji, S., Caldwell, J.W., Temple, C.A., and Wood, F.S., Clinical results of a cross-over treatment with pyridoxine and placebo of the carpal tunnel syndrome, *Am. J. Clin. Nutr.*, 32, 2040, 1979.

634. Shizukuishi, S., Nishii, S., Ellis, J., and Folkers, K., The carpal tunnel syndrome as a probable primary deficiency of vitamin B-6 rather than a deficiency of a dependency state, *Biochem. Biophys. Res. Commun.*, 95, 1126, 1980.

635. Folkers, K., Willis, R., Takemura, K., Escudier, S., and Shorey, R.A., Biochemical correlations of a deficiency of vitamin B-6, the carpal tunnel syndrome and the Chinese restaurant syndrome, *IRCS Med. Sci.*, 9, 444, 1981.

636. Ellis, J., Folkers, K., Levy, M., Takemura, K., Shizukuishi, S., Ulrich, R., and Harrison, P., Therapy with vitamin B-6 with and without surgery for treatment of patients having idiopathic carpal tunnel syndrome, *Res. Commun. Chem. Pathol. Pharmacol.*, 33, 331, 1981.

637. Ellis, J., Folkers, K., Levy, M., Shizukuishi, S., Lewandwski, J., Nishii, S., Schubert, H.A., and Ulrich, R., Response of vitamin B-6 deficiency and the carpal tunnel syndrome to pyridoxine, *Proc. Natl. Acad. Sci. U.S.A.*, 79, 7494, 1982.

638. Wolaniuk, A., Electromyographic data differentiate patients with the carpal tunnel syndrome when double blindly treated with pyridoxine and placebo, *Res. Commun. Chem. Pathol. Pharmacol.*, 41, 501, 1983.

639. Folkers, K., Wolaniuk, A., and Vadhanavikit, S., Enzymology of the response of the carpal tunnel syndrome to riboflavin and to combined riboflavin and pyridoxine, *Proc. Natl. Acad. Sci. U.S.A.*, 81, 7076, 1984.

640. Ellis, J.M., Treatment of carpal tunnel syndrome with vitamin B6, *South. Med. J.*, 80, 882, 1987.

641. Ellis, J., Tenosynovitis including carpal tunnel syndrome (CTS) responsive to vitamin B-6, *FASEB J.*, 2(4), A439, 1988.

642. Ellis, J., Vitamin B6 prevents thenar muscular atrophy in carpal tunnel syndrome (CTS), *FASEB J.*, 3(3), A668, 1989.

643. Folkers, K. and Ellis, J., Successful therapy with vitamin B_6 and vitamin B_2 of the carpal tunnel syndrome and need for determination of the RDAs for vitamins B_6 and B_2 for disease states, *Ann. N. Y. Acad. Sci.*, 585, 295, 1990.

644. Ellis, J.M. and Folkers, K., Clinical aspects of treatment of carpal tunnel syndrome with vitamin B_6, *Ann. N. Y. Acad. Sci.*, 585, 302, 1990.

645. Hamfelt, A., Carpal tunnel syndrome and vitamin B-6 deficiency, *Clin. Chem.*, 28, 721, 1982.

646. Del Tredici, A.M., Bernstein, A.L., and Chinn, K., Carpal tunnel syndrome and vitamin B-6 therapy, in *Vitamin B-6: Its Role in Health and Disease*, Reynolds, R.D. and Leklem, J.E., Eds., Alan R. Liss, New York, 1985, 459.

647. Salkeld, R.M. and Stotz, R., Vitamin B-6 deficiency: an etiological factor of the carpal tunnel syndrome, in *Vitamin B-6: Its Role in Health and Disease*, Reynolds, R.D. and Leklem, J.E., Eds., Alan R. Liss, New York, 1985, 463.

648. Del Tredici, A.M. and Bernstein, A.L., Vitamin B_6 therapy for carpal tunnel syndrome: a double-blind study, *J. Am. Diet. Assoc.*, 86, 150, 1986.

649. Bernstein, A. and Lobitz, C., Treatment of painful diabetic neuropathies with vitamin B_6: a clinical and electrophysiological study, *FASEB J.*, 2(4), A438, 1988.

650. Bernstein, A.L. and Dinesen, J.S., Brief communication: effect of pharmacologic doses of vitamin B6 on carpal tunnel syndrome, electroencephalographic results, and pain, *J. Am. Coll. Nutr.*, 12, 73, 1993.

651. Byers, C.M., DeLisa, J.A., Frankel, D.L., and Kraft, G.H., Pyridoxine metabolism in carpal tunnel syndrome, with and without peripheral neuropathy, *Arch. Phys. Med. Rehabil.*, 64, 512, 1983.

652. Smith, G.P., Rudge, P.J., and Peters, T.J., Biochemical studies of pyridoxal and pyridoxal phosphate status and therapeutic trial of pyridoxine in patients with carpal tunnel syndrome, *Ann. Neurol.*, 15, 104, 1984.

653. Bernstein, A.L., Vitamin B_6 in clinical neurology, *Ann. N.Y. Acad. Sci.*, 585, 250, 1990.

654. Schumacher, H.R., Bernhart, F.W., and György, P., Vitamin B_6 levels in rheumatoid arthritis: effect of treatment, *Am. J. Clin. Nutr.*, 28, 1200, 1975.

655. Kellman, M., Bursitis: a new chemotherapeutic approach, *J. Am. Osteopath. Assoc.*, 61, 896, 1962.

656. Vreugdenhil, G., Wognum, A.W., van Eijk, H.G., and Swaak, A.J.G., Anaemia in rheumatoid arthritis: the role of iron, vitamin B_{12}, and folic acid deficiency, and erythropoietin responsiveness, *Ann. Rheum. Dis.*, 49, 93, 1990.

657. Nardi, G.L. and Zuidema, G.D., The postoperative use of dextro pantothenyl alcohol, *Surg. Gynecol. Obstet.*, 112, 526, 1961.

658. Barton-Wright, E.C. and Elliott, W.A., The pantothenic acid metabolism of rheumatoid arthritis, *Lancet*, 2, 862, 1963.

659. Annand, J.C., *J. Coll. Gen. Practrs.*, 5, 136, 1962.

660. Annand, J.C., Pantothenic acid and osteoarthrosis, *Lancet*, 2, 1168, 1963.

661. General Practitioner Research Group, Calcium pantothenate in arthritic conditions. A report form the General Practitioner Research Group, *Practitioner*, 224, 208, 1980.

662. Schaumburg, H., Kaplan, J., Windebank, A., Vick, N., Rasmus, S., Pleasure, D., and Brown, M.J., Sensory neuropathy from pyridoxine abuse. A new megavitamin syndrome, *N. Engl. J. Med.,* 309, 445, 1983.

663. Schaumburg, H., Sensory neuropathy from pyridoxine abuse. Letter, *N. Engl. J. Med.,* 310, 198, 1984.

664. Berger, A. and Schaumburg, H., More on neuropathy from pyridoxine abuse, *N. Engl. J. Med.,* 1984, 311, 987.

665. Vasile, A., Goldberg, R., and Kornberg, B., Pyridoxine toxicity: report of a case, *J. Am. Osteopath. Assoc.,* 83, 790, 1984.

666. Baer, R.L. and Stillman, M.A., Cutaneous skin changes probably due to pyridoxine abuse, *J. Am. Acad. Dermatol.,* 10, 527, 1984.

667. Parry, G.J. and Bredesen, D.E., Neuropathy due to pyridoxine intoxication, *Neurology,* 35, 1466, 1985.

668. Friedman, M.A., Resnick, J.S., and Baer, R.L., Subepidermal vesicular dermatosis and sensory neuropathy caused by pyridoxine abuse, *J. Am. Acad. Dermatol.,* 14, 915, 1986.

669. Dalton, K. and Dalton, M.J.T., Characteristics of pyridoxine overdose neuropathy syndrome, *Acta Neurol. Scand.,* 76, 8, 1987.

670. Bässler, K.H., Megavitamin therapy with pyridoxine, *Int. J. Vit. Nutr. Res.,* 58, 105, 1988.

671. National Cholesterol Education Program Expert Panel, National Heart, Lung and Blood Institute, Report of the national cholesterol education program expert panel on detection, evaluation and treatment of high blood cholesterol in adults, *Arch. Intern. Med.,* 148, 36, 1988.

672. Knopp, R., Ginsberg, J., Albers, J.J., Hoff, C., Ogilvie, J.T., Warnick, G.R., Burrows, E., Retzlaff, B., and Poole, M., Contrasting effects of unmodified and time release forms of niacin on lipoproteins in hyperlipidemic subjects: clues to mechanism of action of niacin, *Metabolism,* 34, 642, 1985.

673. Bender, D.A., Vitamin C, in *Nutritional Biochemistry of the Vitamins,* Cambridge University Press, Cambridge, 1992, 360.

674. Combs, G.F., Vitamin C, in *The Vitamins. Fundamental Aspects in Nutrition and Health,* Academic Press, San Diego, 1992, 223.

675. Moser, U. and Bendich, A., Vitamin C, in *Handbook of Vitamins. Second Edition, Revised and Expanded,* 2nd ed., Machlin, L.J., Ed., Marcel Dekker, New York, 1991, 195.

676. Sauberlich, H.E., Ascorbic acid, in *Present Knowledge in Nutrition,* 6th ed., Brown, M.L., Ed., International Life Sciences Foundation, Washington, D.C., 1990, 132.

677. Hornig, D.H., Moser, U., and Glatthaar, B.E., Ascorbic acid, in *Modern Nutrition in Health and Disease,* 7th ed., Shils, M.E. and Young, V.R., Eds., Lea & Febiger, Philadelphia, 1988, 417.

678. Schwartz, P.L., Ascorbic acid in wound healing — a review, *J. Am. Diet. Assoc.,* 56, 497, 1970.

679. Dryburgh, D.R., Vitamin C and chiropractic, *J. Manip. Physiol. Ther.,* 8, 95, 1985.

680. Hunt, A.H., The role of vitamin C in wound healing, *Br. J. Surg.,* 28, 436, 1941.

681. Ingalls, T.H. and Warren, H.A., Asymptomatic scurvy. Its relation to wound healing and its incidence in patients with peptic ulcer, *N. Engl. J. Med.,* 217, 443, 1937.

682. Crandon, J.H., Lund, C.C., and Dill, D.B., Experimental human scurvy, *N. Engl. J. Med.,* 223(10), 353, 1940.

683. Bartlett, M., Jones, C.M., Ryan, A.E., Vitamin C and wound healing. II. Ascorbic acid content and tensile strength of healing wounds in human beings, *N. Engl. J. Med.,* 226, 474, 1942.

684. Wolfer, J.A., Farmer, C.J., Carroll, W.W., and Manshardt, D.O., An experimental study in wound healing in vitamin C depleted human subjects, *Surg. Gynecol. Obstet.,* 84, 1, 1947.

685. Crandon, J.H., Lennihan, R., Mikal, S., and Reif, A.E., Ascorbic acid economy in surgical patients, *Ann. N.Y. Acad. Sci.,* 92, 246, 1961.

686. Hodges, R.E., Hood, J., and Canham, J.E., Clinical manifestations of ascorbic acid deficiency in man, *Am. J. Clin. Nutr.,* 24, 432, 1971.

687. Irvin, T.T., Vitamin C requirements in postoperative patients, *Int. J. Vit. Nutr. Res.,* 23, 277, 1982.

688. Shulka, S.P., Plasma and urinary ascorbic acid levels in the postoperative period, *Experentia,* 25, 704, 1969.

689. Fishchenko, A.I., Vitamin C correction in patients with complicated cholecystitis, *Vrach. Delo.,* (11), 21, 1988.

690. Ringsdorf, W.M. and Cheraskin, E., Vitamin C and human wound healing, *Oral Surg.,* 53, 231, 1982.

691. Mallek, H., An investigation of the role of ascorbic acid and iron in the etiology of gingivitis in humans, Ph.D. dissertation, Massachusetts Institute of Technology, Boston, 1978.

692. Woolfe, S.N., Kenney, E.B., Hume, W.R., and Carranza, F.A., Relationship of ascorbic acid levels of blood and gingival tissue with response to periodontal therapy, *J. Clin. Periodontol.,* 11, 159, 1984.

693. Leggott, P.J., Robertson, P.B., Rothman, D.C., Murray, P.A., and Jacob, R.A., The effect of controlled ascorbic acid depletion and supplementation on periodontal health, *J. Periodontal.,* 57, 480, 1986.

694. Jacob, R.A., Omaye, S.T., Skala, J.H., Leggott, P.J., Rothman, D.L., and Murray, P.A., Experimental vitamin C depletion and supplementation in young men, *Ann. N.Y. Acad. Sci.,* 498, 333, 1987.

695. Buzina, R., Ayrer-Kozelj, J., Srdak-Jorgic, K., Buhler, E., and Gey, K.F., Increase in gingival hydroxyproline and proline by improvement of ascorbic acid status in man, *Int. J. Vit. Nutr. Res.,* 53, 367, 1986.

696. Lytle, R.L., Chronic dental pain: possible benefits of food restriction and sodium ascorbate, *J. Appl. Nutr.,* 40, 95, 1988.

697. Hunter, T. and Rajan, K.T., The role of ascorbic acid in the pathogenesis and treatment of pressure sores, *Paraplegia,* 8, 211, 1971.

698. Burr, R.G. and Rajan, K.T., Leucocyte ascorbic acid and pressure sores in paraplegia, *Br. J. Nutr.,* 28, 275, 1972.

699. Afifi, A.M., Ellis, L., Huntsman, R.G., and Said, M.I., High dose ascorbic acid in the management of thalassaemia leg ulcers — a pilot study, *Br. J. Dermatol.,* 92, 339, 1975.

700. Taylor, T.V., Rimmer, S., Day, B., Butcher, J., and Dymock, I.W., Ascorbic acid supplementation in the treatment of pressure sores, *Lancet*, 2, 544, 1974.

701. Greenwood, J., Optimum vitamin C intake as a factor in the preservation of disc integrity, *Med. Ann. DC*, 33, 274, 1964.

702. Injeyan, H.S., Adams, A.H., and Dhami, M.S.I., Nutrition of the invertebral disc, *Nutr. Perspect.*, 6, 7, 1983.

703. Biskind, M.A. and Martin, W.C., The use of citrus flavonoids in infection. II, *Am. J. Digest. Dis.*, 2, 41, 1955.

704. Schwartz, E.R., Metabolic response during early stages of surgically-induced osteoarthritis in mature beagles, *J. Rheumatol.*, 7, 788, 1980.

705. Stout, L.E., A study in vitamin C levels in patients with neuromusculoskeletal disorders and its significance, *Am. Chirop. Assoc. J. Chirop.*, 144, 626, 1973.

705a. Avioli, L.V., Calcium and phosphorus, in *Modern Nutrition in Health and Disease*, 7th ed., Shils, M.E. and Young, V.R., Eds., Lea & Febiger, Philadelphia, 1988, 142.

706. Arnaud, C.D. and Sanchez, S.D., Calcium and phosphorus, 4, in *Present Knowledge in Nutrition*, 6th ed., Brown, M.L., Ed., International Life Sciences Foundation, Washington, D.C., 1990, 212.

707. Riggs, B.L. and Melton, L.J., Involutional osteoporosis, *N. Engl. J. Med.*, 314, 1676, 1986.

708. Compston, J.E., Osteoporosis, *Clin. Endocrinol.*, 33, 653, 1990.

709. Spencer, H. and Kramer, L., NIH consensus conference: osteoporosis. Factors contributing to osteoporosis, *J. Nutr.*, 116, 316, 1986.

710. Resnick, N.M. and Greenspan, S.L., 'Senile' osteoporosis reconsidered, *JAMA*, 261, 1025, 1989.

711. Heaney, R.P., Nutritional factors in osteoporosis, *Ann. Rev. Nutr.*, 13, 287, 1993.

712. Williams, M.H., The role of minerals in physical activity, in *Nutritional Aspects of Human Physical Performance*, 2nd ed., Charles C. Thomas, Springfield, IL, 1985, 186.

713. Sauberlich, H.E., Skala, J.H., and Dowdy, R.P., *Laboratory Tests for the Assessment of Nutritional Status*, 2nd ed., CRC Press, Cleveland, 1977.

714. Houston, M.E., Diet, training and sleep: a survey study of elite Canadian swimmers, *Can. J. Appl. Sport Sci.*, 5, 161, 1980.

715. Perron, M. and Endres, J., Knowledge, attitudes, and dietary practices of female athletes, *J. Am. Diet. Assoc.*, 85, 573, 1985.

716. Welch, P.K., Zager, K.A., Endres, J., and Poon, S.W., Nutrition education, body composition, and dietary intake of female college athletes, *Phys. Sportsmed.*, 15, 63, 1987.

717. Lamar-Hildebrand, N., Saldanha, L., and Endres, J., Dietary and exercise practices of college-aged female bodybuilders, *J. Am. Diet. Assoc.*, 89, 1308, 1989.

718. Barr, S.I., Relationship of eating attitudes to anthropometric variables and dietary intakes of female collegiate swimmers, *J. Am. Diet. Assoc.*, 91, 976, 1991.

719. Nutter, J., Seasonal changes in female athletes' diets, *Int. J. Sport Nutr.*, 1, 395, 1991.

720. Calabrese, L.H., Kirkendall, D.T., Floyd, M., Rapoport, S., Williams, G.W., Welker, G.G., and Bergfeld, J.A., Menstrual abnormalities, nutritional patterns, and body composition in female classical ballet dancers, *Phys. Sportsmed.*, 11, 86, 1983.

721. Moffatt, R.J., Dietary status of elite female high school gymnasts: inadequacy of vitamin and mineral intake, *J. Am. Diet. Assoc.*, 84, 1361, 1984.

722. Cohen, J.L., Potosnak, L., Frank, O., and Baker, H., A nutritional and hematological assessment of elite ballet dancers, *Phys. Sportsmed.*, 13, 43, 1985.

723. Benson, J., Gillien, D.M., Bourdet, K., and Loosli, A.R., Inadequate nutrition and chronic calorie restriction in adolescent ballerinas, *Phys. Sportsmed.*, 13, 79, 1985.

724. Calabrese, L.H., Nutritional and medical aspects of gymnasts, *Clin. Sports Med.*, 4, 23, 1985.

725. Humphries, L.L. and Gruber, J.J., Nutrition behaviors of university majorettes, *Phys. Sportsmed.*, 14, 91, 1986.

726. Huber, L.H., Zeigler, P., Congdon, K., Lindholm, S., and Manfredi, T.G., Nutritional status of college female gymnasts and cross-country runners, *Med. Sci. Sports Exer.*, 18, S64, 1986.

727. Deuster, P.A., Kyle, S.B., Moser, P.B., Vigersky, R.A., Singh, A., and Schoomaker, E.B., Nutritional survey of highly trained women runners, *Am. J. Clin. Nutr.*, 44, 954, 1986.

728. Rucinski, A., Relationship of body image and dietary intake of competitive ice skaters, *J. Am. Diet. Assoc.*, 89, 98, 1989.

729. Bergen-Cico, D.K. and Short, S.H., Dietary intakes, energy expenditures, and anthropometric characteristics of adolescent female cross-country runners, *J. Am. Diet. Assoc.*, 92, 611, 1992.

730. Baer, J.T. and Taper, L.J., Amenorrheic and eumenorrheic adolescent runners: dietary intake and exercise training status, *J. Am. Diet. Assoc.*, 92, 89, 1992.

731. Ruud, J.S. and Grandjean, A.C., Nutritional concerns of female athletes, in *Nutrition in Exercise and Sport*, 2nd ed., Wolinksy, I. and Hickson, J.F., Eds., CRC Press, Boca Raton, FL, 1994, 347.

732. Bucci, L.R., Micronutrient supplementation and ergogenesis — minerals, in *Nutrients as Ergogenic Aids for Sports and Exercise*, CRC Press, Boca Raton, FL, 1993, 63.

733. Myerson, M., Gutin, B., Warren, M.P., May, M.T., Contento, I., Lee, M., Pi-Sunyer, F.X., Pierson, R.N., and Brooks-Gunn, J., Resting metabolic rate and energy balance in amenorrheic and eumenorrheic runners, *Med. Sci. Sports Exer.*, 23, 15, 1991.

734. Brooks-Gunn, J., Warren, M.P., and Hamilton, L.H., The relation of eating problems and amenorrhea in ballet dancers, *Med. Sci. Sports Exer.*, 19, 41, 1987.

735. Sanborn, C.F., Amenorrhea and osteoporosis, presented at the International Sports Nutrition Conference, Colorado Springs, CO, Sept. 1993.

736. Marcus, R., Cann, C., Madvig, P., Minkoff, J., Goddard, M., Bayer, M., Martin, M., Gaudiani, L., Kaskell, W., and Genant, H., Menstrual function and bone mass in elite women distance runners, *Ann. Intern. Med.*, 102, 158, 1985.

737. Nelson, M.E., Fisher, E.C., Catsos, P.D., Meredith, C.N., Turksoy, R.N., and Evans, W.J., Diet and bone status in amenorrheic runners, *Am. J. Clin. Nutr.,* 43, 910, 1986.

738. Schweiger, U., Laessle, R., Schweiger, M., Herrmann, F., Riedel, W., and Pirke, K., Calorie intake, stress and menstrual function in athletes, *Fertil. Steril.,* 49, 447, 1988.

739. Kaiserauer, S., Snyder, A.C., Sleeper, M., and Zierath, J., Nutritional, physiological, and menstrual status of distance runners, *Med. Sci. Sports Exer.,* 21, 120, 1989.

740. Drinkwater, B.L., Bruemmer, B., and Chesnut, C.H., Menstrual history as a determinant of current bone density in young athletes, *JAMA,* 263, 545, 1990.

741. Lloyd, T., Myers, C., Buchanan, J.R., and Demers, L.M., Collegiate women athletes with irregular menses during adolescence have decreased bone density, *Obstet. Gynecol.,* 72, 639, 1988.

742. Grimston, S.K., Engsberg, J.R., Kloiber, R., and Hanley, D.A., Menstrual, calcium, and training history: relationship to bone health in female runners, *Clin. Sports Med.,* 2, 119, 1990.

743. Howat, P.M., Carbo, M.L., Mills, G.Q., and Wozniak, P., The influence of diet, body fat, menstrual cycling, and activity upon the bone density of females, *J. Am. Diet. Assoc.,* 89, 1305, 1989.

744. Warren, M.P., Brooks-Gunn, J., Hamilton, L.H., Warren, L.F., and Hamilton, W.G., Scoliosis and fractures in young ballet dancers, *N. Engl. J. Med.,* 314, 1348, 1986.

745. Bucci, L.R., Osteoporosis treatment: much more than calcium, *Today's Chirop.,* 20(2), 38, 1991.

746. Miller, J.Z., Smith, D.L., Flora, L., Slemenda, C., Jiang, X., and Johnston, C.C., Calcium absorption from calcium carbonate and a new form of calcium (CCM) in healthy male and female adolescents, *Am. J. Clin. Nutr.,* 48, 1291, 1988.

747. Nicar, M.J. and Pak, C.Y.C., Calcium bioavailability from calcium carbonate and calcium citrate, *J. Clin. Endocrinol. Metab.,* 61(2), 391, 1985.

748. Pak, C.Y.C., Harvey, J.A., and Hsu, M.C., Enhanced calcium bioavailability from a solubilized form of calcium citrate, *J. Clin. Endocrinol. Metab.,* 65(4), 801, 1987.

749. Reid, I.R., Hannan, S.F., Schooler, B.A., and Ibbertson, H.K., The acute biochemical effects of four proprietary calcium preparations, *Aust. N.Z. J. Med.,* 16, 193, 1986.

750. Schuette, S.A. and Knowles, J.B., Intestinal absorption of $Ca(H_2PO_4)_2$ and Ca citrate compared by two methods, *Am. J. Clin. Nutr.,* 47, 884, 1988.

751. Mills, T.J., Davis, H., and Broadhurst, B.W., The use of whole bone extract in the treatment of fractures, *Manitoba Med. Rev.,* 45, 92, 1965.

752. Štěpán, J.J., Pospíchal, J., Presl, J., and Pacovský, V., Prospective trial of ossein-hydroxyapatite compound in surgically induced postmenopausal women, *Bone,* 10, 179, 1989.

753. Drivdahl, R.H., Howard, G.A., and Baylink, D.J., Extracts of bone contain a potent regulator of bone formation, *Biochim. Biophys. Acta,* 714, 26, 1982.

754. Štěpán, J.J., Mohan, S., Jennings, J.C., Wergedal, J.E., Taylor, A.K., and Baylink, D.J., Quantitation of growth factors in ossein-mineral-compound, *Life Sci.,* 49, 79, 1991.

755. Küng, H.L., Comparative study of calcium and phosphate balances following administration of whole-bone preparation and other bone substances, *Ann. Paediatr.,* 170, 1, 1948.

756. Heaney, R.P., Recker, R.R., and Weaver, C.M., *Calcif. Tissue Int.,* 46, 300, 1990.

757. Windsor, A.C.M., Misra, D.P., Loudon, J.M., and Staddon, G.E., The effect of whole-bone extract on ^{47}Ca absorption in the elderly, *Age Ageing,* 2, 230, 1973.

758. Buclin, T., Jacquet, A.F., and Burckhardt, P., Absorption intestinale de gluconate de calcium et de complexe osséino-minéral: évaluation par des dosages conventionnels, *Schweiz. Med. Wochenschr.,* 116, 1780, 1986.

759. Küng, H.L., Untersuchungen über die Callusbildungen bei Ratten, *Helv. Chir. Acta,* 18B, 64, 1951.

760. Eschler, J., Experimentelle und klinische Untersuchungen über den Einfluss des Knochen-Vollpräparates Ossopan auf die Frakturheilung, *Dtsch. Zahnärztl. Z.,* 8, 1063, 1953.

761. Fouret, M., Influence de l'Ossopan sur la rapidité de la consolidation osseuse chez le lapin, *Sem. Hop. Thér.,* 34, 744, 1958.

762. Jondet, A. and Leroy, G., Influence de l'ingestion de préparations d'os Ossopan, administrées par voie buccale, sur la formation du cal de fractures chez le rat, *Thérapie,* 14, 304, 1959.

763. Czyzewski, L., Przestalski, S., and Skóra, K., Der Einfluss von Ossopan auf die Aufnahmegrösse von 32-P in frakturierten Röhrenknochen des Kaninchens, *Chir. Narzadów Ruchu Ortop. Pol.,* 25, 205, 1960.

764. Annefeld, M., Caviezel, R., Schacht, E., and Schicketanz, K.H., The influence of ossein-hydroxyapatite compound ('Ossopan') on the healing of a bone defect, *Curr. Res. Med. Opin.,* 10(4), 241, 1986.

765. Durance, R.A., Parsons, V., Atkins, C.J., Hamilton, E.B.D., and Davies, C., Treatment of osteoporotic patients. A trial of calcium supplements (Ossopan) and ashed bone, *Clin. Trials J.,* 10(3), 67, 1973.

766. Galasko, C.S.B., Russell, S., and Rushton, S., Microcrystalline hydroxyapatite in patients with Colles' fractures, in *Osteoporosis,* Christiansen, C., Arnaud, C.D., Nordin, B.E.C., Parfitt, A.M., Peck, W.A., and Riggs, B.L., Eds., Stiftsbogtrykkin, Denmark, 1984, 663.

767. Dambacher, M.A. and Rüegsegger, P., Therapy of osteoporosis with an ossein-hydroxyapatite compound evaluated with quantitative computed tomography, *J. Bone Min. Res.,* 2(Suppl. 2), 325, 1987.

768. Nilsen, K.H., Jayson, M.I.V., and Dixon, A.St.J., Microcrystalline calcium hydroxyapatite compound in corticosteroid-treated rheumatoid patients: a controlled study, *Br. Med. J.,* 2, 1124, 1978.

769. Pines, A., Raafat, H., Lynn, A.H., and Whittington, J., Clinical trial of microcrystalline hydroxyapatite compound ('Ossopan') in the prevention of osteoporosis due to corticosteroid therapy, *Curr. Med. Res. Opin.,* 8, 734, 1984.

770. Stellon, A., Davies, A., Webb, A., and Williams, R., Microcrystalline hydroxyapatite compound in prevention of bone loss in corticosteroid-treated patients with chronic active hepatitis, *Postgrad. Med. J.,* 61, 791, 1985.

771. Dent, C.E. and Davies, I.J.T., Calcium metabolism in bone disease: effects of treatment with microcrystalline calcium hydroxyapatite compound and dihydrotachysterol, *J. R. Soc. Med.,* 73, 780, 1980.

772. Epstein, O., Kato, Y., Dick, R., and Sherlock, S., Vitamin D, hydroxyapatite, and calcium gluconate in treatment of cortical bone thinning in postmenopausal women with primary biliary cirrhosis, *Am. J. Clin. Nutr.,* 36, 426, 1982.

773. Cantin, M. and Seelig, M.S., Eds., *Magnesium in Health and Disease,* SP Medical & Scientific Books, New York, 1980.

774. Seelig, M.S., *Magnesium Deficiency in the Pathogenesis of Disease. Early Roots of Cardiovascular, Skeletal, and Renal Abnormalities,* Plenum Medical Book Co., New York, 1980.

775. Altura, B.M., Durlach, J., and Seelig, M.S., Eds., *Magnesium in Cellular Processes and Medicine,* S. Karger, Basel, 1985.

776. Shils, M.E., Magnesium, in *Modern Nutrition in Health and Disease,* 7th ed., Shils, M.E. and Young, V.R., Eds., Lea & Febiger, Philadelphia, 1988, 159.

777. Shils, M.E., Magnesium, 5, in *Present Knowledge in Nutrition,* 6th ed., Brown, M.L., Ed., International Life Sciences Foundation, Washington, D.C., 1990, 224.

778. Lasserre, B. and Durlach, J., *Magnesium — A Relevant Ion,* John Libbey & Co., London, 1991.

779. Pennington, J.A.T., Young, B.E., Wilson, D.B., Johnson, R.D., and Vanderveen, J.E., Mineral content of foods and total diets: the selected minerals in foods survey, 1982 to 1984, *J. Am. Diet. Assoc.,* 86, 876, 1986.

780. Fogelholm, M., Laakso, J., Lehto, J., and Ruokonen, I., Dietary intake and indicators of magnesium and zinc status in male athletes, *Nutr. Res.,* 11, 1111, 1991.

781. Casoni, I., Guglielmini, C., Graziano, L., Reali, M.G., Mozzotta, D., and Abbasciano, V., Changes of magnesium concentrations in endurance athletes, *Int. J. Sports Med.,* 11, 234, 1990.

782. Deuster, P.A., Dolev, E., Kyle, S.B., Anderson, R.A., and Schoomaker, E.B., Magnesium homeostasis during high-intensity anaerobic exercise in men, *J. Appl. Physiol.,* 62, 545, 1987.

783. Singh, A., Day, B.A., DeBolt, J.E., Trostmann, U.H., Bernier, L.L., and Deuster, P.A., Magnesium, zinc, and copper status of U.S. Navy SEAL trainees, *Am. J. Clin. Nutr.,* 49, 695, 1989.

784. Singh, A., Deuster, P.A., Day, B.A., and Moser-Veillion, P.B., Dietary intakes and biochemical markers of selected minerals: comparison of highly trained runners and untrained women, *J. Am. Coll. Nutr.,* 9(1), 65, 1990.

785. McDonald, R. and Keen, C.L., Iron, zinc and magnesium nutrition and athletic performance, *Sports Med.,* 5, 171, 1988.

786. Stendig-Lindberg, G., Shapiro, Y., Epstein, Y., Galun, E., Schonberger, E., Graff, E., and Wacker, W.E.C., Changes in serum magnesium concentration after exercise, *J. Am. Coll. Nutr.,* 6, 35, 1987.

787. Fogelholm, G.M., Himberg, J.J., Alopaeus, K., Gref, C.G., Laakso, J.T., Lehto, J.J., and Mussalo-Rauhamaa, H., Dietary and biochemical indices of nutritional status in male athletes and controls, *J. Am. Coll. Nutr.,* 11, 181, 1992.

788. Pennington, J.A.T., *Bowes and Church's Food Values of Portions Commonly Used,* 15th ed., J.B. Lippincott, Philadelphia, 1989.

789. Liu, L., Borowski, G., and Rose, L.I., Hypomagnesemia in a tennis player, *Phys. Sportsmed.,* 11, 79, 1983.

790. Cohen, L. and Kitzes, R., Infrared spectroscopy and magnesium content of bone mineral in osteoporotic women, *Isr. J. Med. Sci.,* 17(12), 1123, 1981.

791. Cohen, L., Laor, A., and Kitzes, R., Lymphocyte and bone magnesium in alcohol-associated osteoporosis, *Magnesium,* 4(2–3), 148, 1985.

792. Cohen, L., Bitterman, H., Froom, P., and Aghai, E., Decreased bone magnesium in beta thalassemia with spinal osteoporosis, *Magnesium,* 5(1), 43, 1986.

793. Ditmar, R. and Steidl, L., The significance of magnesium in orthopedics. V. Magnesium in osteoporosis, *Acta Chir. Orthop. Traumatol. Cech.,* 56(2), 143, 1989.

794. Driessens, F.C., Verbeeck, R.M., and van Dijk, J.W., A systemic approach to the oral problem of mandibular resorption, *Bull. Group Int. Rech. Sci. Stomatol. Odontol.,* 32(3), 127, 1989.

795. Miravet, L., Tubiana, M., and Durlach, J., Magnesium and several metabolic osteopathies, *Rev. Rhum. Mal. Osteoartic.,* 46(4), 279, 1979.

796. Reginster, J.Y., Strause, L., Deroisy, R., Lecart, M.P., Saltman, P., and Franchimont, P., Preliminary report of decreased serum magnesium in postmenopausal osteoporosis, *Magnesium,* 8(2), 106, 1989.

797. Saggese, G., Bertelloni, S., Baroncelli, S.I., Federico, G., Calisti, L., and Fusaro, C., Bone demineralization and impaired mineral metabolism in insulin-dependent diabetes mellitus. A possible role of magnesium deficiency, *Helv. Paediatr. Acta,* 43(5–6), 405, 1989.

798. Taylor, W.H., Low serum magnesium concentration in Paget's disease of bone (osteitis deformans), *Ann. Clin. Biochem.,* 22(6), 591, 1985.

799. Angus, R.M., Sambrook, P.N., Pocock, N.A., and Eisman, J.A., Dietary intake and bone mineral density, *Bone Mineral,* 4, 265, 1988.

800. Muenzenburg, K.J. and Koch, W., Mineralogic aspects in the treatment of osteoporosis with magnesium, *J. Am.Coll. Nutr.,* 8, 461, 1989.

801. Abraham, G.E. and Grewal, H., A total dietary program emphasizing magnesium instead of calcium. Effect on the bone mineral density of calcaneous bone in postmenopausal women on hormonal therapy, *J. Reprod. Med.,* 35, 503, 1990.

802. Vikhanski, L., Magnesium may slow bone loss, *Med. Tribune,* July 22, 9, 1993.

803. Clement, D.B. and Sawchuk, L.L., Iron status and performance, *Sports Med.,* 1, 65, 1984.

804. Haymes, E.M., Trace minerals and exercise, 1, in *Nutrition in Exercise and Sport*, 2nd ed., Wolinksy, I. and Hickson, J.F., Eds., CRC Press, Boca Raton, FL, 1994, 223.

805. Biemond, P., Swaak, A.J.G., van Eijk, H.G., and Koster, J.F., Superoxide dependent iron release from ferritin in inflammatory diseases, *Free Radical Biol. Med.*, 4, 185, 1988.

806. Rowley, D.A. and Halliwell, B., Formation of hydroxyl radicals from hydrogen peroxide and iron salts by superoxide- and ascorbate-dependent mechanisms: relevance to the pathology of rheumatoid disease, *Clin. Sci.*, 64, 649, 1983.

807. Pories, W.J. and Strain, W.H., Zinc sulfate therapy in surgical patients, in *Clinical Applications of Zinc Metabolism*, Pories, W.J., Strain, W.H., Hsu, J.M., and Woosley, R.L., Eds., Charles C. Thomas, Springfield, IL, 1974, 139.

808. Solomons, N.W., Zinc and copper, in *Modern Nutrition in Health and Disease*, 7th ed., Shils, M.E. and Young, V.R., Eds., Lea & Febiger, Philadelphia, 1988, 238.

809. Cousins, R.J. and Hempe, J.M., Zinc, in *Present Knowledge in Nutrition*, Brown, M.L., Ed., International Life Sciences Institute, Washington, D.C., 1990, 251.

810. Whitehouse, M.W., Trace element supplements for inflammatory disease, 1, in *Second-Line Agents in the Treatment of Rheumatic Diseases*, Dixon, J.S. and Furst, D.E., Eds., Marcel Dekker, New York, 1992, 549.

811. Evans, G.W., Zinc and its deficiency diseases, *Clin. Physiol. Biochem.*, 4, 94, 1986.

812. Sandstead, H.H. and Shephard, G.H., The effect of zinc deficiency on tensile strength of healing surgical incisions in the integument of the rat, *Proc. Soc. Exp. Biol. Med.*, 128, 687, 1968.

813. Sandstead, H.H., Lanier, V.C., Shephard, G.H., and Gillespie, D.D., Zinc and wound healing. Effects of zinc deficiency and zinc supplementation, *Am. J. Clin. Nutr.*, 23(5), 514, 1970.

814. Abdulla, M., How adequate is plasma zinc as an indicator of zinc status?, in *Zinc Deficiency in Human Subjects*, Prasad, A.S., Cavdar, A.O., and Brewer, G.J., Eds., Alan R. Liss, New York, 1983, 171.

815. Cunnane, S.C., Assessment of zinc nutriture, in *Zinc: Clinical and Biochemical Significance*, CRC Press, Boca Raton, FL, 1988, 11.

816. English, J.L., Hambidge, E.M., and Goodall, M.J., Evaluation of some factors that may affect plasma or serum zinc concentrations, in *Trace Elements in Man and Animals 6*, Hurley, L.S., Keen, C.L., Lönnerdal, B., and Rucker, R.B., Eds., Plenum Press, New York, 1988, 459.

817. Bryce-Smith, D. and Simpson, R.I.D., Anorexic depression and zinc deficiency, *Lancet*, 2, 1162, 1984.

818. Solomons, N.W., Biological availability of zinc in humans, *Am. J. Clin. Nutr.*, 35, 1048, 1982.

819. Patterson, K.Y., Holbrook, J.T., Bodner, J.E., Kelsay, J.L., Smith, J.C., and Veillon, C., Zinc, copper, and manganese intake and balance for adults consuming self-selected diets, *Am. J. Clin. Nutr.*, 40, 1397, 1984.

820. Haralambie, G., Serum zinc in athletes in training, *Int. J. Sports Med.*, 2, 135, 1981.

821. Couzy, F., Lafargue, P., and Guezennec, C.Y., Zinc metabolism in the athlete: influence of training, nutrition and other factors, *Int. J. Sports Med.*, 11, 263, 1990.

822. Barrie, S.A., Wright, J.V., Pizzorno, J.E., Kutter, E., and Barron, P.C., Comparative absorption of zinc picolinate, zinc citrate and zinc gluconate in humans, *Agents Actions*, 21, 223, 1987.

823. Battistone, G.C., Rubin, M.I., Cutright, D.E., and Miller, R.A., Zinc and bone healing: effect of zinc cysteamine-n-acetic acid on the healing of experimentally injured guinea pig bone, *Oral Surg.*, 34, 542, 1972.

824. van Rij, A.M. and Pories, W.J., Zinc and copper in surgery, in *Zinc and Copper in Medicine*, Karcioğlu, Z.A. and Sarper, R.M., Eds., Charles C. Thomas, Springfield, IL, 1980, 535.

825. Pories, W.J. and Strain, W.H., Zinc and wound healing, in *Zinc Metabolism*, Prasad, A.S., Ed., Charles C. Thomas, Springfield, IL, 1966, 378.

826. Pories, W.J., Henzel, J.H., Rob, C.G., and Strain, W.H., Acceleration of wound healing in man with zinc sulfate given by mouth, *Lancet*, 1, 121, 1967.

827. Pories, W.J., Henzel, J.H., Rob, C.G., and Strain, W.H., Acceleration of healing with zinc sulfate, *Ann. Surg.*, 165, 432, 1967.

828. Pories, W.J., Strain, W.H., Peer, R.M., and Landew, M.H., Zinc deficiency as a cause for delayed wound healing, *Curr. Topics Surg. Res.*, 1, 315, 1969.

829. Henzel, J.H., DeWeese, M.S., and Lechti, E.L., Zinc concentration within healing wounds, *Arch. Surg.*, 100, 349, 1970.

830. Barcia, P.J., Lack of acceleration of healing with zinc sulfate, *Ann. Surg.*, 172, 1048, 1970.

831. Buerk, C.A., Chandy, M.G., Pearson, E., MacAuly, A., and Soroff, H.S., Zinc deficiency: effect on healing and metabolism in man, *Surg. Forum*, 24, 101, 1973.

832. Pullen, F.W., Pories, W.J., and Strain, W.H., Delayed healing, the rationale for zinc therapy, *Laryngoscope*, 81, 1638, 1971.

833. Pullen, F.W., Oral zinc and vitamin therapy for laryngotracheal trauma and surgical aftercare, in *Clinical Applications of Zinc Metabolism*, Pories, W.J., Strain, W.H., Hsu, J.M., and Woosley, R.L., Eds., Charles C. Thomas, Springfield, IL, 1974, 237.

834. Flynn, A., Strain, W.H., Pories, W.J., and Hill, D.A., Zinc deficiency with altered adrenocortical function and its relation to wound healing, *Lancet*, 1, 789, 1973.

835. Haley, J., Zinc sulfate and wound healing, *J. Surg. Res.*, 27, 168, 1979.

836. Liszewski, R.F., The effect of zinc on wound healing: a collective review, *J. Am. Osteopath. Assoc.*, 81, 104, 1981.

837. Wacker, W.E.C., Biochemistry of zinc — role in wound healing, in *Zinc and Copper in Clinical Medicine*, Hambidge, K.M. and Nichols, B.L., Eds., SP Medical & Scientific Books, New York, 1978, 15.

838. Abbott, D.F., Exton-Smith, A.N., Millard, P.H., and Temperly, J.M., Zinc sulfate and bed sores, *Br. Med. J.*, 2, 763, 1968.

839. Cohen, C., Zinc sulfate and bed sores, *Br. Med. J.*, 2, 561, 1968.

840. Husain, S.L., Oral zinc sulfate in leg ulcers, *Lancet*, 1, 1069, 1969.

841. Greaves, M.W. and Skillen, A.W., Effects of long-continued ingestion of zinc sulfate in patients with venous leg ulceration, *Lancet*, 2, 889, 1970.

842. Serjeant, G.R., Galloway, R.E., and Gueri, M.C., Oral zinc sulfate in sickle-cell ulcers, *Lancet*, 2, 891, 1970.

843. Myers M.B and Cherry, G., Zinc and the healing of chronic leg ulcers, *Am. J. Surg.*, 120, 77, 1970.

844. Norris, J.R. and Reynolds, R.E., The effect of oral zinc sulfate therapy on decubitus ulcers, *J. Am. Geriat. Soc.*, 19, 793, 1971.

845. Clayton, R.J., Double-blind trial of zinc sulfate in patients with leg ulcers, *Br. J. Clin. Pract.*, 26, 368, 1972.

846. Greaves, M.W. and Ive, F.A., Double-blind trial of zinc sulfate in the treatment of chronic venous leg ulceration, *Br. J. Dermatol.*, 87, 632, 1972.

847. Hallböök, T. and Lanner, E., Serum-zinc and healing of venous leg ulcers, *Lancet*, 2, 781, 1972.

848. Haeger, K., Lanner, E., and Magnusson, P.O., Oral zinc sulfate in the treatment of venous leg ulcers, in *Clinical Applications of Zinc Metabolism*, Pories, W.J., Strain, W.H., Hsu, J.M., and Woosley, R.L., Eds., Charles C. Thomas, Springfield, IL, 1974, 158.

849. Husain, S.L. and Bessant, R.G., Oral zinc sulfate in the treatment of leg ulcers, in *Clinical Applications of Zinc Metabolism*, Pories, W.J., Strain, W.H., Hsu, J.M., and Woosley, R.L., Eds., Charles C. Thomas, Springfield, IL, 1974, 168.

850. Merchant, H.W., Gangarossa, L.P., Glassman, A.B., and Sobel, R.E., Zinc sulfate supplementation for treatment of recurring oral ulcers, *South. Med. J.*, 70(5), 559, 1977.

851. Watkinson, M., Aggett, P.J., and Cole, T.J., Zinc and acute tropical ulcers in Gambian children and adolescents, *Am. J. Clin. Nutr.*, 41(1), 43, 1985.

852. Ågren, M.S., Strömberg, H.E., Rindby, A., and Hallamns, G., Selenium, zinc, iron and copper levels in serum of patients with arterial and venous leg ulcers, *Acta Derm. Venereol.*, 66, 237, 1986.

853. Bruske, K. and Salfeld, K., Zinc and its status in some dermatological diseases — a statistical assessment, *Z. Hautkr.*, 62 (Suppl. 1), 125, 1987.

854. Thomas, A.J., Bunker, V.W., Hinks, L.J., Sodha, N., Mulle, M.A., and Clayton, B.E., Energy, protein, zinc and copper status of twenty-one elderly inpatients: analysed dietary intake and biochemical indices, *Br. J. Nutr.*, 59(2), 181, 1988.

855. Savelev, I.S., The rehabilitation of patients with trophic ulcers of the legs in a polyclinic, *Vestn. Khir.*, 140, 92, 1988.

856. Gasior-Chrzan, B. and Milian, A., Zinc in crural varicose ulcers, *Przegl. Dermatol.*, 76, 152, 1989.

857. Ackerman, Z., Loewenthal, E., Seidenbaum, M., Rubinow, A., and Gorodetsky, R., Skin zinc concentrations in patients with varicose ulcers, *Int. J. Dermatol.*, 29, 260, 1990.

858. Breslow, R., Nutritional status and dietary intake of patients with pressure ulcers: a review of research literature from 1943 to 1989, *Decubitus*, 4(1), 16, 1991.

859. Breslow, R.A., Hallfrisch, J., and Goldberg, A.P., Malnutrition in tubefed nursing home patients with pressure sores, *JPEN*, 15, 663, 1991.

860. Banos, J.E. and Bulbena, O., Zinc compounds as therapeutic agents in peptic ulcer, *Methods Find. Exp. Clin. Pharmacol.*, 11(Suppl. 1), 117, 1989.

861. Cho, C.H. and Pfeiffer, C.J., The developing role of zinc as an antiulcer agent, in *Drugs and Peptic Ulcer*, Vol. 1, Pfeiffer, C.J., Ed., CRC Press, Boca Raton, FL, 1982.

862. Escolar, G., Zinc compounds, a new treatment in peptic ulcer, *Drugs Exp. Clin. Res.*, 15(2), 83, 1989.

863. Fraser, P.M., Doll, R., Langman, M.J.S., Misiewicz, J.J., and Shawdon, H.H., Clinical trial of a new carbenoxolone analog (BX24), zinc sulfate, and vitamin A in the treatment of gastric ulcer, *Gut*, 13, 459, 1972.

864. Frommer, D.J., The healing of gastric ulcers by zinc sulfate, *Med. J. Aust.*, 2, 793, 1975.

865. Orr, K.B., Healing of gastric ulcer by zinc sulfate, *Med. J. Aust.*, 1, 244, 1976.

866. Berger, M.M., Cavadini, C., Bart, A., Mansourian, R., Guinchard, S., Bartholdi, I., Vandervale, A., Krupp, S., Chiolero, R., Freeman, J., and Dirren, H., Cutaneous copper and zinc losses in burns, *Burns*, 18, 373, 1992.

867. Boosalis, M.G., Solem, L.D., McCall, J.T., Ahrenholz, D.H., and McClain, C.J., Serum zinc response in thermal injury, *J. Am. Coll. Nutr.*, 7(1), 69, 1988.

868. Larson, D.L., Maxwell, R., Abston, S., and Dobrkovsky, M., Zinc deficiency in burned children, *Plast. Reconstr. Surg.*, 46, 13, 1970.

869. Larson, D.L., Oral zinc sulfate in the management of severely burned patients, in *Clinical Applications of Zinc Metabolism*, Pories, W.J., Strain, W.H., Hsu, J.M., and Woosley, R.L., Eds., Charles C. Thomas, Springfield, IL, 1974, 229.

870. Kennedy, A.C., Le, P., Dick, W.C., and Buchanan, W.W., Plasma zinc in rheumatoid arthritis. Its relationship to corticosteroid therapy and osteoporosis, *Ann. Rheum. Dis.*, 34, 201, 1975.

871. Kennedy, A.C., Fell, G.S., Rooney, P.J., Stevens, W.H., Dick, W.C., and Buchanan, W.W., Zinc: its relationship to osteoporosis in rheumatoid arthritis, *Scand. J. Rheumatol.*, 4, 243, 1975.

872. Neidermeier, W. and Griggs, J.H., Trace metal composition of synovial fluid and blood serum of patients with rheumatoid arthritis, *J. Chron. Dis.*, 23, 527, 1971.

873. Balogh, Z., El-Ghobarey, A.F., Fell, G.S., Brown, D.H., Dunlop, J., and Dick, W.C., Plasma zinc and its relationship to clinical symptoms and drug treatment in rheumatoid arthritis, *Ann. Rheum. Dis.*, 39, 329, 1980.

874. Svenson, K.L.G., Hällgren, R., Johansson, E., and Lindh, U., Reduced zinc in peripheral blood cells from patients with inflammatory connective tissue diseases, *Inflammation*, 9(2), 189, 1985.

875. Simkin, P.A., Oral zinc sulfate in rheumatoid arthritis, *Lancet,* 1, 539, 1976.

876. Simkin, P.A., Zinc sulfate in rheumatoid arthritis, in *Zinc Metabolism: Current Aspects in Health and Disease,* Brewer, G.J. and Prasad, A.S., Eds., Alan R. Liss, New York, 1977, 343.

877. Simkin, P.A., Oral zinc and rheumatoid arthritis, *Arthritis Rheum.,* 24, 865, 1981.

878. Simkin, P.A., Treatment of rheumatoid arthritis with oral zinc sulfate, *Agents Actions,* Suppl. 8, 587, 1981.

879. Simkin, P.A., Treatment of rheumatoid arthritis with zinc sulfate, in *Inflammatory Diseases and Copper,* Sorenson, J.R.J., Ed., Humana Press, Clifton, NJ, 1982, 483.

880. Clemmensen, O.J., Siggard-Andersen, J., Worm, A.M., Stahl, D., Frost, F., and Bloch, I., Psoriatic arthritis treated with oral zinc sulfate, *Br. J. Dermatol.,* 103, 411, 1980.

881. Frigo, A., Tambalo, C., Bambara, L.M., Biasi, D., Marrella, M., Milanino, R., Moretti, U., Velo, G., and DeSandre, G., Zinc sulfate in the treatment of psoriatic arthritis, *Recenti Prog. Med.,* 80, 577, 1989.

882. Job, C., Menkes, C.J., and Delbarre, F., Zinc sulfate in the treatment of rheumatoid arthritis, *Arthritis Rheum.,* 23, 1408, 1980.

883. Mattingly, P.C. and Mowat, A.G., Zinc sulfate in rheumatoid arthritis, *Ann. Rheum. Dis.,* 41, 456, 1982.

884. Menkes, C.J., Job, C., and Delbarre, F., Traitment de la polyarthrite rhumatoide par le sulfate de zinc per os, *Nouv. Presse Med.,* 7, 760, 1978.

885. Rasker, J.J. and Kardaun, S.H., Lack of beneficial effect of zinc sulfate in rheumatoid arthritis, *Scand. J. Rheumatol.,* 11, 168, 1982.

886. Cimmino, M.A., Mazzucotelli, A., Rovetta, G., Bianchi, G., and Cutolo, M., The controversy over zinc sulfate efficacy in rheumatoid and psoriatic arthritis, *Scand. J. Rheumatol.,* 13, 191, 1984.

887. Heinitz, M., Allgemeiner und Kasuisticher Beitrag zur Zinktherapie der Rheumatoiden Arthritis, *Med. Welt.,* 29, 1772, 1978.

888. Calhoun, N.R., Smith, J.C., and Becker, K.L., The role of zinc in bone metabolism, *Clin. Orthop.,* 103, 212, 1974.

889. Askari, A., Long, C.L., and Blakemore, W.S., Net metabolic changes of zinc, copper, nitrogen, and potassium balances in skeletal trauma patients, *Metabolism,* 31, 1185, 1982.

890. Sugarman, B., Zinc and spinal cord injury: a review, *J. Am. Paraplegia Soc.,* 7(2), 39, 1984.

891. Ohry, A., Shemesh, Y., Zak, R., and Herzberg, M., Zinc and osteoporosis in patients with spinal cord injury, *Paraplegia,* 18(3), 174, 1980.

892. Krebs, J., Schneider, V., Cintron, N., LeBlanc, A., Kuo, M.C., Johnson, P.C., and Leach-Huntoon, C., Zinc balance during bed rest: sodium fluoride supplementation, *Fed. Proc.,* 44, 543, 1985.

893. Higashi, A., Nakamura, T., Nishiyama, S., Matsukura, M., Tomoeda, S., Futagoshi, Y., Shinohara, M., and Matsuda, I., Zinc kinetics in patients with bone demineralization due to physical immobilization, *J. Am. Coll. Nutr.,* 12(1), 61, 1993.

894. Cunnane, S.C., Zinc toxicity, in *Zinc: Clinical and Biochemical Significance,* CRC Press, Boca Raton, FL, 1988, 65.

895. Chandra, R.K., Excess intake of zinc impairs immune responses, *JAMA,* 252, 1443, 1984.

896. Hooper, P.L., Visconti, L., Garry, P.J., and Johnson, G.E., Zinc lowers high-density lipoprotein cholesterol levels, *JAMA,* 244, 1960, 1980.

897. O'Dell, B.L., Copper, in *Present Knowledge in Nutrition,* 6th ed., Brown, M.L., Ed., International Life Sciences Institute, Washington, D.C., 1990, 261.

898. Lontie, R., The structure and mechanism of Cu/Zn-Superoxide dismutase, in *Copper Proteins and Copper Enzymes,* Vol. 2, Lontie, R., Ed., CRC Press, Boca Raton, FL, 1984, 23.

899. Anonymous, Activation of lysyl oxidase by copper, *Nutr. Rev.,* 37, 330, 1979.

900. Buse, G., Cytochrome *c* oxidase, in *Copper Proteins and Copper Enzymes,* Vol. 3, Lontie, R., Ed., CRC Press, Boca Raton, FL, 1984, 119.

901. Rydén, L., Ceruloplasmin, in *Copper Proteins and Copper Enzymes,* Vol. 3, Lontie, R., Ed., CRC Press, Boca Raton, FL, 1984, 37.

902. Strain, J.J., A reassessment of diet and osteoporosis — possible role for copper, *Med. Hypoth.,* 27, 333, 1988.

903. Al-Rashid, R.A. and Spangler, J., Neonatal copper deficiency, *New Engl. J. Med.,* 285(15), 841, 1971.

904. Allen, T.M., Manoli, A., and LaMont, R.L., Skeletal changes associated with copper deficiency, *Clin. Orthop.,* 168, 206, 1982.

905. Ashkenazi, A., Levin, S., Djaldeti, M., Fishel, E., and Benvenisti, D., The syndrome of neonatal copper deficiency, *Pediatrics,* 52, 525, 1973.

906. Cordano, A., Baertl, J.M., and Graham, G.G., Copper deficiency in infancy, *Pediatrics,* 34, 324, 1964.

907. Graham, G.G. and Cordano, A., Copper depletion and deficiency in the malnourished infant, *Johns Hopkins Med. J.,* 124, 139, 1969.

908. Griscom, N.T., Craig, J.N., and Neuhauser, E.B.D., Systemic bone disease developing in small premature infants, *Pediatrics,* 48, 883, 1971.

909. Heller, R.M., Kirchner, S.G., O'Neill, J.A., Hough, A.J., Howard, L., Krammer, S.S., and Green, H.L., Skeletal changes of copper deficiency in infants receiving prolonged total parenteral nutrition, *J. Pediatr.,* 92(6), 947, 1978.

910. Karpel, J.T. and Peden, V.H., Copper deficiency in long-term parenteral nutrition, *J. Pediatr.,* 80, 32, 1972.

911. Tanaka, Y., Hatano, S., Nishi, Y., and Usui, T., Nutritional copper deficiency in a Japanese infant on formula, *J. Pediatr.,* 96(2), 255, 1980.

912. Velin, P., Dupont, D., and Daoud, A., Nutritional copper deficiency. Apropos of a case, *Ann. Pediatr.,* 36(4), 269, 1989.

913. Wiss, D.A. and Ledesma-Medina, J., Skeletal changes in copper deficiency following prolonged total parenteral nutrition, *Orthopedics,* 3, 969, 1980.

914. Yuen, P., Lin, H.J., and Hutchinson, J.H., Copper deficiency in a low birth weight infant, *Arch. Dis. Child.,* 54, 553, 1979.

915. Danks, D.M., Copper deficiency in infants with particular reference to Menke's Disease, in *Copper in Animals and Man*, Vol. 2, Howell, J.M. and Gawthorne, J.M., Eds., CRC Press, Boca Raton, FL, 1987, 29.

916. Paynter, D.I., The diagnosis of copper insufficiency, in *Copper in Animals and Man*, Vol. 1, Howell, J.M. and Gawthorne, J.M., Eds., CRC Press, Boca Raton, FL, 1987, 101.

917. Milne, D.B. and Johnson, P.E., Assessment of copper status: effect of age and gender on reference ranges in healthy adults, *Clin.Chem.*, 39(5), 883, 1993.

918. Klevay, L.M., An appraisal of current human copper nutriture, in *Inflammatory Diseases and Copper*, Sorenson, J.R.J., Ed., Humana Press, Clifton, NJ, 1982, 123.

919. O'Dell, B.L., Dietary carbohydrate source and copper bioavailability, *Nutr. Rev.*, 48(12), 425, 1990.

920. Carnes, W.H., Copper and connective tissue metabolism, *Int. Rev. Connect. Tissue Res.*, 4, 197, 1968.

921. Carnes, W.H., Role of copper in connective tissue metabolism, *Fed. Proc.*, 30(3), 995, 1971.

922. Strause, L., Hegenauer, J., Saltman, P., Cone, R., and Resnick, D., Effects of long-term dietary manganese and copper deficiency on rat skeleton, *J. Nutr.*, 116, 135, 1986.

923. Strause, L., Saltman, P., and Glowacki, J., The effect of deficiencies of manganese and copper on osteoinduction and on resorption of bone particles, *Calcif. Tissue Int.*, 41(3), 145, 1987.

924. Strause, L. and Saltman, P., Role of manganese in bone metabolism, in *Nutritional Bioavailability of Manganese*, Kies, C., Ed., American Chemical Society, Washington, D.C., 1987, 46.

925. Pickart, L., Downey, D., Lovejoy, S., and Weinstein, B., Gly-L-his-L-lys:copper(II) — a human plasma growth factor with superoxide dismutase-like and wound-healing properties, in *Superoxide and Superoxide Dismutase in Chemistry, Biology and Medicine*, Rotilio, G., Ed., Elsevier, Amsterdam, 1986, 555.

926. Sorenson, J.R.J., Antiarthritic, antiulcer, and analgesic activities of copper complexes, in *Trace Elements in Clinical Medicine*, Tomita, H., Ed., Springer-Verlag, Tokyo, 1990, 261.

927. Walker, W.R. and Keats, D.M., An investigation of the therapeutic value of the 'Copper Bracelet' -dermal assimilation of copper in arthritic/rheumatic conditions, *Agents Actions*, 6(4), 454, 1976.

928. Walker, W.R., The results of a copper bracelet clinical trial and subsequent studies, in *Inflammatory Diseases and Copper*, Sorenson, J.R.J., Ed., Humana Press, Clifton, NJ, 1982, 469.

929. Whitehouse, M.W., Ambivalent role of copper in inflammatory disorders, *Agents Actions*, 6, 201, 1976.

930. Hangarter, W. and Lubke, A., Uber die behandlung rheumatischer erkuankungen mite einer kupfernatrium-salicylat-komplexverbindung (Permalon), *Dtsch. Med. Wochenschr.*, 77, 870, 1952.

931. Kushner, I., The phenomenon of the acute phase response, *Ann. N.Y. Acad. Sci.*, 389, 39, 1982.

932. Koskelo, P., Kekki, M., Virkkunen, M., Lassus, A., and Somer, T., Serum ceruloplasmin concentration in rheumatoid arthritis, ankylosing spondylitis, psoriasis and sarcoidosis, *Acta Rheum. Scand.*, 12, 261, 1966.

933. Scudder, P.R., Al-Timimi, D., McMurray, W., White, A.G., Zoob, B.C., and Dormandy, T.L., Serum copper and related variables in rheumatoid arthritis, *Ann. Rheum. Dis.*, 37, 67, 1978.

934. Banford, J.C., Brown, D.H., Hazelton, R.A., McNeil, C.J., Sturrock, R.D., and Smith, W.E., Serum copper and erythrocyte superoxide dismutase in rheumatoid arthritis, *Ann. Rheum. Dis.*, 41, 458, 1982.

935. Oriente, P., Scarpa, R., Cutolo, M., Riccio, A., Pucino, A., and Postiglione, L., Serum copper and caeruloplasmin are higher in seropositive than seronegative rheumatoid arthritis, *Eur. J. Rheum. Inflam.*, 6, 163, 1983.

936. Sorenson, J.R.J., Ed., *Inflammatory Diseases and Copper*, Humana Press, Clifton, NJ, 1982.

937. Milanino, R., Conforti, A., Franco, L., Marrella, M., and Velo, G., Review: copper and inflammation — a possible rationale for the pharmacological manipulation of inflammatory disorders, *Agents Actions*, 16(6), 504, 1985.

938. Garrett, I.R. and Whitehouse, M.W., Copper and inflammation, in *Copper in Animals and Man*, Vol. 1, Howell, J.M. and Gawthorne, J.M., Eds., CRC Press, Boca Raton, FL, 1987, 107.

939. DiSilvestro, R.A., Marten, J., and Skehan, M., Effects of copper supplementation on ceruloplasmin and copper-zinc superoxide dismutase in free-living rheumatoid arthritis patients, *J. Am. Coll. Nutr.*, 11(2), 177, 1992.

940. Sorenson, J.R.J. and Hangarter, W., Treatment of rheumatoid and degenerative diseases with copper complexes, *Inflammation*, 2(3), 217, 1977.

941. Hangarter, W., Copper-salicylate in rheumatoid arthritis and similar degenerative diseases, in *Inflammatory Diseases and Copper*, Sorenson, J.R.J., Ed., Humana Press, Clifton, NJ, 1982, 439.

942. Fenz, E., Le cuivre dans le rhumatisme articulaire, *Munch. Med. Wochenschr.*, 18, 398, 1941.

943. Fenz, E., Kupfer, ein neues mittel gegen chron und subakuten gelenkrheumatismus, *Munch. Med. Wochenschr.*, 41, 1101, 1951.

944. Forestier, J., Les sels organiques de cuivre dans le traitement des rhumatismes chroniques, *Bull. Acad. Med.*, 2, 22, 1944.

945. Forestier, J. and Certonciny, A., Le traitement des rhumatismes chronique par les sels organiques des cuivre, *Presse Med.*, 64, 884, 1946.

946. Forestier, J., La chryso et la cuprotherapies dans le traitement de la polyarthritic chroniques evolution, *Ann. Rheum. Dis.*, 8, 27, 1948.

947. Forestier, J., Comparative results of copper salts and gold salts in rheumatoid arthritis, *Ann. Rheum. Dis.*, 8, 132, 1949.

948. Forestier, J., Certonciny, A., and Jacqueline, F., Therapeutic value of copper salts in rheumatoid arthritis, *Stanford Med. Bull.*, 8, 12, 1950.

949. Kuzell, W.C., Schaffarzick, R.W., Mankle, E.A., and Gardner, G.M., Copper treatment of experimental and clinical arthritis, *Ann. Rheum. Dis.,* 10, 238, 1951.

950. Tyson, T.L., Holmes, H.H., and Ragan, C., Copper therapy of rheumatoid arthritis, *Am. J. Med. Sci.,* 220, 418, 1950.

951. Pullar, T., Wrigley, H., Newton, K., Toothill, C., and Wright, V., A study of adjunctive copper sulfate treatment in patients with rheumatoid arthritis who have relapsed while taking D-penicillamine, *Br. J. Clin. Pharm.,* 31, 105, 1991.

952. Clark, S.F., Gilbert, C., and Thye, F.W., Copper status in multiple trauma patients, *Am. J. Clin. Nutr.,* 51(3), 511, 1990.

953. White, H.S., Inorganic elements in weighed diets of girls and young women, *J. Am. Diet. Assoc.,* 55, 38, 1969.

954. Wolf, W.R., Holden, J., and Greene, F.E., Daily intake of zinc and copper from self selected diets, *Fed. Proc.,* 36, 1175, 1977.

955. Gormican, A., Inorganic elements in foods used in hospital menus, *J. Am. Diet. Assoc.,* 56, 397, 1970.

956. Murphy, P., Wadiwala, I., Sharland, D.E., and Rai, G.S., Copper and zinc levels in "healthy" and "sick" elderly, *J. Am. Geriatr. Soc.,* 33, 847, 1985.

957. Lappalainen, R., Knuuttila, M., Lammi, S., Alhava, E.M., and Olkkonen, H., Zn and Cu content in human cancellous bone, *Acta Orthop. Scand.,* 53 51, 1982.

958. Seymour, C.A., Copper toxicity in man, in *Copper in Animals and Man,* Vol. 2, Howell, J.M. and Gawthorne, J.M., Eds., CRC Press, Boca Raton, FL, 1987, 79.

959. Keen, C.L. and Zidenburg-Cherr, S., Manganese, in *Present Knowledge in Nutrition,* Brown, M.L., Ed., Nutrition Foundation, Washington, D.C., 1990, 279.

960. Leach, R.M., Metabolism and function of manganese, in *Trace Elements in Human Health and Disease,* Vol. 2, Essential and Toxic Elements, Prasad, A.S. and Oberleas, D., Eds., Academic Press, New York, 1976, 235.

961. Leach, R.M. and Lilburn, M.S., Manganese metabolism and its function, *World Rev. Nutr. Diet.,* 32, 123, 1978.

962. Klimis-Tavantzis, D.J., Ed., *Manganese in Health and Disease,* CRC Press, Boca Raton, FL, 1993.

963. Keen, C.L., Lönnerdal, B., and Hurley, L.S., Manganese, in *Biochemistry of the Ultratrace Elements,* Frieden, E., Ed., Plenum Publishing, New York, 1984, 89.

964. Schramm, V.L. and Wedler, F.C., Eds., *Manganese in Metabolism and Enzyme Function,* Academic Press, Orlando, 1986.

965. Hurley, L.S. and Keen, C.L., Manganese, in *Trace Elements in Human Health and Animal Nutrition,* Underwood, E. and Mertz, W., Eds., Academic Press, New York, 1987, 185.

966. Kies, C., Ed., *Nutritional Bioavailability of Manganese,* American Chemical Society, Washington, D.C., 1987.

967. Bucci, L.R., Manganese: its role in nutritional balance, *Today's Chirop.,* 17(2), 23 & 17(3), 45, 1988.

968. Levander, O.A., Manganese, in *Modern Nutrition in Health and Disease,* 7th ed., Shils, M.E. and Young, V.R., Eds., Lea & Febiger, Philadelphia, 1988, 274.

969. Leach, R.M., Role of manganese in mucopolysaccharide metabolism, *Fed. Proc.,* 30(3), 991, 1971.

970. de Rosa, G., Keen, C.L., Leach, R.M., and Hurley, L.S., Regulation of superoxide dismutase activity by dietary manganese, *J. Nutr.,* 110, 795, 1980.

971. Ludwig, M.L., Pattridge, K.A., and Stallings, W.C., Mitochondrial superoxide disantase, in *Manganese in Metabolism and Enzyme Function,* Schramm, V.L. and Wedler, F.C., Eds., Academic Press, Orlando, 1986, 405.

972. Scrutton, M.C., Pyruvate carboxylase, in *Manganese in Metabolism and Enzyme Function,* Schramm, V.L. and Wedler, F.C., Eds., Academic Press, Orlando, 1986, 147.

973. Bond, J.S., Unger, D.F., and Garganta, C.L., Arginase rules and functions, in *Manganese in Metabolism and Enzyme Function,* Schramm, V.L. and Wedler, F.C., Eds., Academic Press, Orlando, 1986, 239.

974. Leach, R.M. and Muenster, A.M., Studies on the role of manganese in bone formation. I. Effect upon the mucopolysaccharide content of chick bone, *J. Nutr.,* 78, 51, 1962.

975. Watts, D.L., The nutritional relationships of manganese, *J. Orthomol. Med.,* 5(4), 219, 1990.

976. National Research Council, *Recommended Dietary Allowances,* 10th ed., National Academy Press, Washington, D.C., 1989.

977. Freeland-Graves, J.H., Bales, C.W., and Behmardi, F., Manganese requirements of humans, in *Nutritional Bioavailability of Manganese,* Kies, C., Ed., American Chemical Society, Washington, D.C., 1987, 90.

978. Kies, C., Aldrich, K.D., Johnson, J.M., Creps, C., Kowalski, C., and Wang, R.H., Manganese bioavailability for humans: effect of selected dietary factors, in *Nutritional Bioavailability of Manganese,* Kies, C., Ed., American Chemical Society, Washington, D.C., 1987, 136.

979. Kies, C., Manganese bioavailability overview, in *Nutritional Bioavailability of Manganese,* Kies, C., Ed., American Chemical Society, Washington, D.C., 1987, 1.

980. Davidsson, L., Lönnerdal, B., Sandström, B., Kunz, K., and Keen, C.L., Identification of transferrin as the major plasma carrier protein for manganese introduced orally or intravenously or after *in vitro* addition in the rat, *J. Nutr.,* 119, 1461, 1989.

981. Kies, C., Creps, C., Kowalski, C., and Fox, H.M., Manganese utilization of humans as affected by iron supplementation, *Fed. Proc.,* 44(6), 1850, 1985.

982. Gruden, N., Iron in manganese metabolism, in *Nutritional Bioavailability of Manganese,* Kies, C., Ed., American Chemical Society, Washington, D.C., 1987, 67.

983. McDermott, S.D. and Kies, C., Manganese usage in humans as affected by use of calcium supplements, in *Nutritional Bioavailability of Manganese,* Kies, C., Ed., American Chemical Society, Washington, D.C., 1987, 146.

984. Bales, C.W., Freeland-Graves, J.H., Lin, P.H., Stone, J.M., and Dougherty, V., Plasma uptake of manganese: influence of dietary factors, in *Nutritional Bioavailability of Manganese*, Kies, C., Ed., American Chemical Society, Washington, D.C., 1987, 112.

985. Freeland-Graves, J.H., Behmardi, F., and Bales, C.W., Metabolic balance of manganese in young men consuming diets containing five levels of manganese, *J. Nutr.*, 118, 764, 1988.

986. Andon, M., Luhrsen, K., Kanerva, R., and Chatzidakis, C., Effects of dietary copper and manganese restriction on serum mineral concentrations and femoral shaft bone density in rats, *J. Am. Coll. Nutr.*, 11(5) (Abstr. 13), 600, 1992.

987. Martin, R.B., Effects of different commercial diets on several orthopedic experiments, *Clin. Orthop.*, 138, 217, 1979.

988. Bolze, M.S., Reeves, R.D., Lindbeck, F.E., Kemp, S.F., and Elders, M.J., Influence of manganese on growth, somatomedin and glycosaminoglycan metabolism, *J. Nutr.*, 115, 352, 1985.

989. Stern, P.H., Biphasic effects of manganese on hormone-stimulated bone resorption, *Endocrinology*, 117(5), 2044, 1985.

990. Schor, R.A., Prussin, S.G., Jewett, D.L., Ludowieg, J.J., and Bhatnagar, R.S., Trace levels of manganese, copper, and zinc in rib cartilage as related to age in humans and animals, both normal and dwarfed, *Clin. Orthop.*, 93, 346, 1973.

991. Fincham, J.E., van Rensburg, S.J., and Marasas, W.F.O., Mseleni joint disease — a manganese deficiency?, *S. Afr. Med. J.*, 60(12), 445, 1981.

992. Mackenzie, D.B., Something fishy about Mseleni joint disease, *S. Afr. Med. J.*, 61, 920, 1981.

993. Xilinas, M.E., Manganese intake and congenital dislocation of the hip, *S. Afr. Med. J.*, 63, 393, 1983.

994. Svensson, O., Engfeldt, B., Reinholt, F.P., and Hjerpe, A., Manganese rickets. A biochemical and stereological study with special reference to the effect of phosphate, *Clin. Orthop.*, 218, 302, 1987.

995. Svensson, O., Hjerpe, A., Reinholt, F.P., Wikstrom, B., and Engfeldt, B., The effect of strontium and manganese on freshly isolated chondrocytes, *Acta Pathol. Microbiol. Immunol. Scand.*, 93, 115, 1985.

996. Donaldson, J., The physiopathologic significance of manganese in brain: its relation to schizophrenia and neurodegenerative disorders, *Neurotoxicology*, 8, 451, 1987.

997. Keen, C.L. and Lönnerdal, B., Manganese toxicity in man and experimental animals, in *Manganese in Metabolism and Enzyme Function*, Schramm, V.L. and Wedler, F.C., Eds., Academic Press, Orlando, 1986, 35.

998. Banta, G. and Markesbery, W.R., Elevated manganese levels associated with dementia and extrapyramidal signs, *Neurology*, 27, 213, 1977.

999. Underwood, E.J., *Trace Elements in Human and Animal Nutrition*, 4th ed., Academic Press, New York, 1977, 436.

1000. Loomis, W.D. and Durst, R.W., Chemistry and biology of boron, *BioFactors*, 3, 229, 1992.

1001. Hunt, C.D., The biochemical effects of physiologic amounts of dietary boron in animal nutrition models, *Environ. Health Perspect.*, in press.

1002. Lovatt, C.J. and Dugger, W.M., Boron, in *Biochemistry of the Ultratrace Elements*, Frieden, E., Ed., Plenum Press, New York, 1984, 389.

1003. Nielsen, F.H., Facts and fallacies about boron, *Nutr. Today*, May/Jun, 6, 1992.

1004. Siegel, E. and Wason, S., Boric acid toxicity, *Pediatr. Clin. N. Am.*, 33, 363, 1986.

1005. Hunt, C.D., Shuler, T.R., and Mullen, L.M., Concentration of boron and other elements in human foods and personal-care products, *J. Am. Diet. Assoc.*, 91(5), 558, 1991.

1006. Hunt, C.D. and Nielsen, F.H., Interaction between boron and cholecalciferol in the chick, in *Trace Element Metabolism in Man and Animals*, Gawthorne, J.M., Howell, J.M, and White, C.L., Eds., Springer-Verlag, Berlin, 1982, 597.

1007. Hunt, C.D. and Nielsen, F.H., Interactions among dietary boron, calcium, magnesium, and cholecalciferol in the chick, *Fed. Proc.*, 44, 1848, 1985.

1008. Qin, X. and Klandorf, H., Effect of dietary boron supplementation on egg production, shell quality, and calcium metabolism in aged broiler breeder hens, *Poult. Sci.*, 70(10), 2131, 1991.

1009. King, N., Odom, T.W., Sampson, H.W., and Yersin, A.G., The effect of in ovo boron supplementation on bone mineralization of the vitamin D-deficient chicken embryo, *Biol. Trace Elem. Res.*, 31(3), 223, 1991.

1010. King, N., Odom, T.W., Sampson, H.W., and Pardue, S.L., In ovo administration of boron alters bone mineralization of the chicken embryo, *Biol. Trace Elem. Res.*, 30(1), 47, 1991.

1011. Pardue, S.L., Odom, T.W., King, N., and Sampson, W., In ovo administration of boron or sodium aluminosilicate alters mineralization in the turkey, *FASEB J.*, 3, A1072, 1989.

1012. Elliot, M.A. and Edwards, H.M., Studies to determine whether an interaction exists among boron, calcium, and cholecalciferol on the skeletal development of broiler chickens, *Poult. Sci.*, 71(4), 677, 1992.

1013. Nielsen, F.H., Shuler, T.R., Zimmerman, T.J., and Uthus, E.O., Magnesium and methionine deprivation affect the response of rats to boron deprivation, *Biol. Trace Elem. Res.*, 17, 91, 1988.

1014. Hegsted, M., Keenan, M., Siver, F., and Wozniak, P., Effect of boron on vitamin D deficient rats, *Biol. Trace Elem. Res.*, 28(3), 243, 1991.

1015. McCoy, H., Montgomery, C., Kenney, M.A., and Williams, L., Effects of boron supplementation on bones from rats fed calcium-deficient diets, *FASEB J.*, 4, A1050, 1990.

1016. Bock, M.A., Powey, M., and Ortiz, M., Fecal and urinary excretion of calcium (Ca), magnesium (Mg) and manganese (Mn) in female rats fed high and low levels of calcium and boron (B), *FASEB J.*, 4, A520, 1990.

1017. Nielsen, F.H. and Shuler, T.R., Studies of the interaction between boron and calcium, and its modification by magnesium and potassium, in rats. Effects on growth, blood variables, and bone mineral composition, *Biol. Trace Elem. Res.*, 35, 225, 1992.

1018. Brown, T.F., McCormick, M.E., Morris, D.R., and Zeringue, L.K., Effects of dietary boron on mineral balance in sheep, *Nutr. Res.,* 9, 503, 1989.

1019. Newnham, R.E., The role of boron in human and animal health, in *Trace Elements in Man and Animals 7,* Momcilovic, B., Ed., IMI, Zagreb, 1991, 8.4.

1020. Nielsen, F.H., The ultratrace elements, in *Trace Minerals in Foods,* Smith, K.T., Ed., Marcel Dekker, New York, 1988, 357.

1021. Shah, S.A. and Vohora, S.B., Boron enhances antiarthritic effects of garlic oil, *Fitoterapia,* 61, 121, 1990.

1022. Schlettwein-Gsell, D., and Mommsen-Straub, S., Übersicht spurelemente in lebensmitteln. IX. Bor, *Int. Z. Vit. Ern. Forschung,* 43, 93, 1973.

1023. Nielsen, F.H., Hunt, C.D., Mullen, L.M., and Hunt, J.R., Effect of dietary boron on mineral, estrogen, and testosterone metabolism in postmenopausal women, *FASEB J.,* 1, 394, 1987.

1024. Ellis, F.R., Holesh, S., and Ellis, J.W., Incidence of osteoporosis in vegetarians and omnivores, *Am. J. Clin. Nutr.,* 25, 555, 1972.

1025. Marsh, A.G., Sanchez, T.V., Chaffee, F.L., Mayor, G.H., and Mickelsen, O., Bone mineral mass in adult lacto-ovo-vegetarian and omnivorous males, *Am. J. Clin. Nutr.,* 37, 453, 1983.

1026. Nielsen, F.H., Dietary boron affects variables associated with copper metabolism in humans, in *6th International Trace Element Symposium 1989 As, B, Br, Co, Cr, F, Fe, Mn, Ni, Sb, Sc, Si, Sn and Other Ultratrace Elements,* Anke, M., Baumann, W., Bräunlich, H., Brückner, C., Groppel, B., and Grün, M., Eds., Fiedrich-Schiller-Universität, Jena, 1989, 1106.

1027. Nielsen, F.H., Mullen, L.M., and Gallagher, S.K., Effect of boron depletion and repletion on blood indicators of calcium status in humans fed a magnesium-low diet, *J. Trace Elem. Exp. Med.,* 3, 45, 1990.

1028. Nielsen, F.H., Biochemical and physiological consequences of boron deprivation in humans, in press.

1029. Nielsen, F.H., Mullen, L.M., and Nielsen, E.J., Dietary boron affects blood cell counts and hemoglobin concentrations in humans, *J. Trace Elem. Exp. Med.,* 4, 211, 1991.

1030. Nielsen, F.H., Gallagher, S.K., Johnson, L.K., and Nielsen, E.J., Boron enhances and mimics some effects of estrogen therapy in postmenopausal women, *J. Trace Elem. Exp. Med.,* 5, 237, 1992.

1031. Kivirikko, K.I., Urinary excretion of hydroxyproline in health and disease, *Int. Rev. Connect. Tissue Res.,* 5, 93, 1970.

1032. Azria, M., The value of biomarkers in detecting alterations in bone metabolism, *Calcif. Tissue Int.,* 45, 7, 1989.

1033. Robins, S.P., Turnover of collagen, in *Collagen in Health and Disease,* Weiss, J. and Jayson, M.I.V., Eds., Churchill Livingstone, Edinburgh, 1982, 160.

1034. Baslé, M.F., Mauras, Y., Audran, M., Clochon, P., Rebel, A., and Allain, P., Concentration of bone elements in osteoporosis, *J. Bone Min. Res.,* 5, 41, 1990.

1035. Moukarzel, A.A., Buchman, A.L., Song, M., and Ament, M.E., Is boron deficiency an etiological factor in osteopenia of parenteral nutrition bone disease of children?, *J. Am. Coll. Nutr.,* 11(5), 601, 1992. (abst. 14).

1036. Darnton, S., Taper, J., and Volpe-Snyder, S., The effects of boron supplementation on bone mineral density, blood and urinary calcium, magnesium, phosphorus and urinary boron in female athletes, *FASEB J.,* 6(4), A1945, 1992.

1037. Ferrando, A. and Green, N.R., The effect of boron supplementation on lean body mass, plasma testosterone levels and strength in male weightlifters, *FASEB J.,* 6(4), A1946, 1992.

1038. Newnham, R.E., Mineral imbalance and boron deficiency, in *Trace Element Metabolism in Man and Animals,* Gawthorne, J.M., Howell, J.M., and White, C.L., Eds., Springer-Verlag, Berlin, 1982, 400.

1039. Travers, R.L. and Rennie, G.C., Clinical trial — boron and arthritis, *Townsend Lett.,* 83, 360, 1990.

1040. Seal, B.S. and Weeth, H.J., Effect of boron in drinking water on the male laboratory rat, *Bull. Environ. Contam. Toxicol.,* 25, 782, 1980.

1041. Nielsen, F.H., Ultratrace minerals mythical elixirs or nutrients of concern?, *Bol. Asoc. Med. P.R.,* 83, 131, 1991.

1042. Nielsen, F.H., Trace and ultratrace elements in health and disease, *Comp. Ther.,* 17, 20, 1991.

1043. Nielsen, F.H., Nutritional requirements for boron, silicon, vanadium, nickel, and arsenic: current knowledge and speculation, *FASEB J.,* 5, 2661, 1991.

1044. Nielsen, F.H., Ultratrace elements of possible importance for human health: an update, in *Essential and Toxic Trace Elements in Human Health and Disease: An Update,* Prasad, A.S., Ed., Wiley-Liss, New York, 1993, 355.

1045. Harrison, J.E., Krishnan, S.S., and Hitchman, A.J.W., Fluoride effects in man, in *Metabolism of Minerals and Trace Elements in Human Disease,* Abdulla, M., Dashti, H., Sarkar, B., Al-Sayer, H., and Al-Naqeeb, N., Eds., Smith-Gordon, London, 1987.

1046. Ophaug, R.H., Fluoride, in *Present Knowledge in Nutrition,* Brown, M.L., Ed., Nutrition Foundation, Washington, D.C., 1990, 274.

1047. McDowell, L.R., Fluorine, in *Minerals in Animal and Human Nutrition,* Academic Press, New York, 1992, 333.

1048. Abdulla, M., Parr, R.M., and Iyengar, G.V., Trace element requirements, intake, and recommendations, in *Essential and Toxic Trace Elements in Human Health and Disease: An Update,* Prasad, A.S., Ed., Wiley-Liss, New York, 1993, 311.

1049. Kleerekoper, M. and Balena, R., Fluorides and osteoporosis, *Ann. Rev. Nutr.,* 11, 309, 1991.

1050. Coombs, G.F., Spallholz, J.E., Levander, O.A., and Oldfield, J.E., Eds., *Selenium in Biology and Medicine,* AVI Van Nostrand Reinhold Co., New York, 1987.

1051. World Health Organization, *Selenium,* World Health Organization, Geneva, 1987.

1052. Wendel, A., Ed., *Selenium in Biology and Medicine,* Springer-Verlag, Berlin, 1988.

1053. Neve, J. and Favier, A., Eds., *Selenium in Medicine and Biology*, Walter de Gruyter, Berlin, 1988.

1054. Levander, O.A. and Burk, R.F., Selenium, in *Present Knowledge in Nutrition*, Brown, M.L., Ed., Nutrition Foundation, Washington, D.C., 1990, 268.

1055. Jiang, Y.F. and Xu, G.L., The relativity between some epidemiological characteristics of Kaschin-Beck Disease and selenium deficiency, in *Selenium in Biology and Medicine*, Wendel. A., Ed., Springer-Verlag, Berlin, 1988, 263.

1056. Li, F.S., Guan, J.Y., Duan, Y.J., Zou, L.M., Yan, X.J., Ma, P., Su, Q., Li, L., and Li, S.Y., The selenium and phospholipid (phosphatidylcholine) deficiency and low temperature of environment may be the pathogenetic basis of Kachin-Beck Disease, in *Selenium in Biology and Medicine*, Wendel, A., Ed., Springer-Verlag, Berlin, 1988, 270.

1057. Burk, R.F., Clinical effects of selenium deficiency, in *Essential and Toxic Trace Elements in Human Health and Disease: An Update*, Prasad, A.S., Ed., Wiley-Liss, New York, 1993, 181.

1058. Ploetz, K. and Wallace, E., Effects of selenium deficiency on mouse articular cartilage, in *Selenium in Biology and Medicine*, Wendel, A., Ed., Springer-Verlag, Berlin, 1988, 137.

1059. Peretz, A., Selenium in inflammation and immunity, *Selenium in Medicine and Biology*, Neve, J. and Favier, A., Eds., Walter de Gruyter, Berlin, 1988, 235.

1060. Aaseth, J., Munthe, E.T., Forre, O., and Steinnes, E., Trace elements in serum and urine of patients with rheumatoid arthritis, *Scand. J. Rheumatol.*, 7, 237, 1978.

1061. Möttönen, T., Hannonen, P., Seppällä, O., Alfthan, G., and Oka, M., *Clin. Rheumatol.*, 3, 195, 1984.

1062. Tarp, U., Overvad, K., Hansen, J.C., and Thorling, E.B., Low selenium level in severe rheumatoid arthritis, *Scand. J. Rheumatol.*, 14, 97, 1985.

1063. Sonne, M. and Jenson, P.T., Selenium status in patients with rheumatoid arthritis, *Scand. J. Rheumatol.*, 14, 318, 1985.

1064. Thorling, E.B., Overvad, K., Heerfordt, A., and Foldspang, A., *Biol. Trace Elem. Res.*, 8, 65, 1985.

1065. Borglund, M., Åkesson, A., and Åkeson, B., *Scand. J. Clin. Lab. Invest.*, 48, 27, 1988.

1066. Peretz, A., Neve, J., Vertongen, F., Fanaey, J.P., and Molle, L., Selenium status in relation to clinical variables and corticosteroid treatment in rheumatoid arthritis, *J. Rheumatol.*, 14, 1104, 1987.

1067. Tarp, U., Hansen, J.C., Overvad, K., Thorling, E.B., Tarp, B.D., and Graudal, H., Glutathione peroxidase activity in patients with rheumatoid arthritis and in normal subjects: effects of long-term selenium supplementation, *Arthritis Rheum.*, 30, 1162, 1987.

1068. Aaseth, J., Alexander, J., and Thomassen, Y., Selenium in rheumatoid arthritis and in liver cirrhosis, in *Inflammatory Diseases and Copper*, Sorenson, J.R.J., Ed., Humana Press, Clifton, NJ, 1982, 600.

1069. Arnaud, J., Imbault-Huart, V., Favier, A., Zagala, A., and Phelip, X., Selenium and other trace elements in patients with rheumatoid arthritis, in *Selenium in Medicine and Biology*, Neve, J. and Favier, A., Eds., Walter de Gruyter, Berlin, 1988.

1070. Anonymous, Rheumatoid arthritis and selenium, *Nutr. Rev.*, 46, 284, 1988.

1071. O'Dell, J.R., Lemley-Gillespie, S., Palmer, W.R., Weaver, A.L., Moore, G.F., and Klassen, L.W., Serum selenium concentrations in rheumatoid arthritis, *Ann. Rheum. Dis.*, 50, 376, 1991.

1072. Munthe, E., Aaseth, J., and Jellum, E., *Acta Pharmacol. Toxicol.*, 59 (Suppl. 2), 365, 1986.

1073. Kondo, M., *Biol. Trace Elem. Res.*, 7, 195, 1985.

1074. Jameson, S., Pain relief and selenium balance in patients with connective tissue disease and osteoarthrosis: a double-blind selenium tocopherol supplementation study, *Nutr. Res., Suppl.*, 1, 391, 1985.

1075. Hill, J. and Bird, H.A., Failure of selenium-ACE to improve osteoarthritis, *Br. J. Rheumatol.*, 29, 211, 1990.

1076. Nielsen, F.H., Other trace elements, 4, in *Present Knowledge in Nutrition*, Brown, M.L., Ed., Nutrition Foundation, Washington, D.C., 1990, 294.

1077. Carlisle, E.M., Silicon as an essential nutrient, *Fed. Proc.*, 33(8), 1758, 1974.

1078. Carlisle, E.M., Silicon as an essential trace element in animal nutrition, *CIBA Found. Symp.*, 121, 123, 1986.

1079. Carlisle, E.M., Silicon as a trace nutrient, *Sci. Total Environ.*, 73(1–2), 95, 1988.

1080. Schwarz, K., A bound form of silicon in glycosaminoglycans and polyuronides, *Proc. Natl. Acad. Sci. U.S.A.*, 70(5), 1608, 1973.

1081. Carlisle, E.M., Everly, J.A., and Amponsah, D., Silicon enhances DNA synthesis in the osteoblast, *FASEB J.*, 6(4), A1947, 1992.

1082. Seaborn, C.D. and Nielsen, F.H., Effect of dietary silicon upon acid and alkaline phosphatase and ^{45}Calcium uptake in bone of rats, *FASEB J.*, 6(4), A1951, 1992.

1083. Mansurova, L.A., Voronkov, M.G., Slutskii, L.I., Dombrovska, L.E., and Bumagina, T.P., Silatranes as stimulators of the development of granulation tissue, *Biull. Eksp. Biol. Med.*, 96(9), 97, 1983.

1084. Mansurova, L.A., Voronkov, M.G., Slutskii, L.I., Dombrovska, L.E., and Bumagina, T.P., Use of silatranes in combination with Vishnevskii'n ointment in wound treatment, *Biull. Eksp. Biol. Med.*, 95(3), 100, 1983.

1085. Taylor, D.E., Cooper, G.J., Evans, V.A., Kenward, C.E., Lawston, I.W., Penhallow, J.E., and Whamond, J.S., Effect of haemorrhage on wound healing and its possible modification by 1-ethoxysilatrane, *J. R. Coll. Surg. Edinburgh*, 31(1), 13, 1986.

1086. Wolf, M. and Ransberger, K., *Enzyme Therapy*, Vantage Press, New York, 1972.

1087. Christie, R.B., The medical uses of proteolytic enzymes, in *Topics in Enzyme and Fermentation Biotechnology*, Vol. 4, Wiseman, A., Ed., Ellis Horwood Ltd., Chichester, 1980, 25.

1088. Felton, G.E., Does kinin released by pineapple stem bromelain stimulate production of prostaglandin E_1-like compounds?, *Hawaii Med. J.*, 36, 39, 1977.

1089. Felton, G.E., Fibrinolytic and antithrombotic action of bromelain may eliminate thrombosis in heart patients, *Med. Hypoth.*, 6, 1123, 1980.

1090. Ito, C., Antiinflammatory actions of proteases, bromelain, trypsin and their mixed preparations, *Folia Pharmacol. Jpn.,* 75, 227, 1979.

1091. Taussig, S.J., The mechanism of the physiological action of bromelain, *Med. Hypoth.,* 6, 99, 1980.

1092. Taussig, S.J. and Batkin, S., Bromelain, the enzyme complex of pineapple (Ananas comosus) and its clinical application. An update, *J. Ethnopharm.,* 22, 191, 1988.

1093. Taussig, S. and Nieper, H., Bromelain: its use in prevention and treatment of cardiovascular disease. Present status, *J. Int. Assoc. Prev. Med.,* 6, 139, 1979.

1094. Ambrus, J.L., Lassman, B.A., and DeMarchi, J.J., Absorption of exogenous and endogenous proteolytic enzymes, *Clin. Pharmacol. Ther.,* 8, 362, 1967.

1095. Avakian, S., Further studies on the absorption of chymotrypsin, *Clin. Pharmacol. Ther.,* 5, 712, 1964.

1096. Izaka, K., Yamada, M., Lawano, T., and Suyama, T., Gastrointestinal absorption and antiinflammatory effect of bromelain, *Jpn. J. Pharmacol.,* 22, 519, 1972.

1097. Kabacoff, B.L., Wohlman, A., Umhey, M., and Avakian, S., Absorption of chymotrypsin from the intestinal tract, *Nature,* 199, 815, 1963.

1098. Miller, J.M. and Opher, A.W., The increased proteolytic activity of human blood serum after the oral administration of bromelain, *Exp. Med. Surg.,* 22, 277, 1964.

1099. Miller, J.M., The absorption of proteolytic enzymes from the gastrointestinal tract, *Clin. Med.,* 75, 35, 1968.

1100. Seifert, J., Ganser, R., and Brendel, W., Die Resorption eines proteolytischen Enzyms pflanzlichen Ursprunges aus dem Magen-Darmtrakt in das Blut und in die Lymphe von erwachsenen Ratten, *Z. Gastroenterol.,* 17, 1, 1979.

1101. Smyth, R.D., Brennan, R., and Martin, G.J., Studies establishing the absorption of the bromelains (proteolytic enzymes) from the gastrointestinal tract, *Exp. Med. Surg.,* 22, 46, 1964.

1102. Pirotta, F. and DeGuili-Morghen, G., Bromelain — a deeper pharmacological study. I. Antiinflammatory and serum fibrinolytic activity after oral administration of bromelain in the rat, *Drugs Exptl. Clin. Res.,* 4, 1, 1978.

1103. Moriya, H., Maniwaki, C., Akimoto, S., Yamaguchi, K., and Iwadare, M., *Chem. Pharm. Bull.,* 15, 1662, 1967.

1104. Blonstein, J.L., The use of 'buccal Varidase' in boxing injuries, *Practitioner,* 185, 78, 1960.

1105. Blonstein, J.L., Oral enzyme tablets in the treatment of boxing injuries, *Practitioner,* 198, 547, 1967.

1106. Blonstein, J.L., Control of swelling in boxing injuries, *Practitioner,* 203, 206, 1969.

1107. Boyne, P.S. and Medhurst, H., Oral antiinflammatory enzyme therapy in injuries in professional footballers, *Practitioner,* 198, 543, 1967.

1108. Bucci, L.R. and Stiles, J.C., Sport injuries and proteolytic enzymes, *Today's Chirop.,* 16(1), 31, 1987.

1109. Buck, J.E. and Phillips, N., Trial of Chymoral on professional footballers, *Br. J. Clin. Prac.,* 24(9), 375, 1970.

1110. Cichoke, A.J. and Marty, L., The use of proteolytic enzymes with soft tissue athletic injuries, *Am. Chirop.,* Sep/Oct, 32, 1981.

1111. Craig, R.P., The quantitative evaluation of the use of oral proteolytic enzymes in the treatment of sprained ankles, *Injury,* 6(4), 313, 1975.

1112. Davidson, E., Prigot, A., and Maynard, A.L., Buccal varidase. An adjunct in the therapy of inflammatory lesions, hematoma and traumatic edema: a preliminary report, *Harlem Hosp. Bull.,* 11, 5, 1958.

1113. Dietrich, R.E., Oral proteolytic enzymes in the treatment of athletic injuries: a double-blind study, *Penn. Med. J.,* 68, 35, 1965.

1114. Donaho, C.R. and Rylander, C.R., Proteolytic enzymes in athletic injuries. A double-blind study of a new anti-inflammatory agent, *Del. Med. J.,* 34(6), 168, 1962.

1115. France, L.H., Treatment of injuries with orally administered Varidase as compared to Chymoral and Tanderil, *Praxis,* 57(19), 683, 1968.

1116. Gordon, K., Sports injuries in the 1970 all blacks team. A special approach to their treatment, *Med. Proc. Med. Bydraes,* June, 193, 1971.

1117. Grillasca, G., Réduction du temps d'indisponiblité au cours de l'entraînement sportif, sous l'action d'un anti-inflammatoire oral, *Rev. Corps Santé.,* 6(3), 395, 1965.

1118. Holt, H.T., Carica papaya as ancillary therapy for athletic injuries, *Curr. Ther. Res.,* 11(10), 621, 1969.

1119. Matta, M. and Mouzas, G.L., Streptokinase-streptodornase in the treatment of minor injuries, *Practitioner,* 209, 343, 1972.

1120. Rathberger, W.F., The use of proteolytic enzymes (Chymoral) in sporting injuries, *S. Afr. Med. J.,* Feb.13, 181, 1971.

1121. Schwinger, O., Ergebnisse der oralen Fermenttherapie bei Verletzungen der Muskeln, Sehnen und Knochen nach Unfällen, *Weiner Med. Wchschr.,* 36(1), 603, 1970.

1122. Stevens, M.A., McCown, I.A., and Campbell, E.A., Control of swelling in sports injuries. A key to prompt recovery, *N.Y. State J. Med.,* June, 1817, 1962.

1123. Trickett, P., Proteolytic enzymes in treatment of athletic injuries, *Appl. Ther.,* 6, 647, 1964.

1124. Weisskirchen, H. and El-Salamouny, A.R., Zur Behandlung posttraumatischer, sowie postoperativ auftrender Schwellungen mit proteolytischen Enzymen, *Med. Welt,* 52, 3211, 1967.

1125. Tsomides, J. and Goldberg, R.I., Controlled evaluation of oral chymotrypsin-trypsin treatment of injuries to the head and face, *Clin. Med.,* 76, 40, 1969.

1126. Kleine, M.W., Introduction to systemic enzyme therapy and results of experimental trials, in *Sports, Medicine and Health,* Hermans, G.P.H. and Mosterd, W.L., Eds., Excerpta Medica, Amsterdam, 1990, 1131.

1127. Rahn, H.D., Efficacy of hydrolytic enzymes in surgery, in *Sports, Medicine and Health,* Hermans, G.P.H. and Mosterd, W.L., Eds., Excerpta Medica, Amsterdam, 1990, 1135.

1128. Baumüller, M., Therapy of ankle joint distortions with hydrolytic enzymes — results from a double blind clinical trial, in *Sports, Medicine and Health,* Hermans, G.P.H. and Mosterd, W.L., Eds., Excerpta Medica, Amsterdam, 1990, 1137.

1129. Pollack, P.J., Oral administration of enzymes from *Carica papaya*: report of a double-blind clinical study, *Curr. Ther. Res.*, 4, 229, 1962.

1130. Schmitz, H.E. and Pavlic, R.S., Control of edema and pain in episiotomy. Use of oral proteolytic enzymes, *Obstet. Gynecol.*, 17, 260, 1961.

1131. Bumgardner, H.D. and Zatuchni, G.I., Prevention of episiotomy pain with oral chymotrypsin, *Am. J. Obst. Gynecol.*, 92, 514, 1965.

1132. Soule, S.D., Wasserman, H.C., and Burstein, R., Oral proteolytic enzyme therapy (Chymoral) in episiotomy patients, *Am. J. Obst. Gynecol.*, 95, 820, 1966.

1133. Zatuchni, G.I. and Colombi, D.J., Bromelains therapy for the prevention of episiotomy pain, *Obstet. Gynecol.*, 29, 275, 1967.

1134. Howat, R.C.L. and Lewis, G.D., The effect of bromelain therapy on episiotomy wounds — a double blind controlled clinical trial, *J. Obstet. Gynaecol. Br. Commonw.*, 79, 951, 1972.

1135. Albright, B.E., Use of antiinflammatory enzymes in 889 episiotomy patients, *Clin. Med.*, 70, 1299, 1963.

1136. De N'Yeurt, A., The use of Chymoral in vasectomy, *J. R. Coll. Gen. Pract.*, 22, 633, 1972.

1137. Shaw, P.C., The use of trypsin-chymotrypsin formulation in fractures of the hand, *Br. J. Clin. Pract.*, 23, 25, 1969.

1138. Sillar, R.W. and Mouzas, G.L., Proteolytic enzymes for minimizing deformities associated with Colles' fracture, *Int. Surg.*, 58, 31, 1973.

1139. Cirelli, M.G., Five years of clinical experience with bromelains in therapy of edema and inflammation in postoperative tissue reaction, skin infections and trauma, *Clin. Med.*, 74, 55, 1967.

1140. Morrison, A.W. and Morrison, M.C.T., Bromelain — a clinical assessment in the post-operative treatment of arthrotomies of the knee and facial injuries, *Br. J. Clin. Pract.*, 19, 207, 1965.

1141. Kapur, B.M.L., Talwar, J.R., and Gulati, S.M., Use of Papase in prevention of experimental peritoneal adhesions, *Surgery*, 65, 629, 1969.

1142. Cohen, A. and Goldman, J., Bromelains therapy in rheumatoid arthritis, *Penn. Med. J.*, 67, 27, 1964.

1143. Hingorani, K., Oral enzyme therapy in severe back pain, *Br. J. Clin. Prac.*, 22(5), 209, 1968.

1144. Gaspardy, G., Balint, G., Mitusova, M., and Lorincz, G., Treatment of sciatica due to invertebral disc herniation with Chymoral tablets, *Rheum. Phys. Med.*, 11, 14, 1971.

1145. Gibson, T., Dilke, T.F.W., and Grahame, R., Chymoral in the treatment of lumbar disc prolapse, *Rheum. Rehabil.*, 14, 186, 1975.

1146. Rathbone, M.P., Christjanson, L., Deforge, S., Deluca, B., Gysbers, J.W., Hindley, S., Jovetich, M., Middlemiss, P., and Takhal, S., Extracellular purine nucleotides stimulate cell division and morphogenesis: pathological and physiological implications, *Med. Hypoth.*, 37, 232, 1992.

1147. Daly, J., Lieberman, M., and Goldfine, J., Enteral nutrition with supplemental arginine, RNA and ω-3 fatty acids — a prospective clinical trial, *JPEN*, 15 (Suppl. 1), 19S, 1991.

1148. Zidenburg-Cherr, S., Keen., C.L., Lonnerdal, B., and Hurley, L.S., Dietary superoxide dismutase does not affect tissue levels, *Am. J. Clin. Nutr.*, 37, 5, 1983.

1149. Giri, S.N. and Misra, H.P., Fate of superoxide dismutase in mice following oral route of administration, *Med. Biol.*, 62, 285, 1984.

1150. Lund-Olesen, K. and Menander, K.B., Orgotein: a new antiinflammatory metalloprotein drug: preliminary evaluation of clinical efficacy and safety in degenerative joint disease, *Curr. Ther. Res.*, 16(7), 706, 1974.

1151. Marklund, S.L., Clinical aspects of superoxide dismutase, *Med. Biol.*, 62, 130, 1984.

1152. Menander-Huber, K.B., Double-blind controlled clinical trials in man with bovine copper-zinc superoxide dismutase, in *Biological and Clinical Aspects of Superoxide Dismutase,* Bannister, W.H. and Bannister, J.V., Eds., Elsevier, New York, 1980, 408.

1153. Menander-Huber, K.B. and Huber, W., Orgotein, the drug version of bovine Cu-Zn superoxide dismutase. II. A summary account of clinical trials in man and animals, in *Superoxide and Superoxide Dismutases,* Michelson, A.M., McCord, J.M., and Fridovich, I., Eds., Academic Press, London, 1977, 537.

1154. Dufourmentel, C., Pailheret, J.P., and Raulo, Y., The double blind clinical trial of a new drug with healing properties, *Ann. Chirop. Plast.*, 19(2), 139, 1974.

1155. Huriez, P. and Leclaire, M., Un nouvea cicatrisant en dermatologie, *Lille Med.*, 17(Suppl. 2), 173, 1972.

1156. Kamaev, M.F., Treatment of wounds with antioxidants, *Khirurgiia*, (4), 52, 1975.

1157. Monteil, R. and Biron, G., Expérimentation d'un cicatrisant nouveau associant une catalase et un antiseptique dans le traitment local des brûlures, *Thérapie*, 26, 535, 1971.

1158. Bucci, L.R., Klenda, B.A., Stiles, J.C., and Sparks, W.S., Truth in labeling for antioxidant enzyme products. Survey of label claims and product potencies, in *Proceedings, Second Symposium on Nutrition and Chiropractic,* Faruqui, S.R. and Ansari, M.S., Eds., Palmer College of Chiropractic, Davenport, IA, 1989, 56.

1159. Morrison, L.M. and Schjeide, O.A., *Coronary Heart Disease and the Mucopolysaccharides (Glycosaminoglycans)*, Charles C. Thomas, Springfield, IL, 1974.

1160. Cullen, J.C., Flint, M.H., and Leider, J., The effect of dried mussel extract on an induced polyarthritis in rats, *N.Z. Med. J.*, 81, 260, 1975.

1161. Rainsford, K.D. and Whitehouse, M.W., Gastroprotective and antiinflammatory properties of green lipped mussel (Perna canaliculus) preparation, *Arzneim. Forsch.*, 30, 2128, 1980.

1162. Highton, T.C. and McArthur, A.W., Pilot study on the effect of New Zealand green mussel on rheumatoid arthritis, *N.Z. Med. J.*, 81, 261, 1975.

1163. Gibson, R.G., Gibson, S.L.M., Conway, V., and Chappell, D., Perna canaliculus in the treatment of arthritis, *Practitioner*, 224, 955, 1980.

1164. Anonymous, Green-lipped mussel extract in arthritis, *Lancet*, 1, 85, 1981.

1165. Gibson, R.G. and Gibson, S.L.M., Green-lipped mussel extract in arthritis, *Lancet*, 1, 439, 1981.

1166. Huskisson, E.C., Scott, J., and Bryans, R., Seatone is ineffective in rheumatoid arthritis, *Br. Med. J.,* 282, 1358, 1981.

1167. Grigor, R.R., Gow, P.J., and Caughey, D.E., Perna-canaliculus New-Zealand green-lipped mussel in the treatment of rheumatic diseases, *Aust. N.Z. J. Med.,* 11(3), 330, 1981.

1168. Gibson, R.G. and Gibson, S.L.M., Seatone in arthritis, *Br. Med. J.,* 282, 1795, 1981.

1169. Gibson, R.G. and Gibson, S.L.M., New Zealand green-lipped mussel extract (Seatone) in rheumatoid arthritis, *N.Z. Med. J.,* 94, 67, 1981.

1170. Caughey, D.E., Grigor, R.R., Caughey, E.B., Young, P., Gow, P.J., and Stewart, A.W., Perna canaliculus in the treatment of rheumatoid arthritis, *Eur. J. Rheumatol. Inflam.,* 6(2), 197, 1983.

1171. Larkin, J.G., Capell, H.A., and Sturrock, R.D., Seatone in rheumatoid arthritis: a six-month placebo-controlled study, *Ann. Rheum. Dis.,* 44(3), 199, 1985.

1172. Morrison, L.M., Treatment of experimental peptic ulcer with a hog stomach extract, *Am. J. Dig. Dis.,* 12, 328, 1945.

1173. Allen, J. and Prudden, J.F., Histologic response to a cartilage powder preparation in a controlled human study, *Am. J. Surg.,* 112, 888, 1966.

1174. Golding, M.R., Oberlander, L.K., and Enquist, I.F., Cartilage speeds healing in diabetic wounds, *Arch. Surg.,* 87, 647, 1963.

1175. Houck, J.C., Jacob, R.A., DeAngelo, L., and Vickers, K., The inhibition of inflammation and the acceleration of tissue repair by cartilage powder, *Surgery,* 51, 632, 1962.

1176. Inoue, T., The "cartilage effect" on healing wounds: a study of the specificity of the phenomenon, *Arch. Surg.,* 82, 432, 1961.

1177. Lattes, R., Martin, J.R., Meyer, K., and Ragan, C., Effect of cartilage and other tissue suspensions on reparative processes of cortisone-treated animals, *Am. J. Pathol.,* 32, 979, 1956.

1178. Moskalewski, S., Increase of rate of wound and ulcer healing under the effect of powdered animal cartilage, *Przegl. Dermatol.,* 55(2), 201, 1968.

1179. Paulette, R.E. and Prudden, J.F., Studies on the acceleration of wound healing with cartilage. II. Histologic observations, *Surg. Gynecol. Obstet.,* 108, 406, 1959.

1180. Prudden, J.F., Nishihara, G., and Baker, L., The acceleration of wound healing with cartilage. I, *Surg. Gynecol. Obstet.,* 105, 283, 1957.

1181. Prudden, J.F., Stimulation of wound healing with heterologous cartilage, *Transplant. Bull.,* 5, 14, 1958.

1182. Prudden, J.F., Inoue, T., and Ocampo, L., Effect of subcutaneous cartilage pellets on wound tensile strength, *Arch. Surg.,* 85, 245, 1962.

1183. Prudden, J.F., Gabriel, O., and Allen, B., Acceleration of wound healing: use of parenteral injections of saline cartilage extract, with a note on the evaluation of electrophoretically separated fractions of the extract by tissue culture, *Arch. Surg.,* 86, 157, 1963.

1184. Prudden, J.F., Teneick, M.L., Svahn, D., and Frueh, B., Acceleration of wound healing in various species by parenteral injection of a saline extract of cartilage, *J. Surg. Res.,* 4, 143, 1964.

1185. Prudden, J.F., Wound healing produced by cartilage preparations; enhancement of acceleration, with a report on the use of a cartilage preparation in clinically chronic ulcers and in primarily closed human surgical incisions, *Arch. Surg.,* 89, 1046, 1964.

1186. Prudden, J.F. and Allen, J., The clinical acceleration of healing with a cartilage preparation, a controlled study, *JAMA,* 192(5), 352, 1965.

1187. Prudden, J.F. and Wolarsky, E., The reversal by cartilage of the steroid-induced inhibition of wound healing, *Surg. Gynecol. Obstet.,* 125, 109, 1967.

1188. Prudden, J.F., Wolarsky, E.R., and Balassa, L., The acceleration of healing, *Surg. Gynecol. Obstet.,* 128, 1321, 1969.

1189. Sabo, J.C., Oberlander, L., and Enquist, I.F., Acceleration of open wound healing by cartilage, *Arch. Surg.,* 90, 414, 1965.

1190. Sabo, J.C. and Enquist, I.F., Wound-stimulating effect of homologous and heterologous cartilage, *Arch. Surg.,* 91, 523, 1965.

1191. Schwartz, M.S., Gump, F., and Prudden, J.F., The influence of cartilage on the time course of wound healing, *Surg. Forum,* 10, 308, 1960.

1192. Wolarsky, E., Ocampo, L., and Ten Eick, M.L., Effect of chondroitin sulfate on tensile strength of healing wounds, *Arch. Surg.,* 91, 521, 1965.

1193. Wolarsky, E., Finke, S.R., and Prudden, J.F., Acceleration of wound healing with cartilage; immunological considerations, *Proc. Soc. Exp. Biol. Med.,* 123, 536, 1966.

1194. Bollet, A.J., Stimulation of protein-chondroitin sulfate synthesis by normal and osteoarthritic articular cartilage, *Arthritis Rheum.,* 11, 663, 1968.

1195. Nevo, Z. and Dorfman, A., Stimulation of chondromucoprotein synthesis in chondrocytes by extracellular chondromucoprotein, *Proc. Natl. Acad. Sci. U.S.A.,* 69(8), 2069, 1972.

1196. Kosher, R.A., Lash, J.W., and Minor, R.R., Environmental enhancement of *in vitro* chondrogenesis. IV. Stimulation of somite chondrogenesis by exogenous chondromucoprotein, *Dev. Biol.,* 35, 210, 1973.

1197. Schwartz, N.B. and Dorfman, A., Stimulation of chondroitin sulfate proteoglycan production by chondrocytes in monolayer, *Connect. Tissue Res.,* 3, 115, 1975.

1198. Prudden, J.F. and Balassa, L.L., The biological activity of bovine cartilage preparations, *Sem. Arthritis Rheum.,* 3(4), 287, 1974.

1199. Andermann, G. and Dietz, M., The influence of the route of administration on the bioavailability of an endogenous macromolecule: chondroitin sulfate (CSA), *Eur. J. Drug Metabol. Pharmacol.,* 7(1), 11, 1982.

1200. Zannotti, A., Bufalino, L., Landi, A., Mantovani, V., and Bianchini, P., Studi sulla stabilita e biodisponibilita di un solfomucopolisaccaride somministrato per via orale, *Farmaco Ed. Prat.,* 29, 264, 1974.

1201. Engel, R.H. and Riggi, S.J., Intestinal absorption of heparin: a study of the interactions of components of oil-in-water emulsion, *J. Pharm. Sci.*, 58, 1372, 1969.

1202. Morrison, L.M. and Schjeide, O.A., Absorption, distribution, metabolism and excretion of acid mucopolysaccharides administered to animals and humans, in *Coronary Heart Disease and the Mucopolysaccharides (Glycosaminoglycans)*, Charles C. Thomas, Springfield, IL 1974, 109.

1203. Morrison, L.M. and Enrick, N.L., Coronary heart disease: reduction of death rate by chondroitin sulfate A, *Angiology*, 24, 269, 1973.

1204. Morrison, L.M. and Schjeide, O.A., Prevention and treatment of ischemic heart disease in human patients, in *Coronary Heart Disease and the Mucopolysaccharides (Glycosaminoglycans)*, Charles C. Thomas, Springfield, IL 1974, 185.

1205. Morrison, L.M., Therapeutic applications of chondroitin-4-sulfate. Appraisal of biological properties, *Folia Angiol.*, 25, 225, 1977.

1206. Morrison, L.M. and Schjeide, O.A., Dietary control of arteriosclerosis, in *Arteriosclerosis. Prevention, Treatment and Regression*, Charles C. Thomas, Springfield, IL, 1984, 159.

1207. Prino, G., Pharmacological profile of Ateroid, *Mod. Probl. Pharmacopsychiatry*, 23, 68, 1989.

1208. Clevidence, B.A., Failla, M.L., Vercellotti, J.R., and Pescador, R., Pharmacokinetics of catalytically tritiated glycosaminoglycans in the rat, *Arzneim. Forsch.*, 33, 228, 1983.

1209. Pescador, R., Diamantini, G., Mantovani, M., Malandrino, S., Riva, A., Casu, B., and Oreste, P., Absorption by the rat intestinal tract of fluorescein-labelled pig duodenal glycosaminoglycans, *Arzneim. Forsch.*, 30, 1893, 1980.

1210. Niada, R., Mantovani, M., and Pescador, R., Antithrombotic activity of glycosaminoglycans of mammalian origin. *In vivo* experiments in the rabbit, *Pharmacol. Res. Commun.*, 11, 349, 1979.

1211. Santini, V., A general practice trial of Ateroid 200 in 8,776 patients with chronic senile cerebral insufficiency, *Mod. Probl. Pharmacopsychiatry*, 23, 95, 1989.

1212. Burger, M., Sherman, B.S., and Sobel, A.E., Observations of the influence of chondroitin sulfate on the rate of bone repair, *J. Bone Jt. Surg.*, 44B, 675, 1962.

1213. Moss, M., Kruger, G.O., and Reynolds, D.C., The effect of chondroitin sulfate on bone healing, *Oral Surg.*, 20(6), 795, 1965.

1214. Herold, H.Z. and Tadmor, A., Chondroitin sulfate in treatment of experimental bone defects, *Isr. J. Med. Sci.*, 5, 425, 1969.

1215. Skinner, R.A., Toto, P.D., and Gargiulo, A.W., Xenogeneic implants in primates. Collagen and chondroitin sulfate, *J. Periodontol.*, 47(4), 196, 1976.

1216. Bouget, P. and Guenaud, D., Packing of a preformed bone cavity with biodegradable material: value of chondroitin sulfuric acid in the osteogenic process, *Inf. Dent.*, 63, 19, 1981.

1217. Hansbrough, J.F., Boyce, S.T., Cooper, M.L., and Foreman, T.J., Burn wound closure with cultured autologous keratinocytes and fibroblasts attached to a collagen-glycosaminoglycan substrate, *JAMA*, 262(15), 2125, 1989.

1218. Frolova, O.A. and Isakova, V.I., The therapeutic effect of a biogenic paste in experimental chronic periodontitis, *Stomatologiya (Moscow)*, 69(1), 20, 1990.

1219. Limberg, M.B., McCaa, C., Kissling, G.E., and Kaufman, H.E., Topical application of hyaluronic acid and chondroitin sulfate in the treatment of dry eyes, *Am. J. Ophthalmol.*, 103(2), 194, 1987.

1220. Alpar, J.J., Alpar, A.J., Baca, J., and Chapman, D., Comparison of Healon and Viscoat in cataract extraction and intraocular lens implantation, *Ophthalmic Surg.*, 19(9), 636, 1988.

1221. Burke, S., Sugar, J., and Farber, M.D., Comparison of the effects of two viscoelastic agents, Healon and Viscoat, on postoperative intraocular pressure after penetrating keratoplasty, *Ophthalmic Surg.*, 21(12), 821, 1990.

1222. Lane, S.S., Naylor, D.W., Kullerstrand, L.J., Knauth, K., and Lindstrom, R.L., Prospective comparison of the effects of Occucoat, Viscoat, and Healon on intraocular pressure and endothelial cell loss, *J. Cataract Refract. Surg.*, 17(1), 21, 1991.

1223. Suyama, T., Iga, Y., and Shirakawa, H., The acceleration of wound healing with chondroitin sulfate A and its acidic hydrolysates, *Jpn. J. Exp. Med.*, 36(4), 449, 1966.

1224. Ashby, M.W. and Nose, Y., Successful use of chondroitin-4-sulfate in prolonging survival of skin allografts of adult mice, *Transplantation*, 11(1), 107, 1971.

1225. Fialkova, M.A., Smirnova, T.I., Ivanova, G.I., Aboiants, R.K., and Golubeva, V.F., The effect of chondroitin sulfate preparations on wound healing and the strength of the surgical scar, *Biull. Eksp. Biol. Med.*, 108(9), 350, 1989.

1226. Oelsner, G., Graebe, R.A., Pan, S.B., Haseltine, F.P., Barnea, E.R., Fakih, H., and DeCherney, A.H., Chondroitin sulfate. A new intraperitoneal treatment for postoperative adhesion prevention in the rabbit, *J. Reprod. Med.*, 32, 812, 1987.

1227. Kajihara, Y., The use of chondroitin sulfuric acid for the prevention of peritoneal adhesions, *J. Kurume Med. Assoc.*, 23, 4641, 1960.

1228. Baggi, G., Massa, G., Laguzzi, B., and Ballario, F., The influence of chondroitin sulphuric acid on the scar formation process in experimentally produced skin wounds, *Min. Chirop.*, 25, 181, 1970.

1229. Graebe, R.A., Oelsner, G., Cornelison, T.L., Pan, S.B., Haseltine, F.P., and DeCherney, A.H., An animal study of different treatments to prevent postoperative pelvic adhesions, *Microsurgery*, 10(1), 53, 1989.

1230. Meyers, S.A., Seaber, A.V., Glisson, R.R., and Nunley, J.A., Effect of hyaluronic acid/chondroitin sulfate on healing of full-thickness tendon lacerations in rabbits, *J. Orthop. Res.*, 7(5), 683, 1989.

1231. Maier, R. and Wilhelmi, G., Influence of antiinflammatory drugs on spontaneous osteoarthrosis in mice, in *A New Antirheumatic-analgesic Agent: Pirprofen (Rengasil®)*, van der Korst, J.K., Ed., Hans Huber Publishers, Bern, 1979, 87.

1232. Viernstein, K., Über die Wirkung von Eleparon bei intraartikulärer Anwendung, *Med. Klin.,* 59, 305, 1964.

1233. Greiling, H. and Stuhlsatz, H.W., Biochemical studies on the mode of action of a polysaccharide sulfate on degenerative articular disease, *Z. Rheumaforsch.,* 25(3/4), 3, 1966.

1234. Kerzberg, E.M., Roldan, E.J.A., Castelli, G., and Huberman, E.D., Combination of glycosaminoglycans and acetylsalicylic acid in knee osteoarthritis, *Scand. J. Rheum.,* 16, 377, 1987.

1235. Thilo, G., Untersuchung von 35 Arthrosefallen, behandelt mit Chondroitinschwefelsaure, *Schweiz. Rundschau Med. (Praxis),* 66, 1896, 1977.

1236. Pipitone, V.R., Chondroprotection with chondroitin sulfate, *Drugs Exp. Clin. Res.,* 17(1), 3, 1991.

1237. Oliviero, U., Sorrentino, G.P., DePaola, P., Tranfaglia, E., D'Alessandro, A., Carifi, S., Porfido, F.A., Cerio, R., Grasso, A.M., and Policicchio, D., Effects of the treatment with Matrix on elderly people with chronic articular degeneration, *Drugs Exp. Clin. Res.,* 17(1), 45, 1991.

1238. Rovetta, G., Galactosaminoglycuronoglycan sulfate (Matrix) in therapy of tibiofibular osteoarthritis of the knee, *Drugs Exp. Clin. Res.,* 17(1), 53, 1991.

1239. Morrison, L.M. and Schjeide, O.A., Toxicity studies on acid mucopolysaccharides, in *Coronary Heart Disease and the Mucopolysaccharides (Glycosaminoglycans)*, Charles C. Thomas, Springfield, IL 1974, 159.

1240. Balazs, E.A., Laurent, T.C., and Jeanloz, R.W., Nomenclature of hyaluronic acid, *Biochem. J.,* 235, 903, 1986.

1241. Morrison, L.M. and Schjeide, O.A., General biological roles of chondromucoproteins and acid mucopolysaccharides, in *Coronary Heart Disease and the Mucopolysaccharides (Glycosaminoglycans)*, Charles C. Thomas, Springfield, IL, 1974, 58.

1242. Berenson, G.S. and Dalferes, E.R., Identification of acid mucopolysaccharides from granulation tissue in rats, *Br. J. Exp. Pathol.,* 41, 422, 1960.

1243. Delaunay, A. and Bazin, S., Mucopolysaccharides, collagen and nonfibrillar proteins in inflammation, in *International Review of Connective Tissue Research*, Vol. 2, Hall, D.A., Ed., Academic Press, New York, 1964, 301.

1244. Smith M.M. and Ghosh, P., The synthesis of hyaluronic acid is influenced by the nature of hyaluronate in the extracellular environment, *Rheumatol. Int.,* 7, 113, 1987.

1245. Tobetto, K., Nakai, K., Akatsuka, M., Yasui, T., Ando, T., and Hirano, S., Inhibitory effects of hyaluronan on neutrophil-mediated cartilage degradation, *Connect. Tissue Res.,* 29, 181, 1993.

1246. Sato, H., Takahashi, T., Ide, H., Fukushima, T., Tabata, M., Sekine, F., Kobayashi, K., Negishi, M., and Niwa, Y., Antioxidant activity of synovial fluid, hyaluronic acid, and two subcomponents of hyaluronic acid, *Arthritis Rheum.,* 31(1), 63, 1988.

1247. Hutadilok, N., Ghosh, P., and Brooks, P.M., Binding of haptoglobin, inter-α-trypsin inhibitor, and α_1 proteinase inhibitor to synovial fluid hyaluronate and the influence of these proteins on its degradation by oxygen derived free radicals, *Ann. Rheum. Dis.,* 47, 377, 1988.

1248. Wiig, M., Amiel, D., and Kitabayashi, L., Potential use of hyaluronan in the healing of ACL, *Med. Sci. Sports Exer.,* 20(2)Suppl., S37, 1988.

1249. Abatangelo, G., Botti, P., Gei, G., Samson, J.C., Cortivo, R., De Galateo, A., and Martelli, M., Intraarticular sodium hyaluronate injections in the Pond-Nuki experimental model of osteoarthritis in dogs. I. Biochemical results, *Clin. Orthop.,* 241, 278, 1989.

1250. Schiavinato, A., Lini, E., Guidolin, D., Pezzoli, G., Botti, P., Martelli, M., Cortivo, R., De Galateo, A., and Abatangelo, G., Intraarticular sodium hyaluronate injections in the Pond-Nuki experimental model of osteoarthritis in dogs. II. Morphological findings, *Clin. Orthop.,* 241, 286, 1989.

1251. Amiel, D., Frey, C., Woo, S.L.Y., Harwood, F., and Akeson, W., Value of hyaluronic acid in the prevention of contracture formation, *Clin. Orthop.,* 196, 306, 1985.

1252. Thomas, S.C., Jones, L.C., and Hungerford, D.S., Hyaluronic acid and its effect on postoperative adhesions in the rabbit flexor tendon, *Clin. Orthop.,* 206, 281, 1986.

1253. Namiki, O., Toyoshima, H., and Morisaki, N., Therapeutic effect of intra-articular injection of high molecular weight hyaluronic acid on osteoarthritis of the knee, *Int. J. Clin. Pharmacol. Ther. Toxicol.,* 20(11), 501, 1982.

1254. Punzi, L., Schiavon, F., Ramonda, R., Malatesta, V., Gambari, P., and Todesco, S., Intra-articular hyaluronic acid in the treatment of inflammatory and noninflammatory knee effusions, *Curr. Ther. Res.,* 43(4), 643, 1988.

1255. Dixon, A.S., Jacoby, R.K., Berry, H., and Hamilton, E.B.D., Clinical trial of intra-articular injection of sodium hyaluronate in patients with osteoarthritis of the knee, *Curr. Med. Res. Opin.,* 11, 205, 1988.

1256. Peyron, J.G. and Balazs, E.A., Preliminary clinical assessment of sodium hyaluronate injection into human arthritic joints, *Pathol. Biol.,* 22, 731, 1974.

1257. Oshima, Y., Azuma, H., Namiki, O., Aoki, T., Azuma, M., Irei, K., Iwata, H., Kegeyama, T., Kudo, H., Shichikawa, K., Sugawara, Y., Sugiura, S., Sugiyama, H., Suzuki, A., Susuki, T., Tsukamoto, I., Toyoshima, H., Shirano, A., Matsumoto, J., Mitani, S., Mitomo, N., Yamamoto, M., and Yoshizawa, H., Intra-articular injection therapy of high molecular weight sodium hyaluronate (SPH) on osteoarthritis of the knee joint. Phase II: clinical study, *Yakuri to Chiryo,* 11, 2253, 1983.

1258. Shichikawa, K., Igarashi, M., Sugawara, S., and Iwasaki, Y., Clinical evaluation of high molecular weight sodium hyaluronate (SPH) on osteoarthritis of the knee. Multicenter well controlled study, *Rinsho Yakuri,* 14, 545, 1983.

1259. Shichikawa, K., Maeda, A., and Ogawa, N., Evaluation of drug effectiveness of sodium hyaluronate (SPH) for osteoarthritis deformans of the knee, *Rheumatism,* 23, 280, 1983.

1260. Bragantini, A., Cassini, M., De Bastiani, G., and Perbellini, A., Controlled single-blind trial of intra-articularly injected hyaluronic acid (Hyalgan) in osteoarthritis of the knee, *Clin. Trials J.,* 24, 330, 1987.

1261. Grecomoro, G., Martorana, U., and Di Marco, C., Intra-articular treatment with sodium hyaluronate in gonarthrosis: a controlled clinical trial versus placebo, *Pharmatherapeutica,* 5, 137, 1987.

1262. Leardini, G., Franceschini, M., Mattara, L., Bruno, R., and Perbellini, A., Intra-articular sodium hyaluronate (Hyalgan) in gonarthritis. A controlled study comparing methylprednisolone acetate, *Clin. Trials J.,* 24, 341, 1987.

1263. Leardini, G., Perbellini, A., Franceschini, M., and Mattara, L., Intra-articular injections of hyaluronic acid in the treatment of painful shoulder, *Clin. Ther.,* 10(5), 521, 1988.

1264. Mazzocato, G., Melanotte, P.L., and Perbellini, A., Efficacia terapeutica dello ialuronato di sodio nell'artrosi di ginocchio. Risultati di uno studio in aperto, *Ortop. Traumatol. Oggi.,* 7, 333, 1987.

1265. Weiss, C., Balazs, E.A., St. Onge, R., and Denlinger, J.L., Clinical studies of the intra-articular injection of Healon (sodium hyaluronate) in the treatment of osteoarthritis of human knees, *Sem. Arthritis Rheum.,* 11, 143, 1981.

1266. Stenfors, L.E., Treatment of tympanic membrane perforations with hyaluronan in an open pilot study of unselected patients, *Acta Oto-Laryngol. (Stockholm),* 442 (Suppl.), 81, 1987.

1267. Stenfors, L.E., Repair of traumatically ruptured tympanic membrane using hyaluronan, *Acta Oto-Laryngol. (Stockholm),* 442 (Suppl.), 88, 1987.

1268. Kopp, S., Wenneberg, B., Haraldson, T., and Carlsson, G.E., The short-term effect of intra-articular injections of sodium hyaluronate and corticosteroid on temporomandibular joint pain and dysfunction, *J. Oral Maxillofac. Surg.,* 43, 429, 1985.

1269. Yasui, T., Akatsuka, M., Tobetto, K., Hayaishi, M., and Ando, T., The effect of hyaluronan on interleukin-1α-induced prostaglandin E_2 production in human osteoarthritic synovial cells, *Agents Actions,* 37, 155, 1992.

1270. Punzi, L., Schiavon, F., Cavasin, F., Ramonda, R., Gambari, P.F., and Tudesco, S., The influence of intra-articular hyaluronic acid on PGE_2 and cAMP of synovial fluid, *Clin. Exp. Rheumatol.,* 7, 247, 1989.

1271. Henderson, E.B., Grootveld, M., Farrell, A., Smith, E.C., Thompson, P.W., and Blake, D.R., A pathological role for damaged hyaluronan in synovitis, *Ann. Rheum. Dis.,* 50, 196, 1991.

1272. Burkhardt, D. and Ghosh, P., Laboratory evaluation of antiarthritic drugs as potential chondroprotective agents, *Sem. Arthritis Rheum.,* 17(2) (Suppl.1), 3, 1987.

1273. Rejholec, V., Long-term studies of antiosteoarthritic drugs: an assessment, *Sem. Arthritis Rheum.,* 17(2) (Suppl.1), 35, 1987.

1274. Altman, R.D., Kapila, P., Dean, D.D., and Howell, D.S., Future therapeutic trends in osteoarthritis, *Scand. J. Rheum. Suppl.,* 77, 37, 1988.

1275. Burkhardt, D. and Ghosh, P., Laboratory evaluation of glycosaminoglycan polysulfate ester for chondroprotective activity: a review, *Curr. Ther. Res.,* 40(6), 1034, 1986.

1276. Ghosh, P., Anti-rheumatic drugs and cartilage, *Bailleres Clin. Rheum.,* 2(2), 309, 1988.

1277. Ghosh, P., Smith, M., and Wells, C., Second-line agents in osteoarthritis, in *Second-Line Agents in the Treatment of Rheumatic Diseases,* Dixon, J.S. and Furst, D.E., Eds., Marcel Dekker, New York, 1992, 363.

1278. Jimenez, R., Innovative therapeutic agents, in *Therapeutic Controversies in the Rheumatic Diseases,* Willkens, R.F. and Dahl, S.L., Eds., Grune & Stratton, Orlando, 1987, 213.

1279. Peliskova, Z., Trnavsky, K., and Krajickova-Trnavska, J., The present state of chondroprotective therapy in osteoarthrosis, *Acta Chirop. Orthop. Traumatol. Cech.,* 56, 185, 1989.

1280. Pinals, R.S., Pharmacologic treatment of osteoarthritis, *Clin. Ther.,* 14(3), 336, 1992.

1281. Wagenhäuser, F.J., Amira, A., Borrachero, J., Brummer, L., Clausen, C., and Winer, J., The treatment of arthroses with cartilage-bone marrow extract. Results of a multi-center trial, *Schweiz. Med. Wochenschr.,* 98, 904, 1968.

1282. Adler, E., Wolf, E., and Taustein, I., A double-blind trial with cartilage and bone marrow extract in degenerative gonarthrosis, *Acta Rheum. Scand.,* 16, 6, 1970.

1283. Schiavetti, L., Tuzi, T., and Galeazzi, M., Trattamento a lungo termine dell'artrosi con Arumalon, *Min. Med.,* 68, 1263, 1977.

1284. Denko, C.W., Restorative chemotherapy in degenerative hip disease, *Agents Actions,* 8, 268, 1978.

1285. Rejholec, V. and Králová, M., Langzeitbehandlung der Coxarthrose mit Rumalon, *Aktual. Rheumatol.,* 9, 139, 1984.

1286. Dinkel, R., Der ökonomische Nutzen der Langzeitbehandlung von Coxarthrose-Patienten mit Arumalon, *Aktual. Rheumatol.,* 9, 149, 1984.

1287. Wägenhauser, F.J., Die medikamentöse Basisbehandlung der Arthrosen, *Fortbildungskurse Rheumatol.,* 5, 57, 1978.

1288. Verbruggen, G. and Veys, E.M., Influence of oversulfated heparinoid upon hyaluronate metabolism of the human synovial cell *in vivo, J. Rheumatol.,* 6, 554, 1979.

1289. Tsuyama, N., Hara, T., Akasaka, Y., Ogino, M., Furuya, M., Mikami, R., Inoue, H., Takahashi, H., Chin, E., Moro, K., Aoki, T., Suzuki, T., Kuriya, N., and Otani, Y., Clinical study of the intraarticular injection of Arteparon for osteoarthritis of the knee joint — double blind controlled study, *Jpn. J. Pharmacol. Ther.,* 12, 39, 1981.

1290. Ishikawa, K., Kitagawa, T., Tanaka, T., Terayama, K., Kuriya, N., Iwata, H., Niwa, S., and Sakurai, M., Clinical evaluation of the intra-articular injection of glycosaminoglycanpolysulfate for osteoarthrosis of the knee joint: a multicentric double blind controlled study, *Z. Orthop.,* 120, 708, 1982.

1291. Anderson, I.F., Intramuscular Arteparon on osteoarthrosis of the knee — a double blind trial, *Aktual. Rheumatol.,* 7, 164, 1982.

1292. Siegmuth, W. and Radi, I., Vergliech von Glykosaminoglykanpolysulfat (Arteparon) und physiologischer Kochsalzlosung bei Arthrosen grosser Gelenke ergebnisse einer multizentrischen Doppelblindstudie, *Z. Rheumatol.,* 42, 223, 1983.

1293. Pastinen, O., Forsskähl, B., and Marklund, M., Local glycosaminoglycan polysulfate injection therapy in osteoarthritis of the hand. A placebo-controlled clinical study, *Scand. J. Rheumatol.,* 17, 197, 1988.

1294. Sarkozi, A.M., Nemeth-Csoka, M., and Bartosiewicz, G., Effects of glycosaminoglycan polysulfate in the treatment of chondrocalcinosis, *Clin. Exp. Rheumatol.,* 6, 3, 1988.

1295. Hess, H. and Thiel, W., The treatment of posttraumatic cartilage damages by intra-articular injections, in *Current Topics in Sports Medicine,* Bachl, N., Prokop, L., and Suckert, R., Eds., Urban & Schwarzenberg, Vienna, 1984, 794.

1296. Kvist, M., Jarvinen, M., Kujala, U., and Forsskahl, B., Comparison of Arteparon and indomethacin in the treatment of apicites patellae and peritendinitis of ligamentum patellae in athletes, in *Current Topics in Sports Medicine,* Bachl, N., Prokop, L., and Suckert, R., Eds., Urban & Schwarzenberg, Vienna, 1984, 825.

1297. Lysholm, J., The relation between pain and torque in an isokinetic strength test of knee extension, *Arthroscopy,* 3(3), 182, 1987.

1298. Sprengel, H., Franke, J., and Sprengel, A., Personal experiences in the conservative therapy of patellar chondropathy, *Beitr. Orthop. Traumatol.,* 37(5), 259, 1990.

1299. Greinacher, A., Michels, I., Schafer, M., Kiefel, V., and Mueller-Eckhardt, C., Heparin-associated thrombocytopenia in a patient treated with polysulfated chondroitin sulfate: evidence for immunological crossreactivity between heparin and polysulfated glycosaminoglycan, *Br. J. Haematol.,* 81, 252, 1992.

1300. Huskisson, E.C., Ed., *Anti-Rheumatic Drugs,* Praeger Scientific, New York, 1983.

1301. McCarty, D.J. and Koopman, W.J., Eds., Clinical pharmacology of antirheumatic drugs, Section III, in *Arthritis and Allied Conditions. A Textbook of Rheumatology,* Vol. 2, McCarty, D.J. and Koopman, W.J., Eds., Lea & Febiger, Philadelphia, 1993, 567.

1302. Prudden, J.F., Migel, P., Hanson, P., Friedrich, L., and Balassa, L., The discovery of a potent pure chemical wound-healing accelerator, *Am. J. Surg.,* 119, 560, 1970.

1303. Vidal y Plana, R.R., Bizzarri, D., and Rovati, A.L., Articular cartilage pharmacology. I. *In vitro* studies on glucosamine and non steroidal antiinflammatory drugs, *Pharm. Res. Commun.,* 10(6), 557, 1978.

1304. Rodén, L., Effect of hexosamines on the synthesis of chondroitin sulphuric acid *in vitro,* *Ark. Kemi.,* 10, 345, 1956.

1305. Tesoriere, G., Dones, F., Magistro, D., and Castagnetta, L., Intestinal absorption of glucosamine and N-acetylglucosamine, *Experentia,* 28(7), 770, 1972.

1306. Setnikar, I., Giachetti, C., and Zanolo, G., Absorption, distribution and excretion of radioactivity after a single intravenous or oral administration of [^{14}C] glucosamine to the rat, *Pharmatherapeutica,* 3(8), 538, 1984.

1307. Setnikar, I., Giacchetti, C., and Zanolo, G., Pharmacokinetics of glucosamine in the dog and man, *Arzneim. Forsch.,* 36(2), 729, 1986.

1308. Setnikar, I., Cereda, R., Pacini, M.A., and Revel, L., Antireactive properties of glucosamine sulfate, *Arzneim. Forsch.,* 41(2), 157, 1991.

1309. Setnikar, I., Pacini, M.A., and Revel, L., Antiarthritic effects of glucosamine sulfate studied in animal models, *Arzneim. Forsch.,* 41(5), 542, 1991.

1310. Vetter, G., Lokale therapie der Arthrosen mit Glukosaminen (Dona 200), *Munch. Med. Wochenschr.,* 111, 1499, 1969.

1311. Mund-Hoym, W.D., Konservative Behandlung von Wirbensäulen-Arthrosen mit Glusoaminsulfat und Phenylbutazon. Eine kontrollierte Studie, *Therapiewoche,* 30, 5922, 1980.

1312. Mund-Hoym, W.D., Die Behandlung von Hüft-und Kniegelenk-arthrosen, *Z. Allg. Med.,* 56, 2153, 1980.

1313. Crolle, G. and D'Este, E., Glucosamine sulfate for the management of arthrosis: a controlled clinical investigation, *Curr. Res. Med. Opin.,* 7(2), 104, 1980.

1314. Pujalte, J.M., Llavore, E.P., and Ylescupidez, F.R., Double-blind clinical evaluation of oral glucosamine sulfate in the basic treatment of osteoarthrosis, *Curr. Res. Med. Opin.,* 7(2), 110, 1980.

1315. Drovanti, A., Bignamini, A.A., and Rovati, A.L., Therapeutic activity of oral glucosamine sulfate in osteoarthritis: a placebo-controlled double-blind investigation, *Clin. Ther.,* 3(4), 260, 1980.

1316. Vajaradul, Y., Double-blind clinical evaluation of intra-articular glucosamine in outpatients with gonarthrosis, *Clin. Ther.,* 3(5), 336, 1981.

1317. D'Ambrosio, E., Casa, B., Bompani, R., Scali, G., and Scali, M., Glucosamine sulfate: a controlled clinical investigation in arthrosis, *Pharmatherapeutica,* 2(8), 504, 1981.

1318. Vaz, A.L., Double-blind clinical evaluation of the relative efficacy of ibuprofen and glucosamine sulfate in the management of osteoarthrosis of the knee in outpatients, *Curr. Med. Res. Opin.,* 8(3), 145, 1982.

1319. Tapadinhas, M.J., Rivera, I.C., and Bignamini, A.A., Oral glucosamine sulfate in the management of arthrosis: report on a multi-centre open investigation in Portugal, *Pharmatherapeutica,* 3(3), 157, 1982.

1320. Böhmer, D., Ambrus, P., Szögy, A., and Haralambie, G., Treatment of chondropathia patellae in young athletes with glucosamine sulfate, in *Current Topics in Sports Medicine,* Bachl, N., Prokop, L., and Suckert, R., Eds., Urban & Schwarzenberg, Vienna, 1984, 799.

1321. Havsteen, B., Flavonoids, a class of natural products of high pharmacological potency, *Biochem. Pharmacol.,* 32(7), 1141, 1983.

1322. Kuhnau, J., The flavonoids. A class of semi-essential food components: their role in human nutrition, *World Rev. Nutr. Diet.,* 24, 117, 1976.

1323. Middleton, E., The flavonoids, *Trends Pharm. Sci.,* 5, 335, 1984.

1324. Cody, V., Middleton, E., and Harborne, J., Eds., *Plant Flavonoids in Biology and Medicine*, Vol. 1, Alan R. Liss, New York, 1986.

1325. Cody, V., Middleton, E., Harborne, J., and Beretz, A., Eds., *Plant Flavonoids in Biology and Medicine*, Vol. 2, Alan R. Liss, New York, 1988.

1326. Anonymous, Flavonoids, *Agents Actions,* 27 (Suppl.), 137, 1989.

1327. Farkas, L., Gábor, M., and Kállay, F., Eds., *Flavonoids and Bioflavonoids, 1985,* Elsevier, Amsterdam, 1985.

1328. Affany, A., Salvayre, R., and Blazy, L., Comparison of the protective effect of various flavonoids against lipid peroxidation of erythrocyte membranes induced by cumene hydroperoxide, *Fund. Clin. Pharmacol.,* 1, 451, 1987.

1329. Monboisse, J.C., Braquet, P., Randoux, A., and Borel, J.P., Non-enzymatic degradation of acid-soluble calf skin collagen by superoxide ion: protective effect of flavonoids, *Biochem. Pharmacol.,* 32(1), 53, 1983.

1330. Pincemail, J. and Dupris, M., Superoxide scavenging effect and superoxide dismutase activity of Gingko biloba extract, *Experentia,* 45, 708, 1989.

1331. Salvayre, R., Comparison of the scavenger effect of bilberry anthocyanosides with various flavonoids, *Stud. Org. Chem.,* 11, 437, 1982.

1332. Takacs, O., Benko, S., Varga, L., Autal, A., and Gabor, M., Metabolism of flavonoids, *Angiologica,* 9, 175, 1972.

1333. Gugler, R., Leschik, M., and Dengler, H.J., Disposition of quercetin in man after single oral and intravenous doses, *Eur. J. Clin. Pharmacol.,* 9, 229, 1975.

1334. Tarayre, J.P. and Lauressergues, H., Advantages of a combination of proteolytic enzymes, flavonoids and ascorbic acid in comparison with non-steroid antiinflammatory agents, *Arzneim. Forsch.,* 27(6), 1144, 1977.

1335. Tarayre, J.P. and Lauressergues, H., The anti-edematous effect of an association of proteolytic enzymes, flavonoids, sterolic heteroside of Ruscus aculeatus and ascorbic acid, *Ann. Pharm. Fr.,* 37(5–6), 191, 1979.

1336. Czernicki, Z., Treatment of experimental brain oedema following sudden decompression, surgical wound, and cold lesion with vasoprotective drugs and the proteinase inhibitor Trasylol, *Acta Neurochir.,* 50(3-4), 311, 1979.

1337. Cragin, R.B., The use of bioflavonoids in the prevention and treatment of athletic injuries, *Med. Times,* 90, 529, 1962.

1338. Miller, M.J., Injuries to athletes, *Med. Times,* 88, 313, 1960.

1339. MacGregor, J., Genetic and carcinogenic effects of plant flavonoids: an overview, in *Nutritional and Toxicological Aspects of Food Safety,* Friedman, M., Ed., Plenum Press, New York, 1984, 497.

1340. Orloff, S., Rao, H.V., and Bose, S.M., Effect of flavonoids on the manifestations of experimental osteolathyrism, *Indian J. Biochem. Biophys.,* 11(4), 318, 1974.

1341. Srinivasan, K.R., A chromatographic study of the curcuminoids in *Curcuma longa,* L., *J. Pharm. Pharmacol.,* 5, 448, 1953.

1342. Govindarajan, V.S., Turmeric — chemistry, technology, and quality, *CRC Crit. Rev. Food Sci. Nutr.,* 12, 199, 1980.

1343. Nadkarni, K.M. and Nadkarni, A.K., Eds., *Indian Materia Medica,* Popular Prakashan, Bombay, 1976.

1344. Tripathi, R.M., Gupta, S.S., and Chandra, D., Antitrypsin and anti-hyaluronidase activity of *Curcuma longa, Indian J. Pharm.,* 5, 260, 1973.

1345. Bhatia, A., Singh, G.A., and Khanna, N.M., Effect of Curcumin, its alkali salts and *Curcuma longa* oil in histamine-induced gastric ulceration, *Indian J. Exp. Biol.,* 2, 158, 1964.

1346. Arora, R.B., Basu, N., Kapoor, V., and Jain, A.P., Antiinflammatory studies on Curcuma longa (Turmeric), *Indian J. Med. Res.,* 59(8), 1289, 1971.

1347. Chandra, D. and Gupta, S.S., Antiinflammatory and anti-arthritic activity of volatile oil of Curcuma longa (Haldi), *Indian J. Med. Res.,* 60(1), 138, 1972.

1348. Srimal, R.C. and Dhawan, B.N., Pharmacology of diferuloyl methane (curcumin), a non-steroidal antiinflammatory agent, *J. Pharm. Pharmacol.,* 25, 447, 1973.

1349. Yegnanarayan, R., Saraf, A.P., and Balwani, J.H., Comparison of antiinflammatory activity of various extracts of Curcuma longa (Linn), *Indian J. Med. Res.,* 64(4), 601, 1976.

1350. Rao, T.S., Basu, N., and Siddiqui, H.H., Antiinflammatory activity of curcumin analogs, *Indian J. Med. Res.,* 75, 574, 1982.

1351. Famaey, J.P., Fontaine, J., and Reuse, J., The effects of non-steroidal antiinflammatory drugs on cholinergic and histamine-induced contractions of guinea pig isolated ileum, *Br. J. Pharmacol.,* 60, 165, 1977.

1352. Mukhopadhay, A., Basu, N., Ghatak, N., and Gujral, P.K., Antiinflammatory and irritant activities of curcumin analogs in rats, *Agents Actions,* 12(4), 508, 1982.

1353. Srivastava, R., Puri, V., Srimal, R.C., and Dhawan, B.N., Effect of curcumin on platelet aggregation and vascular prostacyclin synthesis, *Arzneim. Forsch.,* 36(4), 715, 1986.

1354. Wagner, H., Wierer, M., and Bauer, R., *In vitro* inhibition of prostaglandin biosynthesis by essential oils and phenolic compounds, *Planta Med.,* 0(3), 184, 1986.

1355. Deodhar, S.D., Sethi, R., and Srimal, R.C., Preliminary study on antirheumatic activity of curcumin (diferuloyl methane), *Indian J. Med. Res.,* 71, 632, 1980.

1356. Satoskar, R.R., Shah, S.J., and Shenoy, S.G., Evaluation of antiinflammatory property of curcumin (diferuloyl methane) in patients with postoperative inflammation, *Int. J. Clin. Pharmacol. Ther. Toxicol.,* 24(12), 651, 1986.

1357. Kiso, Y., Suzuki, Y., Watanabe, N., Oshima, Y., and Hikino, H., Antihepatotoxic principles of Curcuma longa rhizomes, *Planta Med.,* 49, 185, 1983.

1358. Reddy, A.C. and Lokesh, B.R., Studies on spice principles as antioxidants in the inhibition of lipid peroxidation of rat liver microsomes, *Mol. Cell. Biochem.,* 111(1-2), 117, 1992.

1359. Salimath, B.P., Sundaresh, C.S., and Srinivas, L., Dietary components inhibit lipid peroxidation in erythrocyte membrane, *Nutr. Res.,* 6, 1171, 1986.

1360. Shalini, V.K. and Srinivas, L., Lipid peroxide induced DNA damage: protection by turmeric (Curcuma longa), *Mol. Cell. Biochem.,* 77, 3, 1987.

1361. Sharma, O.P., Antioxidant activity of curcumin and related compounds, *Biochem. Pharmacol.,* 26, 1811, 1976.

1362. Srinivas, L. and Shalini, V.K., DNA damage by smoke: Protection by turmeric and other inhibitors of ROS, *Free Radical Biol. Med.,* 11, 227, 1991.

1363. Toda, S., Miyase, T., Arichi, H., Tanizawa, H., and Takino, Y., Natural antioxidant. III. Antioxidative components isolated from rhizome of Curcuma longa L., *Chem. Pharm. Bull.,* 33, 1725, 1985.

1364. Zhao, B., Li, X., He, R., Cheng, S., and Wenjuan, X., Scavenging effects of green tea and natural antioxidants on active oxygen radicals, *Cell. Biophys.,* 14(2), 175, 1989.

1365. Huang, M.T., Smart, R.C., Wong, C.Q., and Conney, A.H., Inhibitory effect of curcumin, chlorogenic acid, caffeic acid, and ferulic acid on tumor promotion in mouse skin by 12-O-tetradecanoylphorbol-13-acetate, *Cancer Res.,* 48, 5941, 1988.

1366. Kuttan, R., Bhanumathy, P., Nirmala, K., and George, M.C., Potential anticancer activity of turmeric (*Curcuma longa*), *Cancer Lett.,* 29, 197, 1985.

1367. Azuine, M.A. and Bhide, S.V., Chemopreventive effects of turmeric against stomach and skin tumors induced by chemical carcinogens in Swiss mice, *Nutr. Cancer,* 17, 77, 1992.

1368. Nagabhusan, M. and Bhide, S.V., Curcumin as an inhibitor of cancer, *J. Am. Coll. Nutr.,* 11, 192, 1992.

1369. Srivastava, R., Puri, V., Srimal, R.C., and Dhawan, B.N., Effect of curcumin on platelet aggregation and vascular prostacyclin synthesis, *Arzneim. Forsch.,* 36, 715, 1986.

1370. Freyberg, R.H., The joints, in *Pathologic Physiology. Mechanisms of Disease,* 3rd ed., Sodeman, W.A., Ed., W.B. Saunders, Philadelphia, 1961, 1036.

1371. Kelsey, J.L., Pastides, H., and Bisbee, G.E., *Musculo-Skeletal Disorders. Their Frequency of Occurrence and Their Impact on the Population of the United States,* Prodist, New York, 1978.

1372. Fassbender, H.G., Annefeld, M., Wilhelmi, G., and Maier, R., Eds., *Articular cartilage and osteoarthrosis,* Hans Huber Publishers, Bern, 1983.

1373. Peyron, J.G., Ed., *New Research Developments in Osteoarthrosis,* Hans Huber, Bern, 1983.

1374. Russell, R.G.G. and Dieppe, P.A., Eds., *Osteoarthritis: Current Research and Prospects for Pharmacological Intervention,* IBC Technical Services, London, 1991.

1375. Moskowitz, R.W., Howell, D.S., Goldberg, V.M., and Mankin, H.J., Eds., *Osteoarthritis. Diagnosis and Medical/Surgical Management,* 2nd ed., W.B. Saunders, Philadelphia, 1992, 71.

1376. McCarty, D.J. and Koopman, W.J., Eds., Osteoarthritis, Section IX, in *Arthritis and Allied Conditions. A Textbook of Rheumatology,* Vol. 2, McCarty, D.J. and Koopman, W.J., Eds., Lea & Febiger, Philadelphia, 1993, 567.

1377. Hamerman, D., The biology of osteoarthritis, *N. Engl. J. Med.,* 320, 1322, 1989.

1378. Reimann, I., Christensen, S.B., and Diemer, N.H., Observations of reversibility of glycosaminoglycan depletion in articular cartilage, *Clin. Orthop.,* 168, 258, 1982.

1379. Radin, E.L. and Burr, D.B., Hypothesis: joints can heal, *Sem. Arthritis Rheum.,* 13, 293, 1984.

1380. Bland, J.H. and Cooper, S.M., Osteoarthritis: a review of the cell biology involved and evidence for reversibility. Management rationally related to known genesis and pathophysiology, *Sem. Arthritis Rheum.,* 14, 106, 1984.

1381. Altman, R.D., Howell, D.S., and Gottlied, N.L., New directions in therapy of osteoarthritis, *Sem. Arthritis Rheum.,* 17 (Suppl. 1), 1, 1987.

INDEX

A

Abetalipoproteinemia, 70

Abrasions, 220, 222, see also Dietary protocols

Accretion, bone, 145, see also Bone; Magnesium

Achlorhydria, 144

Achromotrichia, 135

Actin, 3

Activity factor, 23

Actomyosin, 16

Acute Phase Response, 119, 137

Adenosine triphosphate (ATP), 59

S-Adenosyl methionine (SAM), 41–42, 46

Adequan, see Arteparon

Adhesions, 7, 19, 182, 186

Adipose tissue, 4

Aescorin, 207

Aggrecan, 8, 9, 177

ALA, see α-Linolenate

β-Alanyl-L-histidine, see Carnosine

Albumin

    calcium binding, 103

    -globulin ratios, 73

    medium-chain triglycerides carrier, 58

    protein status assessment, 27–29

    zinc deficiency relation, 118–119

Alkaline phosphatase, 130, 147, 165

Alkalinity, 144

Allicin, 138

Alopecia, 118, 122

Alzheimer's disease, 71

Amenorrhea, athletic, 103–106, 223–224, see also
    Calcium; Dietary protocols

Amino acids

    arginine, 34–36

    aspartates, 36–37

    branched chain, 37

    dietary essentials, 33–34, see also Individual entries

    glutamine, 37–39

    glycine, 39

    histidine and carnosine, 39–40

    metabolic demands and muscle catabolism, 27

    ornithine and ornithine-α-ketoglutarate, 42–43

    phenylalanine, 43–44

    proline and hydroxyproline, 43

    roles and functions, 26–27

    sulfhydryl, 40–42

    summary and guidelines for use, 46–48

    tryptophan, 44–46

Aminosugars, 8, see also Glycosaminoglycans

Anabolism, 36, see also Bone

Analgesics, see also Individual entries

    glucosamine salt cotherapy, 200–202

    phenylalanine, 43–44

proteases, 173

rheumatoid arthritis, 55–56

tryptophan, 44, 46

vitamin B_6, 89

Ananase, see Bromelain

Anemia

    copper deficiency, 133–134

    vitamin B_{12} deficiency, 89

    vitamin E deficiency, 70

    wound healing, 117

    zinc toxicity, 131

Aneurysms, 135–136

Angiogenesis, 16

Ankle sprains, 171, see also Protease; Sprains

Ankylosing spondylitis, 137, 139, see also Degenerative
    joint diseases

Anorexia, 118, 122, 144

Antacids, 144

Anthropometric measurements, 24, 28

Antibiotics, 78, see also Vitamin K

Anticonvulsants, 68

Antioxidant enzymes, 176, see also Antioxidants; Free
    radicals

Antioxidants, see also Individual entries

    bioflavinoids, 205

    carotenoids, 66

    ceruloplasmin, 137

    hyaluronan, 185

    ideal formulation for healing, 218

    manganese, 142

    n3 fatty acid shelf-life, 59

    selenium, 163, 165

    vitamin C, 95

    vitamin E, 70, 72, 74, 76

Aphthous ulcers, see Ulcers

Apicitis patellae, 193

Aponeuroses, 3–4

Apple cider vinegar, 137

Arachidonate, 52, 54

Areolar connective tissue, 3, see also Connnective
    tissue

Arginine, 34–36, 46, see also Amino acids

Arteparon, see also Glycosaminoglycans

    human studies, 190–194

    overview, 188

    roles and functions, 188–190

    safety, 194

    summary, 194–195

Arthritis, see also Osteoarthritis; Rheumatoid arthritis

    adjuvant-induced and curcumin therapy, 209

    boron role, 153, 158–160

    cartilage and healing, 19

    copper, 136–140

    hyaluronan, 185